Problems of High Altitude Medicine and Biology

NATO Science for Peace and Security Series

This Series presents the results of scientific meetings supported under the NATO Programme: Science for Peace and Security (SPS).

The NATO SPS Programme supports meetings in the following Key Priority areas: (1) Defence Against Terrorism; (2) Countering other Threats to Security and (3) NATO, Partner and Mediterranean Dialogue Country Priorities. The types of meeting supported are generally "Advanced Study Institutes" and "Advanced Research Workshops". The NATO SPS Series collects together the results of these meetings. The meetings are coorganized by scientists from NATO countries and scientists from NATO's "Partner" or "Mediterranean Dialogue" countries. The observations and recommendations made at the meetings, as well as the contents of the volumes in the Series, reflect those of participants and contributors only; they should not necessarily be regarded as reflecting NATO views or policy.

Advanced Study Institutes (ASI) are high-level tutorial courses intended to convey the latest developments in a subject to an advanced-level audience

Advanced Research Workshops (ARW) are expert meetings where an intense but informal exchange of views at the frontiers of a subject aims at identifying directions for future action

Following a transformation of the programme in 2006 the Series has been re-named and re-organised. Recent volumes on topics not related to security, which result from meetings supported under the programme earlier, may be found in the NATO Science Series.

The Series is published by IOS Press, Amsterdam, and Springer, Dordrecht, in conjunction with the NATO Public Diplomacy Division.

Sub-Series

A.	Chemistry and Biology	Springer
B.	Physics and Biophysics	Springer
C.	Environmental Security	Springer
D.	Information and Communication Security	IOS Press
E.	Human and Societal Dynamics	IOS Press

http://www.nato.int/science
http://www.springer.com
http://www.iospress.nl

Series A: Chemistry and Biology

Problems of High Altitude Medicine and Biology

Edited by

Almaz Aldashev

Kirghiz Institute of Cardiology,
Bishkek, Kyrgyz Republic

Robert Naeije

Free University of Brussels,
Belgium

Springer

Proceedings of the NATO Advanced Research Workshop on
Problems of High Altitude Medicine and Biology
Issyk-Kul, Kyrgyz Republic
5–6 June 2006

A C.I.P. Catalogue record for this book is available from the Library of Congress.

ISBN 978-1-4020-6298-8 (HB)
ISBN 978-1-4020-6299-5 (PB)
ISBN 978-1-4020-6300-8 (e-book)

Published by Springer,
P.O. Box 17, 3300 AA Dordrecht, The Netherlands.

www.springer.com

Printed on acid-free paper

CONTENTS

CHAPTER 1

INTRODUCTION: 45 YEARS OF MOUNTAIN MEDICINE

Talk to NATO Conference on Mountain Medicine
Cholpon-Ata, Kyrgyz Republic. June 6th, 2006

JAMES S. MILLEDGE

Chorleywood; United Kingdom

Keywords: altitude; physiology; medicine; mountain erring

Beginnings

In November 1959 I read in the newspaper that Sir Edmund Hillary and Dr Griffith Pugh were going to lead a scientific and mountaineering expedition the following year to the Everest region of Nepal to study the long-term effects of high altitude. I wrote to Griff, having never met him, asking if there happened to be a place for me on his team. I was at the time a resident in Respiratory Medicine in Southampton and had done some climbing and skiing but had no expedition experience. He replied that the team was actually made up but if I was in London I should come and see him. Well, I immediately asked for a day off and "happened to be in London" the next day! Someone dropped out and I was invited to join what subsequently became known as "The Silver Hut Expedition". Thus, I found myself on my first major expedition and at the start of what became my professional hobby of Mountain Medicine and Physiology. Although my job, throughout my career, has been that of a general physician with a special interest in respiratory medicine, I have been fortunate to have been able to take time off to go on many expeditions to the great ranges, through the kind understanding of colleagues and family.

The Silver Hut Expedition, 1960–61 (Figures 1–6)

The 1960–61 Himalayan and Scientific Expedition, to give it its official title, was a unique enterprise. It was dreamed up by Sir Edmund Hillary and Dr Griffith Pugh when they were together in the Antarctic. Griff Pugh had been with Ed on Cho Oyu in 1952, Everest in 1953 and in Antarctica in 1956/7. The idea for this long Himalayan expedition was based on the pattern, common in Antarctica, of leaving a party of scientists on the ice to "winter over". The idea was to study the long-term effect of really high altitude on

A. Aldashev and R. Naeije (eds.), Problems of High Altitude Medicine and Biology, 1–9.

human lowland subjects. So the plan was to go out from Kathmandu after one monsoon, spend the whole winter at high altitude and in the spring to attempt an 8,000m peak, returning just before the next monsoon. Some members came only for the autumn, others for the spring part and some, including myself, were able to spend the whole nine months in the field. Our winter station was a pre-fabricated wooden hut, painted silver, which we set up at 5800m on the Mingbo Glacier in the Everest region of Nepal. This became known as the Silver Hut.

Our program of research included numerous studies in ourselves as we acclimatized. Many of these examined the changes which took place at the various points of the oxygen transport cascade from air to tissues. The project for which I was particularly responsible was on the changes in the chemical control of breathing with acclimatization. I was also involved in a large study of the ventilation, heart rate and cardiac output on exercise at various altitudes. This was especially Griff Pugh's interest. I also did a project on the changes in the ECG with increasing altitude.

We found that the height of 5800m was too high for optimum acclimatization. We all continued to be anorexic and to lose weight at this altitude. This weight loss was reversed by descent to Base Camp at the still considerable height of 4500m.

In the spring, some physiology was continued as we attempted to climb Mt Makalu (8481m). Exercise studies including measurement of VO_2 max, were conducted up to the Makalu Col (7440m) by Mike Ward and John West.

The Sixties, after "Silver Hut"

Immediately after the Silver Hut Expedition I came back to Oxford where Dan Cunningham and Brian Lloyd, my mentors in the control of breathing project, were based in the Physiology Department. They were hosting the Haldane Centenary Symposium that summer, honouring the birth of JS Haldane the great Oxford physiologist. All the leading cardio-respiratory physiologists were there. One of Haldane's classic contributions was in the field of control of breathing and altitude. He led a famous expedition to Pikes Peak in 1911, so our work, "hot off the press" was very well received. It was my first scientific presentation. I decided to try and make a career in academic medicine and was thinking of applying for a post in a British medical school when we received a pressing invitation to join the staff of Christian Medical College, Vellore in South India. My wife, Betty, as an anaesthesiologist was probably even more welcome. We worked there for the next ten years with a year's sabbatical, in the middle, in San Francisco. There I had a research fellowship working with John Severinghaus.

In 1964 Dr. Sukhamay Lahiri, who had been on the Silver Hut Expedition, invited me to join him in a small physiological team as part of Sir Edmund Hillary's Second Schoolhouse Expedition to Solo Khumbu, Nepal. While Ed and his team built two schoolhouses, a bridge and the Lukla Airstrip as part of his aid to Sherpas, we studied the differences between ourselves, lowlanders and Sherpa highlanders at a camp high above Lukla at 4880 m. We found that Sherpas had a much lower hypoxic ventilatory response than did lowlanders both at rest and exercise. John Severinghaus and colleagues almost simultaneously found the same thing in Andean highlanders.

The Seventies

In 1972 we returned from India and I was fortunate in getting a job at Northwick Park Hospital, where the Medical Research Council had established its Clinical Research Centre. There I began working in Dr John Nunn's division of anaesthesia. A year later I got a combined MRC and NHS appointment. In the '70s we were unable to get to the Great Ranges but did a series of field studies on the effect of long continued exercise (hill walking) on fluid balance and related hormones. These were stimulated by the accounts of high altitude pulmonary edema, in which strenuous exercise seemed to be a risk factor. We first studied the effect of hill-walking at low altitude (<1000m in the hills of the UK) on fluid balance and related hormones. We then repeated the studies in Switzerland adding altitude to the exercise. We found the effect of abrupt change from semi-sedentary to exercising life style was to retain some water, a lot of sodium and increased plasma and extra-cellular fluid volumes.

Thc Eightics

In 1981 I was invited by Mike Ward, whom I had known from the Silver Hut Expedition, to join him and a team of four elite climbers led by Chris Bonington who were attempting to make the first assent of Mt. Kongur (7719 m) in Xinjiang (China). We compared the climbers with us more averagely fit scientists and found evidence that their physiology had moved some way towards that of Sherpas, in that their HVR on exercise was lower than ours. Also on this expedition we collected blood samples for the analysis of erythropoietin. The immunological method had recently become available and was being carried out by Mary Coates in the CRC. The figure in our paper of 1985 showing the altitude, haematocrit and Epo levels against days of the expedition has been reproduced more than any other illustration of my work.

Also in 1981 I had been invited to join John West's American Medical Research Expedition to Everest (AMREE). John had also been on the Silver Hut expedition, Twenty years after Silver Hut we extended much of the work of that expedition with studies on exercise and gas exchange, including alveolar gas measurements up to the summit. There were many other projects in this expedition and I looked at the angiotensin response to renin, which I found to be even more blunted than at more modest altitude in Switzerland.

In 1987 and '89 I had two expeditions with the Royal Navy Mountaineering Club to Mount Kenya and to Bolivia. On these trips we studied fluid and salt balance in relation to acute mountain sickness (AMS). We showed that there was a correlation between sodium retention and aldosterone levels on the day of ascent and the subsequent AMS scores. We also showed that there was no correlation between AMS and fitness (VO_2max) or with the hypoxic ventilatory response. These studies took place during the first 4–5 days at altitude and then we went off in twos and fours to climb a number of peaks.

High Altitude Medicine & Physiology: a Textbook

Mike Ward, who sadly died last year, had been the prime mover of the 1951 Everest Reconnaissance Expedition, which found the route from the South. He had been Medical Officer for the 1953 Everest Expedition and had also been in the Silver Hut (when he and three others made the first ascent of Ama Dablam). He had also been one of the team on our four hill-walking fluid balance studies as well as leader of the Kongur Expedition. In 1975 he had published the first ever text book on Mountain Medicine and I had helped with some of the chapters. In the mid-eighties I asked him if he was thinking of a second edition. He invited me to join him as co-author and we later recruited John West so that in 1989 we published the first edition of our textbook, "High Altitude Medicine and Physiology". There have since been two more editions and we are now revising it for the fourth edition, with "Brownie" Schoene taking Ward's place as third author. We hope it will be published early next year.

The Nineties

I had a number of treks or minor expeditions to the Himalayas of Nepal and India in 1991, '94, '96 and to the Karakoram in '95. In August '95, on my 65th birthday I retired from the NHS and MRC and could now spend more time on Mountain Medicine.

In 1992 I became involved with a group of young British doctors who mounted an Everest Expedition in 1994. This group has evolved into the charity, "Medical Expeditions". We have had two further major expeditions in 1998 to Kangchenjunga and in 2003 to Chamlang Base Camp, all in Nepal. The pattern of these quite large expeditions has been to have a small climbing group attempting the major peak and up to about 50 trekking members going to the base camps in small groups. The science has been done in London before departure and at the base camps with some simple observations on the trek.

Medical Expeditions has two charitable aims, to support research and education in altitude medicine and physiology. The research has mostly been done on the major expeditions and the educational aim has been covered by running weekend courses in Mountain Medicine at intervals in North Wales for the past 14 years. Three years ago we began offering courses for a Diploma in the subject. This was the first such course in English, though courses in Europe have been running for a number of years. The course, which is approved by the UIAA and Leicester University, has elements of practical mountaineering skills, safety and rescue, as well as lectures and workshops in altitude physiology and medicine. There are four modules of a week each, two in North Wales and one each in Scotland in the winter and in Switzerland in the summer.

I have been so very fortunate to have been involved with our subject for so long. I have seen incredible changes in the technology available to us and considerable advances in both the physiology of high altitude and understanding of the medical conditions of mountainous regions. My own contribution to these has been very small. I hope that I have been able to disseminate these advances by talks, lectures and writing; contributing, I hope, to a wider understanding of the subject and possibly fewer deaths. My main delight, however, has been the many friends I have made through mountaineering and expeditions and the abiding memories over this long time.

References to the work mentioned can be found in the relevant chapters of:

Ward MP, Milledge JS and West JB (2000). High Altitude Medicine and Physiology 3rd edition, Arnold, London.

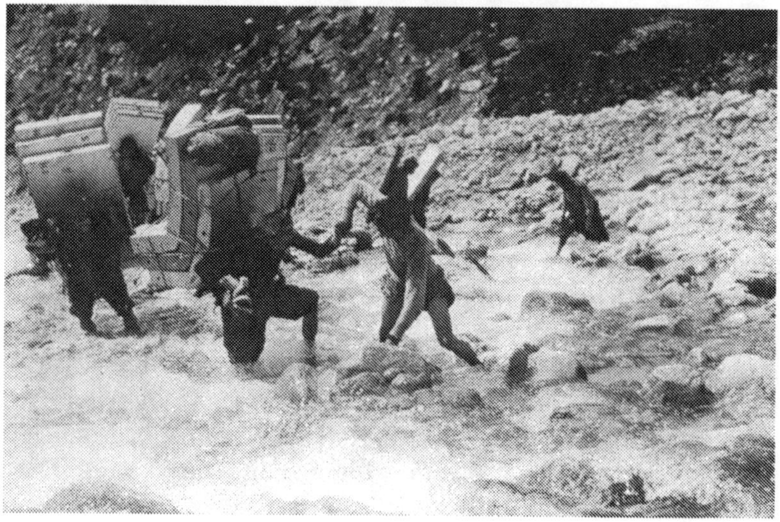

Figure 1. Porters crossing a stream with some of the silver hut panels en route to the Mingbo valley, October 1960.

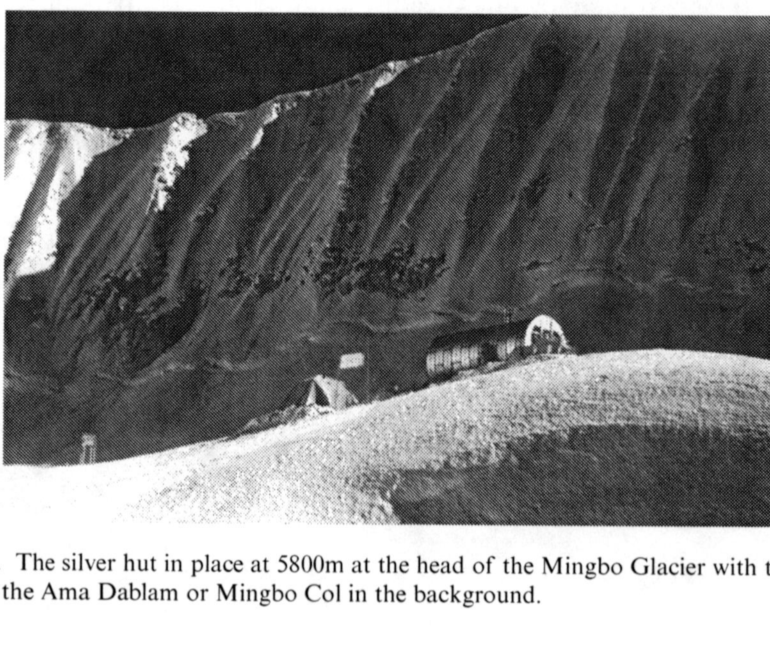

Figure 2. The silver hut in place at 5800m at the head of the Mingbo Glacier with the fluted walls of the Ama Dablam or Mingbo Col in the background.

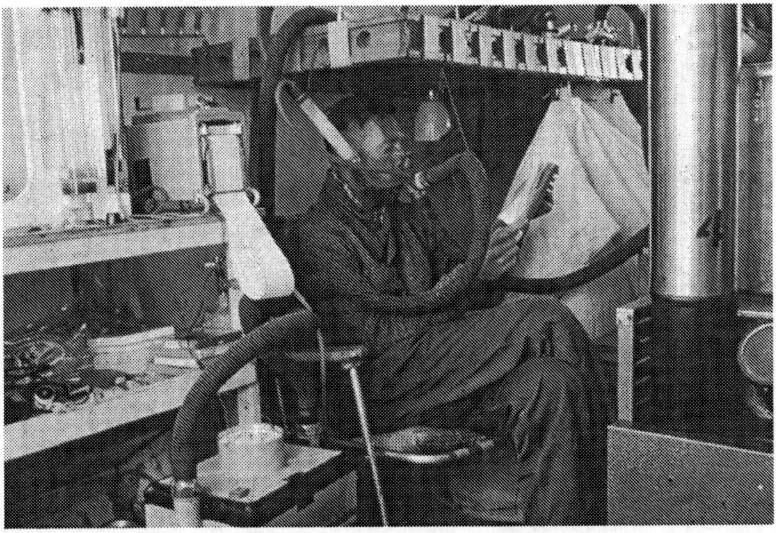

Figure 3. John West as subject for one of my control of breathing experiments inside the Silver Hut during the winter of 1960–61.

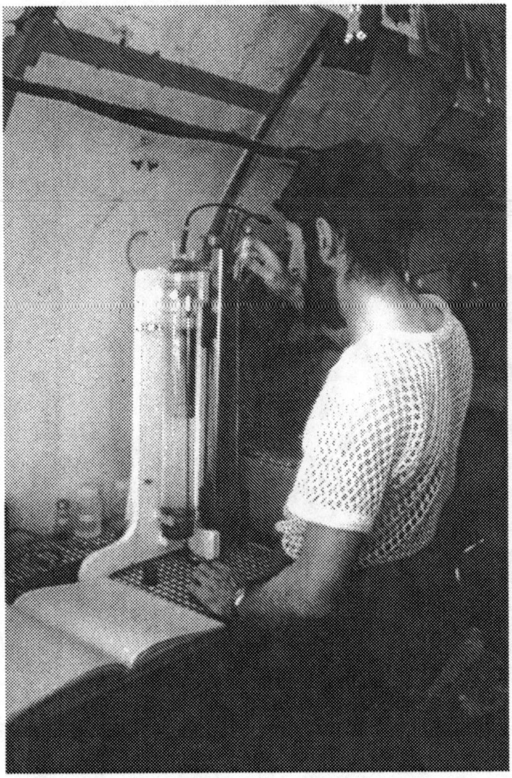

Figure 4. Me analysing alveolar gas samples using the Lloyd-Haldane apparatus in the Silver Hut after a control of breathing experiment.

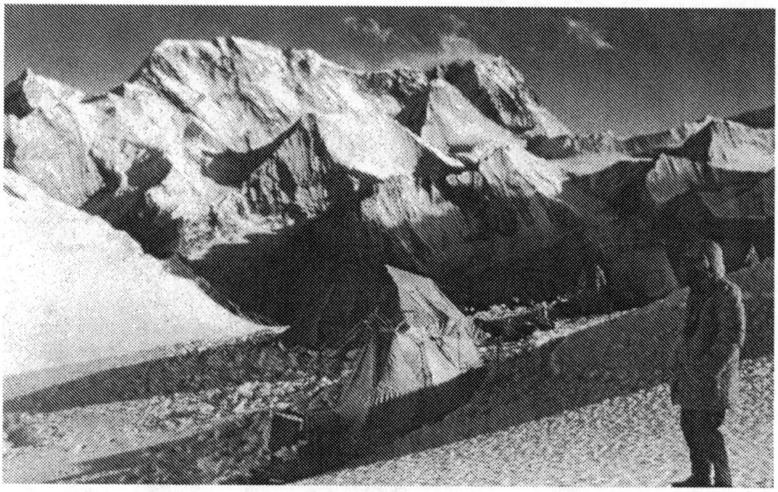

Figure 5. Makalu advanced Base Camp (6,300m) Spring 1961. The route from Silver Hut over to the Barun valley and Makalu is in background. The high, long summit of Chamlang fills the background to the left.

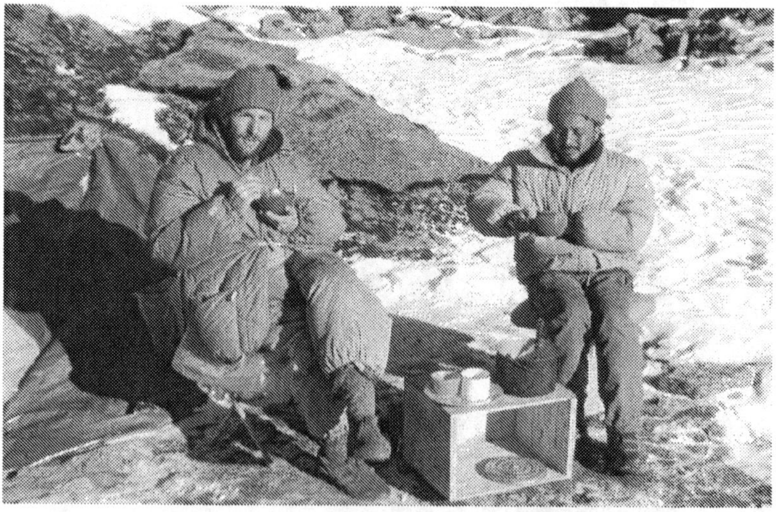

Figure 6. Sukhamay Lahiri and myself breakfasting at our science camp, 4,800m on the Second Schoolhouse Expedition, Physiology wing, late November 1964.

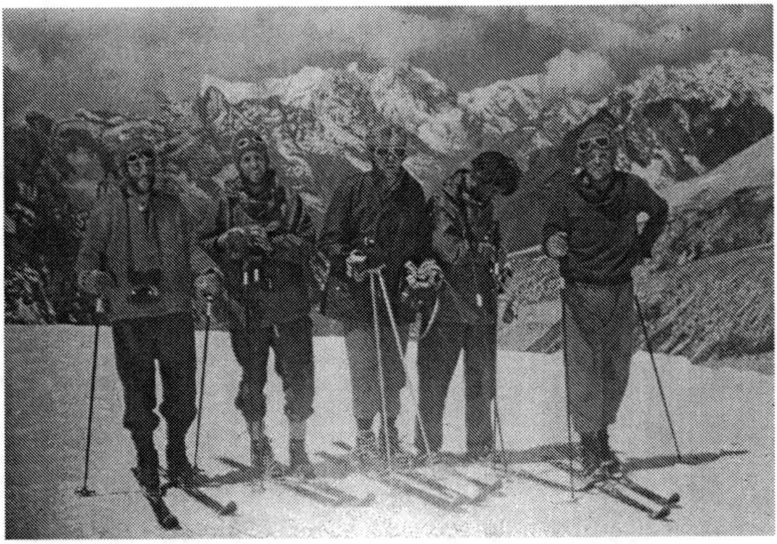

Figure 7. "Silver Hut Ski School". Winter 1960–61. Left to right, Myself, John West Griffith Pugh, Michael Ward, and Michael Gill.

CHAPTER 2

HIGH ALTITUDE PULMONARY HYPERTENSION AND CHRONIC MOUNTAIN SICKNESS - REAPPRAISAL OF THE CONSENSUS ON CHRONIC AND SUBACUTE HIGH ALTITUDE DISEASES

DANTE PENALOZA

University Cayetano Heredia, Lima, Peru

Abstract: An expert consensus workshop group of the International Society for Mountain Medicine recently proposed a new classification of high altitude diseases. Chronic mountain disease or Monge's disease was defined as a separate entity on the assumption that pulmonary hypertension was not always identified in these patients. This may have to be revised. Healthy high altitude natives living above 3500 m have pulmonary hypertension and right ventricular hypertrophy associated to hypoxemia and polycythemia. There is a direct relation between the level of altitude and the degree of pulmonary hypertension, with exception of Tibetan natives who have the oldest altitude ancestry. After many years of residence at high altitude, some healthy highlanders may lose their adaptation and develop chronic mountain sickness, a clinical entity associated with marked hypoxemia, exaggerated polycythemia and increased pulmonary hypertension, evolving in some cases to heart failure. Other chronic high altitude diseases, such as high altitude heart diseases described in China and high altitude cor pulmonale described in Kyrgystan, have a clinical picture similar to chronic mountain sickness, with lesser degrees of hypoxemia and polycythemia which, however, are often measured at lower levels during the recovery. A systematic review of world-wide literature has demonstrated that pulmonary hypertension is a common feature, in different magnitudes, to healthy highlanders and high altitude diseases. Differences of mean pulmonary artery pression amongst chronic mountain sickness, high altitude heart diseases and high altitude cor pulmonale are no significant and it is highly probable that they are the same disease with different shades. Therefore, chronic high altitude diseases should be integrated in one group and consequently, any scoring system should be applicable to all of them. On the other hand, subacute mountain sickness and high altitude pulmonary edema, clinical entities with a distinct time course, should be considered separately.

A. Aldashev and R. Naeije (eds.), Problems of High Altitude Medicine and Biology, 11–37.

Keywords: high altitude diseases; Monge's disease; pulmonary hypertension; polycythemia; heart failure; cor pulmonale; high altitude pulmonary edema

Introduction

Healthy high altitude natives living above 3500 m have pulmonary hypertension (PH) and right ventricular hypertrophy (RVH) associated with hypoxemia and polycythemia and, however, they are able to perform heavy physical exercise. After many years of residence at high altitude, some of these subjects gradually lose their adaptation and develop chronic mountain sickness (CMS). In these patients there is an exaggerated increase of hypoxemia, polycythemia and pulmonary hypertension associated in some cases with right ventricular enlargement and heart failure. This paper deals with pulmonary hemodynamics in healthy high altitude natives and patients with CMS and related diseases. Following this, a reappraisal of the consensus on chronic and subacute high altitude diseases is proposed.

Pulmonary Hypertension in Healthy High Altitude Natives

PULMONARY ARTERY PRESSURE AS RELATED TO AGE

Pioneering studies were performed by Peruvian investigators in healthy natives born and living at high altitudes (HA). Cardiac catheterization was undertaken in newborns, children and adults at 4540 m altitude (Morococha, Peru) and the results were compared with those already described at sea level (SL) [17,52,68]. The mean pulmonary artery pressure (mPAP) in newborns was around 60 mm Hg, a value similar to that described in SL newborns. After birth, the mPAP decreases slowly and persistent PH, of mild or moderate degree, is observed in adolescents and adults, contrasting with the fast decline of mPAP described in the postnatal period at sea level (Figure 1). HA children from 1 to 5 years have an average mPAP of 45 mm Hg, decreasing to 28 mm Hg in adolescents and adults. Table 1 shows the pulmonary hemodynamics in children and adults living at HA.

Histological studies of the distal pulmonary arterial branches were also performed at HA and SL in newborns, children and adults who had died in accidents or from acute non- cardiopulmonary diseases [8,10]. The postnatal changes of the "fetal pattern" differ at SL and HA. At SL the thick medial coat of smooth muscle cells (SMC) suffers a prompt remodeling and consequential thinning of the vessel wall and widening of the lumen. This is in contrast to a delayed maturation at HA, which implies persistence of a

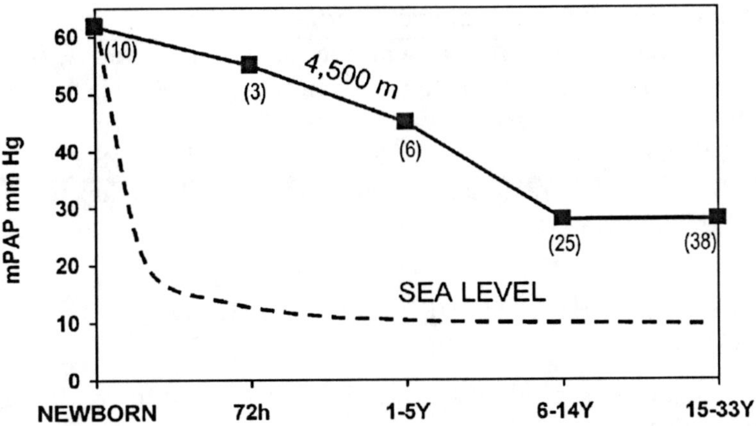

Figure 1. Pulmonary artery pressure related to age. The mPAP in newborns at HA and at SL is around 60 mm Hg. After birth, the mPAP declines rapidly at SL in contrast to the slow decline observed at HA, so that there is persistent PH in children and adults at the altitude of 4500 m. Numbers in parenthesis indicate the number of cases. Reproduced from Penaloza and Arias-Stella [46].

TABLE 1. Hemodynamic values in healthy highlanders by comparison to sea level residents studied at their respective location

	Altitude Children 1–5 years (n=7)	Altitude Children 6–14 years (n=32)	Altitude Adults 18–33 years (n=38)	Sea Level Adults 17–23 years (n=25)	Adults Altitude vs Sea Level P
Hct, %	43.9 ± 3.87	48.0 ± 3.25	59.1 ± 7.20	44.1 ± 2.59	< 0.001
Hb, g/dL	14.1 ± 0.66	15.7 ± 1.07	19.5 ± 1.97	14.7 ± 0.88	< 0.001
SaO_2, %	78.2 ± 2.76	77.3 ± 5.76	78.4 ± 4.81	95.7 ± 2.07	< 0.001
CI, L • min • m^{-2}	4.4 ± 0.60	4.5 ± 1.39	3.7 ± 1.64	3.9 ± 0.97	NS
RAP, mm Hg	2.8 ± 1.57	1.8 ± 1.46	2.6 ± 1.69	2.6 ± 1.31	NS
mPAP, mm Hg	45 ± 16.6	28 ± 10.2	28 ± 10.5	12 ± 2.2	< 0.001
PWP, mm Hg	6.7 ± 2.21	5.0 ± 1.00	5.4 ± 1.96	6.2 ± 1.71	NS
PVR, dyne • s • cm^{-5}	–	459 ± 273.7	332 ± 212.6	69 ± 25.3	< 0.001

Values are mean ± SD. CI indicates cardiac index; RAP, right atrial pressure; mPAP, mean value of PAP;PWP, pulmonary wedge pressure; PVR, pulmonary vascular resistance. Original data from Penaloza et al. [52,68].
Table reproduced from Penaloza and Arias-Stella [46].

thick medial muscular coat and narrowing of the lumen. Therefore, the main factor responsible for PH in healthy HA natives is the increased amount of SMC in the distal pulmonary arterial branches, which increases the pulmonary vascular resistances (PVR) [7,42,53,60].

The hemodynamic and histological findings of the pulmonary circulation in HA natives were in concordance with the electrocardiographic pattern and the anatomical characteristics of the heart in these people. There was persistent postnatal RVH, contrasting with the rapid transition from the right to the left ventricular predominance in SL subjects [9,50,51,58]. The delay of the cardiopulmonary transition in HA infants and children has recently been confirmed by noninvasive methodology [6,39,65].

PULMONARY ARTERY PRESSURE AS RELATED TO LEVEL OF ALTITUDE

Early electrocardiographic observations at six levels of altitude in the Peruvian Andes showed that as the altitude increases there is a greater degree of RVH in HA natives, particularly above 3000 m. Table 2 displays the combined effect of age and the level of altitude on the degree of RVH as assessed by the electrocardiogram ($\hat{A}$QRS>90°) [50,51,54]. Subsequent hemodynamic research demonstrated a highly significant difference of mPAP between SL residents and HA natives living at 4540 m. A mPAP value of 12 ± 2.2 mm Hg was found at SL in contrast to 28 ± 10.5 mm Hg at HA, with a range from 13 to 62 mm Hg. Most of the natives living at 4540 m had mild to moderate PH, 10% had normal PAP and 10% had severe PH (more than 40 mm Hg) [52]. Table 1 exhibits the mPAP and related hemodynamic data of healthy people living at 4540 m, in comparison to sea level residents.

Afterwards, hemodynamic studies were carried out in healthy residents of other high-altitude cities located in South America, North America and Asia. The mPAP in residents of cities located below 3000 m was normal. This was the case in Denver, Colorado [19], Mexico City, Mexico [35], Bogota, Colombia [40] and Xining, China [34]. mPAP values around 22 mm Hg, were found in cities between 3600–3700 m, such as La Paz, Bolivia [4], La Oroya, Peru [22] and Yushu, China [86]. Higher values of mPAP between 23 and nearly 30 mm Hg. were described in cities located around 4000 m or above, such as Chengdou, China [87], Madou, China [86], Cerro de Pasco, Peru [49] and Morococha, Peru [52] (Table 3). When mPAP values are plotted against the corresponding altitudes, a direct relationship is represented by a parabolic curve, so that mild or moderate increases of altitude above 3000 m are associated with significant increases of mPAP (Figure 2). In summary, above 3000 m most healthy natives have mild to moderate PH and at the highest altitudes some cases may have a severe degree of PH.

TABLE 2. Combined effect of age and the level of altitude on the right ventricular hypertrophy assessed by ECG (ÂQRS > 90°)

Altitude	New Born	1 Week 3 Months	4–11 Months	1–5 Years	6–14 Years	15–20 Years	21–40 Years	41–60 Years
Lima (sea level)	145 ± 20.1	110 ± 27.2	65 ± 22.3	51 ± 27.4	57 ± 27.7	55 ± 22.3	45 ± 32.4	30 ± 32.7
Arequipa (2400 m)	149 ± 25.2	124 ± 23.1	88 ± 34.1**	52 ± 26.3	64 ± 18.9	56 ± 31.1	47 ± 9.8	44 ± 29.2*
Huancayo (3200 m)	148 ± 28.5	145 ± 29.3**	129 ± 47.1**	74 ± 37.3*	73 ± 18.8**	75 ± 34.5**	54 ± 36.8	52 ± 29.8*
La Oroya (3700 m)	150 ± 22.3	147 ± 31.0**	141 ± 34.1**	97 ± 31.2**	85 ± 33.4**	68 ± 35.3*	45 ± 40.2	49 ± 39.0*
Cerro De Pasco (4300 m)	142 ± 24.1	147 ± 30.3**	156 ± 41.3**	132 ± 39.7**	102 ± 21.3**	97 ± 36.8**	81 ± 39.1**	79 ± 69.1**
Morococha (4540 m)	133 ± 28.5	152 ± 32.1**	155 ± 38.1**	155 ± 44.9**	137 ± 46.2**	125 ± 46.1**	105 ± 70.2**	108 ± 78.5**

Figures in bold mean ÂQRS > 90°. The statistical significance between the altitude locations and sea level is shown for each age group. *$p < 0.01$; **$p < 0.001$

Lima (sea level) n = 550. Morococha (4540 m) n = 400. Other levels, n = 550. Adapted from Penaloza et. al. [50,51,54].

TABLE 3. Pulmonary arterial pressure and arterial oxygen saturation at various altitudes

First author (Ref.)	Location	Altitude, m	mPAP, mm Hg (n)	SaO_2, % (n)
Penaloza (52)	Lima Peru	150	12 ± 2 (25)	96 ± 2.1 (25)
Grover (19)	Denver Colorado	1500	15 ± 3 (56)	94 (19)
Michelli (35)	Mexico City Mexico	2240	15 ± 2 (21)	92 (21)
Miao (34)	Xining Qinghai, China	2261	14 ± 2 (34)	93 (34)
Ordoñez (40)	Bogota Colombia	2600	13 ± 3 (18)	90 (18)
Grover (19)	Leadville Colorado	3100	24 ± 7 (50)	89 (50)
Antezana (4)	La Paz Bolivia	3600	22 ± 1 (11)	90 ± 0.8 (11)
Groves (18)	Lhasa Tibet	3600	15 ± 1 (5)	88 ± 1.8 (5)
Yang JS (86)	Yushu Qinghai, China	3680	22 ± 4 (17)	–
Hultgren (22)	La Oroya Peru	3700	22 ± 4 (26)	85 (27)
Yang Z (87)	Chengdou Qinghai, China	3950	26 ± 2 (22)	–
Yang JS (86)	Madou Qinghai, China	4280	23 ± 3 (12)	–
Penaloza (49)	Cerro de Pasco Peru	4300	23 ± 5 (12)	81 ± 4.6
Penaloza (52)	Morococha Peru	4540	28 ± 11 (38)	78 ± 4.8 (38)

Values for mPAP are mean ± SD. Values for SaO_2 are mean or mean ± SD.
Reproduced from Penaloza and Arias-Stella [46].

PULMONARY ARTERY PRESSURE AS RELATED TO ALTITUDE ANCESTRY

There are two notable exceptions to the relation of altitude to mPAP (Figure 2). A mPAP value higher than expected was found in Leadville, Colorado (3100 m) in native adolescents of European ancestry and relative newcomers to HA [19,72]. On the other hand, unexpected normal mPAP was found in Lhasa, Tibet (3600 m), in natives with the oldest altitude ancestry in the world [18]. These findings suggest that in addition to the level of altitude itself and the degree of hypoxia, the number of generations and millennia living at HA is a determinant genetic factor of the degree of PH. This hypothesis was pointed out by Grover four decades ago and the findings in Lhasa confirm this visionary insight [19,72].

The normal mPAP in Tibetan natives is associated with normal structure of the distal pulmonary arterial branches [20]. Coincident observations have

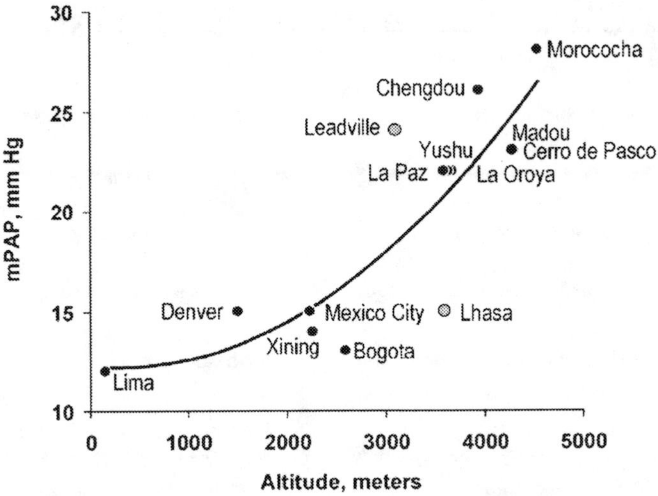

Figure 2. Pulmonary artery pressure related to level of altitude. When mPAP values are plotted against altitudes, a direct relationship is represented by a parabolic curve, so that mild or moderate increases of altitude above 3000 m are associated with significant increases of mPAP. There are two exceptions to this correlation (large symbols), which are discussed in the text. Reproduced from Penaloza and Arias-Stella [46].

been made in native animals to HA, such as yak and camelids, which have normal mPAP and pulmonary vasculature in contrast to domestic animals transported to the Andean mountains by the Spanish conquerors, such as cows and pigs, which have PH and thick pulmonary arterioles [21]. Normal mPAP and pulmonary vasculature at HA would indicate optimal adaptation in humans and animals [18,21].

Pulmonary Hypertension in Chronic Mountain Sickness and Related Diseases

CHRONIC MOUNTAIN SICKNESS
DEFINITION, CLINICAL PICTURE AND PATHOGENESIS

CMS is a clinical syndrome that occurs in native or long-life residents above 2500 m. It is characterized by excessive erythrocytosis (females Hb ≥ 19 g/dL; males Hb ≥ 21 g/dL), severe hypoxemia, and in some cases moderate or severe PH, which may evolve to cor pulmonale, leading to congestive HF. The clinical picture of CMS gradually disappears after descending to low altitude and reappears after returning to HA [26]. CMS was first described by Professor Monge, who placed emphasis on excessive polycythemia [37] Afterwards, Professor Hurtado pointed out that alveolar ventilation is the primary mechanism in CMS leading to severe hypoxemia and hence, to exaggerated polycythemia [23].

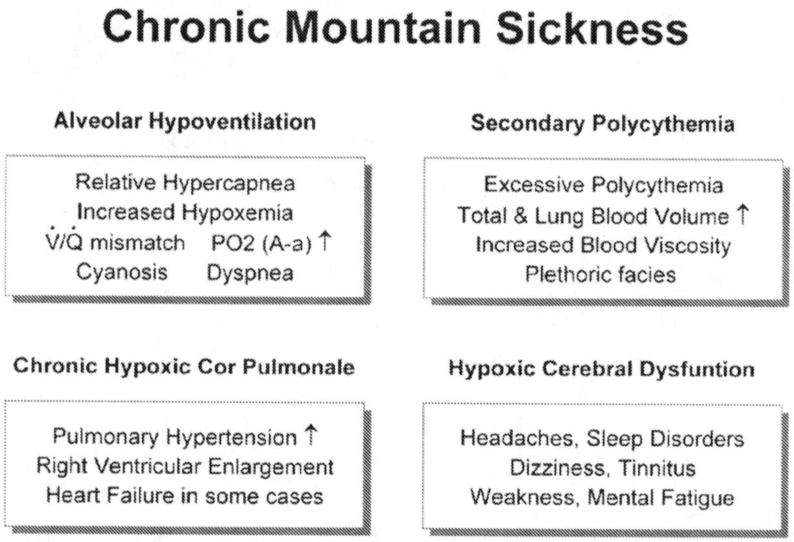

Figure 3. CMS is a variety of chronic alveolar hypoventilation that results in a complex syndrome integrating four main components. Respiratory features result in accentuated hypoxemia. Exaggerated polycythemia is the main expression of the hematological features. There is moderate to severe PH and accentuated RVH, which may evolve to hypoxic cor pulmonale and HF. Neuropsychic symptoms include sleep disorders, headaches, dizziness and mental fatigue.

CMS is a variety of chronic alveolar hypoventilation that results in a complex syndrome integrating four main components. Respiratory features are characterized by alveolar hypoventilation, relative hypercapnea, V/Q mismatch, widened (A-a) PO_2 gradient and increased hypoxemia. Hematological features are excessive polycythemia, increased blood viscosity and expanded total and lung blood volume. Cardiopulmonary abnormalities include moderate or severe PH and RVH, which may evolve to hypoxic cor pulmonale and HF. Neuropsychic symptoms include sleep disorders, headaches, dizziness and mental fatigue (Figure 3).

HEMODYNAMICS

Peruvian investigators were pioneers in this field. Rotta et al. were the first to perform a cardiac catheterization in one case of CMS living in Morococha, Peru, at 4540 m. This patient had mPAP 35 mmHg, Hb 26 g/dL and SaO_2 78% [64]. Afterwards, we performed cardiac catheterization studies in 10 cases of CMS residing in Cerro de Pasco (4340 m) and the mean values of SaO_2, Hb and Hct were 70 ± 5.0%, 25 ± 2.0 g/dL and 79 ± 4.0% respectively.

The mPAP was 47 ± 17 mm Hg and the individual values were all higher than 25 mm Hg, the highest value being 85 mm Hg (range 31 to 85 mm Hg) [49,55]. Table 4 shows hemodynamic data obtained in CMS at 4,540 m in comparison with healthy highlanders of Cerro de Pasco (4340 m) and sea level residents.

Bolivian investigators carried out two studies with cardiac catheterization in La Paz, Bolivia (3600 m). Ergueta et al. studied 20 patients and two of them were submitted to a cardiac catheterization with the following results: mPAP 51 mm Hg, Hb 26 g/dL and SaO2 84% [16]. Manier et al. studied 8 patients with a mean Hb of 21 g/dL and a mPAP of 27 mm Hg [32].

Chinese investigators performed important clinical and epidemiological studies in the last two decades [75,82]. However, there are limited observations with cardiac catheterization. Pei et al. studied 17 patients of CMS in Lhasa, Tibet (3600 m), most of them men of Chinese Han origin and all were smokers. Five patients had cardiac catheterization and the average mPAP was 39.6 ± 11.1 mmHg, greatly exceeding the normal value for healthy highlanders [41]. Yang et al. reported a mPAP of 31 mmHg in six Han male patients studied at Chengdou (3950 m), in contrast to 26 mm Hg found in healthy natives at the same altitude [87].

Hemodynamic investigations carried out with cardiac catheterization at the altitude of residence. The investigations just described are summarized in Table 5. There were two studies performed in Peru, two in Bolivia and two in China. The average of the mPAP values in these studies was 39 mmHg

TABLE 4. Hemodynamic values in chronic mountain sickness in comparison with healthy highlanders and sea level subjects

	Sea-Level Controls (n=25; age 17–23 y)	Healthy Highlanders Controls (n=12; age 19–38 y)	CMS Subjects (n=10; age 22–51 y)	CMS vs Highlanders P
Hb, g/dL	14.7 ± 0.88	20.1 ± 1.69	24.7 ± 2.36	< 0.001
Hct, %	44.1 ± 2.59	59.4 ± 5.4	79.3 ± 4.2	< 0.001
SaO_2, %	95.7 ± 2.07	81.1 ± 4.61	69.6 ± 4.92	< 0.001
RAP, mm Hg	2.6 ± 1.31	2.9 ± 1.4	3.9 ± 1.8	NS
mPAP, mm Hg	12 ± 2.2	23 ± 5.1	47 ± 17.7	< 0.001
PWP, mm Hg	6.2 ± 1.71	6.9 ± 1.4	5.7 ± 2.3	NS
PVR, dyne • s • cm^{-5}	69 ± 25.3	197 ± 57.6	527 ± 218.1	< 0.001
CI, L • min^{-1} • m^{-2}	3.9 ± 0.97	3.8 ± 0.62	4.0 ± 0.93	NS

Values are mean ± SD. Abbreviations are as in Table 1.1. Original data from Penaloza et al. [49, 52]. Table reproduced from Penaloza and Arias-Stella [46]

TABLE 5. Pulmonary Arterial Pressure in Chronic Mountain Sickness. Data obtained by Cardiac Catheterization at the Altitude of Residence

First Author (Ref.)	Location	Altitude, m	mPAP, mm Hg (n)	Hemoglobin g/dL
Rotta (64)	Morococha Peru	4540	35 (1)	26 (1)
Penaloza (49)	Cerro de Pasco Peru	4340	47 ± 17 (10)	25 ± 2 (10)
Ergueta (16)	La Paz Bolivia	3600	51 (2)	26 (2)
Manier (32)	La Paz Bolivia	3600	27 ± 10 (8)	21 ± 2 (8)
Pei (41)	Lhasa Tibet	3600	40 ± 11 (5)	23 ± 2 (5)
Yang Z (87)	Chengdou Qinghai, China	3950	31 (6)	22 (6)

Values for mPAP are mean or mean ± SD.

with a range from 27 to 51 mm Hg. The degree of PH was mild in one study, moderate in two studies and severe in three. There was no relation between the level of altitude and the degree of PH. The lower values of mPAP were found in patients with the lower values of Hb.

Hemodynamic studies during the recovery period at lower altitudes. This kind of study has been performed by Chinese investigators. There are two studies in patients with CMS coming from the Guolok area (3700–4200 m) and studied in Xining (2100 m). One of the studies was carried out with cardiac catheterization and the mPAP was 18 mm Hg, an unexpectedly low value, in contrast to the RVH found by ECG and chest X-ray in the same patients. The authors ascribed the low mPAP value to the lower altitude where the study was undertaken [84]. The second study was performed with a non-invasive procedure ("an equation related to the alveolar air") and the calculated mPAP was 39 mm Hg [81]. There is a significant discrepancy between both studies carried out in patients coming from the same HA and studied at the same lower altitude.

Hemodynamic studies with Doppler-echocardiography. These investigations were carried out by Bolivian investigators and are displayed in Table 6. From the systolic PAP (sPAP) values reported in these publications we calculated the corresponding mPAP values by using a new formula proposed by European investigators [12]. Antezana et al. studied a group of patients with an average age of 40 years and excessive polycythemia (Hb 22g/dL), and the mPAP was 26 mm Hg (sPAP 42 mm Hg) [5]. Vargas and Spielvogel studied two groups of patients with CMS, old and young patients, with Hb values of 24 and 19 g/dL respectively. The mPAP in both groups was 22 mm Hg (sPAP 35 mm Hg), a value similar to the mPAP of healthy people living

TABLE 6. Pulmonary arterial pressure in CMS vs Controls. Data obtained by Doppler-echocardiography at the Altitude of Residence, La Paz, Bolivia (3600 m)

First Author (Ref.)	Group P vs N	Number of cases	Age y	Hemoglobin g/dL	sPAP mm Hg	mPAP* mm Hg
Antezana (5)	P (old)	17	40	22	42	26
	N (young)	14	28	17	43	27
Vargas (71)	P (old)	28	47	24	35	22
	N (old)	27	43	17	29	18
	P (young)	30	22	19	35	22
	N (young)	30	22	17	28	18

P: Polycythemia. N: Normocythemia. *Calculated mPAP values (12).

in La Paz. This result is not congruent with the finding in the same patients of moderate or definite RVH in comparison with the control subjects [71].

An unexpected finding in these studies from Bolivia was the quite opposite mPAP values in the normocythemic and asymptomatic control groups (Table 6). The mPAP value was 27 mm Hg in the first study [5] and 18 mm Hg in the second one [71]. The mPAP of 27 mm Hg is too high and the second one is lower in comparison with the mPAP of 22 mm Hg found in healthy people of La Paz in several studies, as reported by Vargas and Spielvogel [71]. The mPAP of 27 mm Hg is found in healthy people living above 4000 m and is usually associated with definite signs of RVH in the ECG, which was recorded but not described by Antezana et al. [5]. On the other hand, an mPAP of 18 mmHg is found in healthy people living below 3000 m of altitude. The discrepancy between both studies may be ascribed to a probable inaccuracy of sPAP values obtained with Doppler echocardiography.

HIGH ALTITUDE HEART DISEASE (HAHD) DEFINITION AND CLINICAL PICTURE

Chinese investigators have described the adult variety of HAHD as a chronic disease of maladaptation to altitude, mainly occurring in lowlanders who have migrated to high altitudes for prolonged residence [79]. The chronicity of the adult HAHD is in contrast to the subacute evolution of the pediatric HAHD. Epidemiological studies performed by Chinese investigators pointed out that the prevalence of adult HAHD increases with the level of altitude, is higher in Han immigrants than in Tibetan natives and is half of that described in pediatric HAHD [62,78] The prevalence of adult HAHD is six times lower than the 6% reported for CMS in China [82]. Wu was the first to describe the adult HAHD in 1965 [77] and was also the author of the last original paper on this entity in 1990 [80]. In the period of 25 years that elapsed between the two articles, there were numerous publications in Chinese on the clinical and epidemiological aspects of this entity, including studies with great numbers of cases. [13,29,78,79].

According to Chinese authors, the adult type of HAHD is characterized by clinical evidence of PH, RVH and HF without accentuated hypoxemia and polycythemia [62,79]. A review article on adult HAHD pointed out that levels of hemoglobin and hematocrit are in general lower than 20 g/dL and 65% respectively [62]. However, initial descriptions of adult HAHD were confused and there was a great overlap with the polycythemic variety of HA disease (CMS). Under the name of HAHD were included many studies with a variable degree of polycythemia. The original description included 22 cases with average values of Hb 21.1 g/dL and Hct 73% [77] and the last original publication recorded 202 cases with an average Hb of 23.3 g/dL [80].

Wu et al. early supposed that cases with excessive polycythemia were the counterpart of CMS described in the Andes [74] and then realized that CMS was a real entity in China, both in Han immigrants and Tibetan natives [81]. Wu et al. have recognized that publications on adult HAHD, most of them from their own group, actually correspond to CMS [81]. Lastly, Wu has recently published a comprehensive review on CMS in the Qinghai-Tibetan Plateau [75]. On the other hand, publications on HAHD have declined and in the last 15 years only some review papers have been published [62,63]. A proposal for delimitation between adult HAHD and CMS was attempted by the Chinese Association for High Altitude Medicine in 1996 [15].

HEMODYNAMICS

Review articles on HAHD mention that a diagnostic criterion is a mPAP > 24 mm Hg [63,79]. However, Chinese investigators comment that there are no reliable measurements of PAP obtained by cardiac catheterization in adult HAHD. There are only two reports of PAP obtained by Doppler echocardiography after one week of residence at the lower altitude of Xining (2261 m) and the calculated mPAP values in these studies were 36±3 and 28±4 mm Hg respectively (Table 7) [14,80], values similar to or somewhat lower than most of those reported in CMS. In concordance, the ECG, VCG and chest X-ray findings described in patients with adult HAHD are similar to those described in patients with CMS in Peru [49,55] and China [75,81]. In short, the clinical picture of adult HAHD resembles that of CMS with lesser degrees of hypoxemia and polycythemia which, however, are often measured at the lower altitude where the hemodynamic study is carried out.

TABLE 7. Pulmonary arterial pressure in High Altitude Heart Disease (HAHD) and High Altitude Cor Pulmonale (HACP) obtained during recovery at lower altitudes

First Author (Ref.)	Diagnosis	Location	Altitude of Residence, m	Altitude of Study, m	mPAP, mm Hg (n)
Wu (80)	HAHD	Qinghai-Tibetan Plateau, China†	3000–5000	2260	36 ± 3 (108)
Cheng (14)	HAHD	Qinghai-Tibetan Plateau, China†	3000–5000	2260	28 ± 4 (10)
Saryvaeb (67)	HACP	Tien-Shan & Pamir Mountains, Kyrgyzstan‡	3200–4200	760	38 ± 3 (8)
Aldashev (1)	HACP	Tien-Shan & Pamir Mountains, Kyrgyzstan‡	2800–3100	760	32 ± 4 (11)

Values for mPAP are mean ± SD.
†Doppler echocardiography in Xining, 2260 m.
‡Cardiac catheterization in Bishkek, 760 m.

HIGH ALTITUDE COR PULMONALE DEFINITION AND CLINICAL PICTURE

Kyrgyzian investigators do not have any publications under the name of CMS. Five decades ago they described a clinical picture named High Altitude Pulmonary Hypertension (HAPH), which may evolve to High Altitude Cor Pulmonale (HACP) and HF [36]. This clinical entity is observed in people living at the high altitudes of the Tien-Shan and Pamir Mountains (2800–4200 m) and its prevalence is 4.6% in the male population. HACP is characterized by a variable degree of PH, RVH and HF in the absence of significant hypoxemia and polycythemia [1,67]. Cardiac auscultation and the findings obtained by ECG and chest-X rays resemble those found in patients with CMS [49,55,81] and adult HAHD [62,79,80].

HEMODYNAMICS

From 1989 to 1999, cardiac catheterization studies were carried out in 136 symptomatic highlanders (2800–3600 m) and resting PH with a mPAP value of 37 ± 3 mm Hg was found in 27 subjects (20%) [1]. Sarybaev and

Mirrakhimov found a mPAP of 38 ± 3.2 mm Hg in a group of patients with HACP living at 3200–4200 m [67]. Recently, Aldashev et al. reported a mPAP of 32 ± 4 mm Hg (range 20–64 mm Hg) in 11 subjects with HACP living at 2800–3100 m [1]. It should be noted that all cardiac catheterization studies reported by Kyrgyzian investigators were performed after one week of residence at low altitude (Bishkek, 750 m) (Table 7), which may explain, at least in part, the absence of significant hypoxemia and polycythemia. There is little data on SaO2, Hb and Hct in Kyrgyzian investigations. SaO2 improves promptly after descending to low levels and becomes normal or near normal in reported cases [1].

SUBACUTE MOUNTAIN SICKNESS DEFINITION, CLINICAL PICTURE AND PATHOGENESIS

Five decades ago, Chinese investigators described in humans the counterpart of cattle brisket disease, with the name of High Altitude Heart Disease (HAHD) of the pediatric type [73]. This entity is mainly observed in infants of Chinese Han origin who are born at low altitude and then brought to high altitude where they develop PH and HF within a few weeks or months with a fatal outcome if the infants are not moved down to lower places. Pediatric HAHD is also observed in children from 2 to 14 years of age but the prevalence is lower than in infants. Prevalence of pediatric HAHD is higher in Han infants than in Tibetan infants [78]. The mechanism of SMS is ascribed to exaggerated hypoxic pulmonary reactivity of distal pulmonary arterial branches, which are muscularized in excess.

HEMODYNAMICS AND PATHOLOGY

In 1963, with the name of “primary pulmonary hypertension in children living at high altitude”, Khoury and Hawes reported their findings in 11 infants from 6 to 23 months living in Leaville, Colorado (3,100 m). Five of them were moved to Denver, Colorado (1500 m) and had cardiac catheterization with an average mPAP of 44 mm Hg and a range of 28–72 mm Hg. Post-mortem studies in two patients showed severe RVH and marked hypertrophy of the medial muscular coat and intimal proliferation, but not occlusive lesions [25]. In the following years Tibetan investigators described similar pathological findings in 57 infants who died with the diagnosis of pediatric HAHD [28] and several years later, the same authors extended their investigations to 100 infants with HAHD [27]. Lin and Wu published their clinical observations in 286 cases of pediatric HAHD [30].

TABLE 8. Pulmonary arterial pressure in infants with subacute mountain sickness while recovering at lower altitudes

First Author (Ref.)	Location	Altitude of Residence, m	Altitude of Study, m	mPAP, mm Hg (n)
Khoury (25)	Leadville Colorado‡	3100	1500	44 (5)
Wu (76)	Qinghai-Tibetan Plateau, China†	3000–4200	2260	33 ± 11 (8)
Ru-Yan (66)	Qinghai-Tibetan Plateau, China†	2440–3700	2260	72 ± 17 (55)

Values for mPAP are mean or mean ± SD.
†Doppler echocardiography in Xining, 2260 m.
‡Cardiac catheterization in Denver, 1500 m.

The first report in English with the name of Subacute Mountain Sickness (SMS) was published in 1988 by Asian and British investigators who placed emphasis on the subacute evolution of this disease and reported the post-mortem findings in 15 infants. Extreme medial hypertrophy of the small pulmonary arteries and massive hypertrophy and dilatation of the right ventricle were the main factors [70]. Some hemodynamic studies have been undertaken in SMS.

Wu and Miao reported an average mPAP of 33 mm Hg in 8 infants living at 3000–4000 m and recovering from SMS in Xining (2261 m) [76]. Recently, a moderate to severe PH with a mPAP of 72 mmHg was assessed by Doppler-echocardiography in 55 infants coming from high altitudes and recovering from SMS in Xining [66] (Table 8). SMS in adults has also been described in soldiers patrolling at very high altitudes of the Himalayan mountains, with prompt recovery after moving down to lower levels [2]. A comprehensive review of SMS has recently been published [3]. SMS is not frequent in the Andes but some observational cases have been described in Peru and Bolivia [24,44,56].

COMPARATIVE HEMODYNAMICS OF CHRONIC MOUNTAIN SICKNESS AND RELATED DISEASES

CHRONIC HIGH ALTITUDE DISEASES

Currently, there are no hemodynamic publications demonstrating significant differences of PH amongst chronic HA diseases as CMS, HAHD and HACP. However, most publications on PH in CMS reveal values somewhat greater than in HAHD and HACP. The average mPAP of six studies of CMS displayed in Table 5 is 39 mm Hg (range 27 to 51 mm Hg) in comparison with 33.5 mm Hg (range 28 to 38 mm Hg) of four studies of HAHD and HACP shown in Table 7. Severe degrees of PH (mPAP $\geq$ 40 mm Hg) have only been reported in CMS. The magnitude of clinical PH as assessed by auscultation, ECG, VCG and chest X-ray do not show differences amongst CMS, HAHD and HACP. Lower degrees of hypoxemia and polycythemia have been reported in HAHD and HACP; however these features are ascribed, at least in part, to the low altitude at which the studies were performed. It appears that CMS, HAHD and HACP are basically the same entity with some different shades.

SUBACUTE MOUNTAIN SICKNESS

On the other hand, SMS is a very definite disease, which has fundamental differences, on clinical and pathophysiological grounds, from the group of chronic high altitude diseases (CMS, HAHD and HACP). While these are chronic diseases occurring in adults after long residence at HA, SMS is a disease with a characteristic subacute evolution, weeks or months, and mainly occurring in infants from low levels after their arrival at HA. SMS is an entity with a strong basis on clinical, hemodynamic and pathological grounds. Most patients with SMS have exaggerated degrees of PH, RVH and HF, while hypoxemia and polycythemia are only of slight degree. The primary mechanism in SMS is vasoconstriction due to exaggerated hypoxic pulmonary vasoreactivity of the small pulmonary arteries, which are excessively muscularized. The primary mechanism in SMS is vascular, in contrast to the respiratory mechanism described in some chronic HA diseases, such as CMS (Figure 4).

Reappraisal of the Consensus on Chronic and Subacute High Altitude Diseases

BACKGROUND

During the VI World Congress on Mountain Medicine and High Altitude Physiology, which was held in Xining, Qinghai, China in 2004, a Consensus Statement on Chronic and Subacute High Altitude Diseases was achieved by an ad hoc committee of the International Society for Mountain Medicine (ISMM). The Consensus Statement was published in 2005 and in the introduction to this document, a cautious warning was included on the possible evolution of this consensus as result of further research [26].

The Consensus recognizes two main groups of chronic and subacute high altitude diseases. A) Chronic Mountain Sickness (CMS) or Monge's

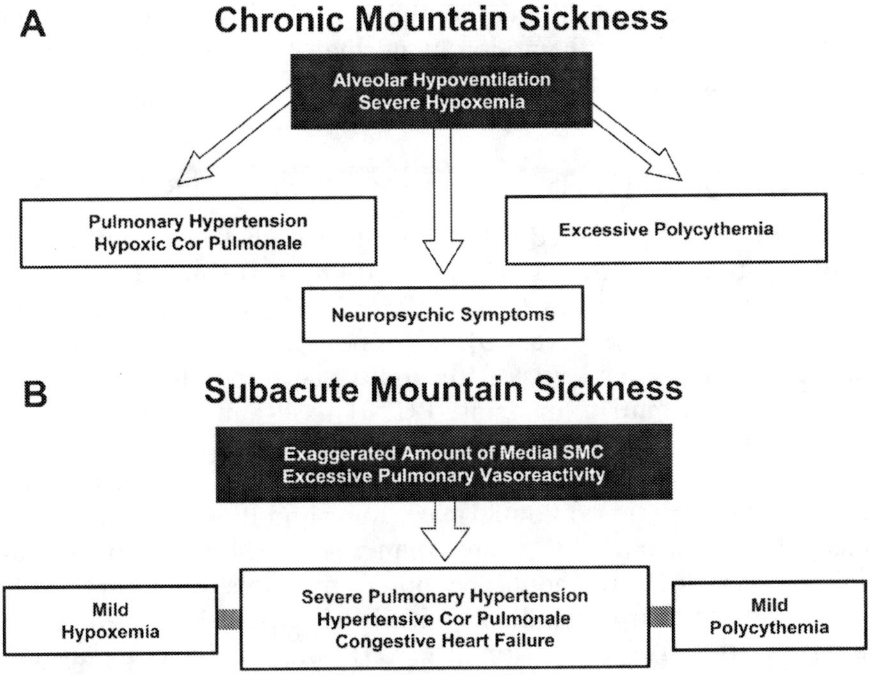

Figure 4. **A**, Pathogenesis of CMS. Development of alveolar hypoventilation in life-long residents at HA induces severe hypoxemia, exaggerated polycythemia and neuropsychic symptoms. There is moderate or severe PH and some cases evolve to hypoxic cor pulmonale and HF. **B**, Pathogenesis of SMS. In some infant newcomers to HA there is an excessive amount of SMC in the distal pulmonary arterial branches and exaggerated vasoconstriction, which induces severe PH, hypertensive cor pulmonale and HF. Hypoxemia and polycythemia of mild degree are found in these cases. HF indicates heart failure. Reproduced from Penaloza and Arias-Stella [46].

disease and B) High Altitude Pulmonary Hypertension (HAPH), which includes several entities: 1) High Altitude Heart Disease (HAHD) of adult chronic type, described in China, 2) High Altitude Cor Pulmonale (HACP) described in Kyrgyzstan, and 3) Subacute Mountain Sickness (SMS), also named subacute High Altitude Heart Disease (subacute HAHD) of infantile and adult types.

The main rationale for this classification was the assumption of definite PH in diseases of group B in contrast to CMS. This assumption motivated us to carry out a review of world-wide literature of hemodynamic studies on high altitude diseases with the exclusion of High Altitude Pulmonary Edema (HAPE), an acute HA disease characterized by excessive PH, which has a well-known role as an initiating factor of this entity. In addition, and for comparative purposes, we reviewed the hemodynamic studies undertaken in healthy highlanders at different altitudes. Before discussing our findings, it is important to clarify the notion of normal PAP values at sea level and consequently the definition of PH.

PROPOSALS FOR DEFINITION OF PULMONARY HYPERTENSION

Reeves and Groves published a literature review that involved 70 normal individuals at sea level and found a mPAP of 14 ± 3 mm Hg, and consequently an upper limit (mean + 2SD) of 20 mm Hg for people, from 6 to 45 years of age, living at sea level [59]. It has been a common clinical practice to consider the following levels of PH and the corresponding mPAP values: mild PH, 21 to 30 mmHg, moderate PH, 31 to 40 mm Hg and severe PH, over 40 mmHg.

On the other hand, the Primary Pulmonary Hypertension (PPH) Registry initiated by the National Heart, Lung and Blood Institute in 1981, defined PH as a mean PAP greater than 25 mm Hg at rest or 30 mmHg during exercise [61]. It should be noted that this criterion has been derived from a registry of patients with PPH (currently named Idiopatic Pulmonary Arterial Hypertension or IPAH), who usually have exaggerated degrees of PH and complex lesions associated with vascular occlusion [57]. Despite this, the proposed criterion was maintained for all varieties of PH in the Third World Symposium on Pulmonary Arterial Hypertension held in Venice, Italy (2004) [11].

HIGH ALTITUDE PULMONARY HYPERTENSION: A COMMON FEATURE OF HIGH ALTITUDE DISEASES SUMMARY OF THE LITERATURE REVIEW

The world-wide research of hemodynamic studies in healthy highlanders and high altitude diseases may be summarized as follows.

Healthy people living above 3000 m have mild to moderate PH, with a mPAP range from 22 to near 30 mm Hg, and at the highest altitudes some individual cases may have severe PH, with values of mPAP greater than 40 mm Hg (Table 3 and Figure 2).

Patients with CMS, in six studies with cardiac catheterization at their altitude of residence, had an average mPAP of 39 mmHg with a range from 27 to 51 mm Hg. The degree of PH was mild in one study, moderate in two studies and severe in three studies (Table 5). In an additional study carried out with Doppler-echocardiography at 3600 m, the calculated mPAP was 26 mmHg (Table 6).

Patients with HAHD and HACP, living at HA and studied at low altitudes, had an average mPAP of 33.5 mm Hg, with a range from 28 to 38 mm Hg.

The degree of PH was mild in one study and moderate in three. No study with severe PH has been reported (Table 7).

Infants with SMS, coming from HA and studied during recovery at lower places, had an average mPAP of 50 mm Hg with a range from 33 to 72 mm Hg. The degree of PH was moderate in one study and severe in two (Table 8).

ANALYSIS BASED ON CURRENT EVIDENCE

The preceding analysis based on current evidence indicates that HAPH is a distinctive feature, in different magnitude, of healthy highlanders and high altitude diseases. Maggiorini and Leon-Velarde envisioned this important concept [31] which, however, was modified in a subsequent publication, excluding CMS from the group entitled HAPH [26]. We envisage HAPH as a true pathophysiological spectrum. At one end of the spectrum are healthy highlanders with mild PH and at the other end is infantile SMS (pediatric HAHD) with severe PH. HAPE, an acute HA disease, is also at this end of the spectrum, particularly in HA natives with reentry HAPE [48]. In the middle of the spectrum are the high altitude diseases with chronic evolution, such as CMS, HAHD (described in China) and HACP (described in Kyrgyzstan). There are no significant differences in mPAP amongst these HA chronic entities, however severe PH has been described only in CMS.

EXPERT OPINIONS

In addition to the analysis based on evidence, it is of interest to be aware of the opinion of the experts living in the Andes and Asia with experience in pulmonary hemodynamics in patients with CMS. Rotta et al. commented "it is evident that the pulmonary pressures found in CMS exceed largely those corresponding to the healthy altitude natives" [64]. Penaloza et al. found severe PH in 50% of their cases and arrived at a similar conclusion [49]. Authorities in altitude medicine like Hurtado [23] as well as Monge M. and Monge C. [38] defined CMS as a disease associated with accentuated degree of PH, based on the findings of Rotta and Penaloza. Other authorities who worked in Peru for long periods such as Heath [21] and Hultgren [22] expressed similar opinions.

Bolivian investigators have also associated CMS with PH. Vargas et al. mention that "clinical and radiological signs of PH" are components of the clinical picture in CMS [71]. Zubieta Sr and Zubieta Jr commented: "diverse etiopathogenesis lead to a sustained low oxygen saturation and cyanosis, giving rise to PH and increased polycythemia" [88]. Outstanding Chinese investigators have also emphasized the presence of PH in CMS. Pei et al. wrote: "It is clear that our patients had a pulmonary arterial pressure greatly exceeding the norm for the altitude" [41]. Wu et al. commented "An aggravating hypoxemia is the pathophysiological basis of CMS from start to finish, which leads to excessive polycythemia and marked PH" [83]. Ge Ri-Li and Helun stated "the most striking features in patients with CMS are severe hypoxemia, excessive polycythemia and marked PH" [62].

REAPPRAISAL OF THE CONSENSUS STATEMENT

The classification proposed by the Consensus Statement, excluding CMS from the group of HA diseases associated with HAPH, is not in concordance with the analysis based on current evidence nor with expert opinion. There are no data in the current literature indicating that CMS is not associated with PH of variable magnitude and there are no data demonstrating that adult HAHD and HACP have greater degrees of PH than CMS. Differences of mPAP amongst these three chronic high altitude diseases are not significant, however the evidence demonstrates that mPAP in CMS is somewhat greater that in HAHD and HACP and that severe degrees of PH have only been reported in CMS. It is surprising that in the Consensus Statement there is no reference to any original research dealing with PH in HAHD [26]. There are ten references from Wu, an outstanding Chinese investigator, but none of them deals with PH in HAHD.

Chronic HA diseases (CMS, HAHD, HACP) and subacute HA diseases are associated with HAPH in different magnitudes. Therefore, the presence or absence of PH should not be the rationale for a classification of HA diseases. Instead, the time course of the disease, following a chronic, subacute or acute evolution, should be the natural and logical criterion for any classification of HA diseases. Chronic HA diseases, all of them associated with PH, should be integrated in one group. It is highly probable that CMS, HAHD and HACP are the same disease with different tints. SMS and HAPE should be considered separately.

PROPOSAL FOR CLASSIFICATION OF HIGH ALTITUDE PULMONARY HYPERTENSION

A revised clinical classification of PH was proposed by Simonneau et al. during the Third World Symposium on Pulmonary Arterial Hypertension, and HAPH was considered in item 3.5 as "Chronic exposure to high altitude" [69]. For those interested in high altitude medicine, we propose a more detailed classification of HAPH with the corresponding clinical conditions, as follows:

High Altitude Pulmonary Hypertension.

1. Healthy highlanders living above 3000m
2. Chronic high altitude diseases
   2.1. Chronic mountain sickness (CMS)
   2.2. Adult high altitude heart disease (HAHD described in China)
   2.3. High altitude cor pulmonale (HACP described in Kyrgyz)
3. Subacute mountain sickness (subacute HAHD)
   3.1. Infantile subacute mountain sickness (or pediatric HAHD)
   3.2. Adult subacute mountain sickness
4. High altitude pulmonary edema

SCORING SYSTEM FOR DIAGNOSIS OF CHRONIC MOUNTAIN SICKNESS

In the last two decades, epidemiological studies of CMS have been performed in Peru, China and Kyrgyzstan and several scoring systems for its diagnosis have been proposed. However, it is not easy to develop a unique scoring system because of the individual characteristics (ethnicity, gender, age) and dissimilar geographical areas and altitudes. Nevertheless, the Qinghai score proposed by Chinese investigators was approved by the CMS Consensus Group during the VI World Congress on Mountain Medicine (Xining, China, 2004) [26]. This scoring system is based on the level of Hb ≥ 21 for men and ≥ 19 for females, the presence of cyanosis and subjective symptoms such as breathlessness, sleep disorders, headache, tinnitus and paresthesias. Each symptom is scored as 0, 1, 2, 3 based on absent, mild, moderate and severe symptoms, respectively. Hb is scored 3 if it equals or exceeds the limits pointed out. According to the overall scoring, CMS is defined as follows: absent (0–5), mild (6–11), moderate (10–14) and severe (>15) [26]. Some comments related to this scoring system are pertinent [45].

HEMOGLOBIN THRESHOLD VALUES

The Hb threshold value of 21 g/dl, selected at 4340 m in Peru, may not be valid for lower altitudes and the diagnosis of CMS may be missed. A review of the epidemiological Chinese study in more than 5000 subjects at three levels of altitude demonstrates that the Hb values vary significantly according to the level of altitude and ethnicity and consequently, the threshold values are not the same [83]. Similar reasoning may be applicable to the range of altitudes between 2500 m and 4500 m in Peru and Bolivia.

HYPOXEMIA LEVELS

This key feature of CMS has not been included in the scoring system despite it being previously considered in all proposed scoring systems. Variable threshold values for SaO2 as <82%, <85% and <90% were proposed by Peruvian, Chinese and Kyrgyzian investigators respectively. These values could be scored as 3, 2 and 1 respectively.

PULMONARY HYPERTENSION

PH, a major component of CMS, was mentioned in most previous scoring systems, however was not included in the approved scoring system. The clinical evidence of PH, easily assessed by auscultation, chest X-ray and ECG, has been advised as the initial methodology for diagnosis of PH in the recently approved guidelines [11,33]. Following these guidelines, the clinical evidence of PH in CMS could be scored as 0 (absent), 1 (mild), 2 (moderate) and 3 (severe), based on simple objective diagnostic procedures (ECG, chest X-ray) and the clinical signs. Quantification of PH by Doppler-echocardiography or right heart catheterization could be carried out in selected cases of CMS, when these procedures are available in the altitude of residence [45].

LIMITATIONS AND EXPANSION OF THE SCORING SYSTEM FOR DIAGNOSIS OF CHRONIC MOUNTAIN SICKNESS

Subacute mountain sickness and high altitude pulmonary edema are clinical entities associated with moderate or severe PH but with a distinct time course. Therefore, these diseases should be out of the scope of the Scoring System for CMS. On the other hand, the Scoring System should not be limited to CMS and should be extended to other chronic high altitude diseases such as HAHD and HACP, since PH is a common feature to all of them, without significant differences. Moreover, most of the symptoms and signs are also similar with exception of the levels of hemoglobin and hypoxemia which, however, should be considered at the place of residence and not during the recovery at lower altitudes.

Acknowledgments

The author is indebted to the late Professor Alberto Hurtado, pioneer of the scientific research in Peru, for his valuable support to our classic investigation on chronic mountain sickness. I would also like to express my gratitude to all who were my collaborators at the Cardiovascular Laboratory of the High Altitude Research Institute, Peruvian University Cayetano Heredia. I am grateful to Hector Villagarcia, BSc, for his diligence in the diagramming support for this article.

References

1. Aldashev A, Sarybaev AS, Sydkykov AS, Kalmyrzaev BB, Kim EV, Mamanova LB, Maripov R, Kojonazarov BK, Mirrakhimov MM, Wilkins MR, Morrell NW (2002) Characterization of high-altitude pulmonary hypertension in the Kyrgyz: Association with angiotensin-converting enzyme genotype. Am J Respir Crit Care Med 166:1396–1402
2. Anand IS, Malhotra R, Chandershekhar Y, Bali HK, Chauhan SS, Jindal SK, Bhandar RK, Wahi PL (1990) Adult subacute mountain sickness: A syndrome of congestive heart failure in man at very high altitude. Lancet 335:561–565
3. Anand IS, Wu TY (2004) Syndromes of subacute mountain sickness. High Alt Med Biol 5:156–170
4. Antezana G, Barragan L, Coudert J, Cudkowitz L, Durand J, Lockhart A, Mensch-Dechene J, Paz Zamora M, Spielvogel H, Vargas E, Zelter M (1982) The pulmonary circulation of high altitude natives. In: High Altitude Physiology and Medicine. Brendel W, Zink RA, (eds) Springer Verlag, New York, pp 142–149
5. Antezana AM, Antezana G, Aparicio O, Noriega I, Leon-Velarde F, Richalet JP (1998) Pulmonary hypertension in high-altitude chronic hypoxia: response to nifedipine. Eur Respir J 12:1181–1185
6. Aparicio O, Romero F, Harris P, Anand I (1991) Echocardiography shows persistent thickness of the wall of the right ventricle in infants at high altitude. Cardioscience 2:63–68
7. Arias-Stella J. Morphological patterns: Mechanism of pulmonary arterial hypertension. In: Life at High Altitudes. Pan American Health Organization, Scientific Publication No. 140, Washington DC, 1966: 9–12
8. Arias-Stella J, Castillo Y (1966) The muscular pulmonary arterial branches in stillborn natives of high altitudes. Laboratory Investigation 15:1951–1959
9. Arias Stella J, Recavarren S (1962) Right ventricular hypertrophy in native children living at high altitude. Am J Pathol 41:55–64
10. Arias Stella J, Saldaña M (1963) The terminal portion of the pulmonary arterial tree in people native to high altitude. Circulation 28:915–925
11. Barst RJ, McGoon M, Torbicki A, Sitbon O, Krowka MJ, Olschewsky H, Gaine S (2004) Diagnosis and differential assessment of pulmonary arterial hypertension. J Am Coll Cardiol 43:40S–47S
12. Chemla D, Castelain V, Humbert M, Hébert JL, Simmoneau G, Lecarpentier Y, Hervé P (2004) New formula for predicting mean pulmonary artery pressure using systolic pulmonary artery pressure. Chest 126:1313–1317
13. Chen YC, Wong LZ, Mung ZH, Fung GY (1982) An analysis of 300 cases of high altitude heart diseases in adults (in Chinese). Chin J Cardiol 10:256–258
14. Cheng DS, Yang YX, Bian HP, Lu YZ, Liu PF, Zhou HL, Go BH. A study on altitude hypoxic pulmonary hypertension by Doppler echocardiography (1996) Chin J High Alt Med. (Chinese with English abstract) 6:28–31
15. Chinese Medical Association for High Altitude Medicine (1996) Recommendation for the classification and the diagnostic criteria of high altitude diseases in China (in Chinese). Chin J High Alt Med 6:2–4
16. Ergueta J, Spielvogel H, Cudkowitz L (2002) Cardio-respiratory studies in chronic mountain sickness (Monge's Syndrome). Respiration 28:485–517
17. Gamboa R, Marticorena E (1971) Presión arterial pulmonar en el recién nacido en la grandes alturas. Arch Inst Biol Andina 4:55–66
18. Groves BM, Droma T, Sutton JR, McCullough RG, McCullough RE, Zhuang J, Rapmund G, Sun S, Janes C, Moore LG (1993) Minimal hypoxic pulmonary hypertension in normal Tibetans at 3658m. J Appl Physiol 74:312–318
19. Grover RF (1990) Chronic hypoxic pulmonary hypertension. In: Fishman AP (ed) The Pulmonary Circulation: Normal and Abnormal. University of Pennsylvania, Philadelphia, pp 283–299

20. Gupta ML, Rao KS, Anand IS, Banerjee AK, Boparai MS (1992) Lack of smooth muscle in the small pulmonary arteries of the native Ladakh- is the Himalayan highlander adapted? Am Rev Respir Dis 145:1201–1204
21. Heath D, Williams DR (1995) High-altitude medicine and pathology. Adaptation to hypobaric hypoxia. Oxford University Press, Oxford, pp 403–415
22. Hultgren HN, Kelly J, Miller H (1965) Pulmonary circulation in acclimatized man at high altitude. J Appl Physiol 20:233–238
23. Hurtado A (1964) Animals in high altitude: Resident man. In: Handbook of Physiology. Sect 4, Vol 1, Chapter 54. Adaptation to the Environment. Am Physiol Soc, Washington DC, pp 843–860
24. Hurtado GL, Calderon RG (1965) Hipoxia de la altura en la insuficiencia cardiaca del lactante. Bolet Soc Boliv Pediatr IX:11–23
25. Khoury GH, Hawes CR (1963) Primary pulmonary hypertension in children living at high altitude. J Pediatrics 62:177–185
26. León-Velarde F, Maggiorini M, Reeves JT, Aldashev A, Asmus I, Bernardi L, Ri-Li Ge, Hackett P, Kobayashi T, Moore L, Penaloza D, Richalet JP, Roach R, Wu T, Vargas E, Zubieta-Castillo G, Zubieta-Calleja G (2005) Consensus statement on chronic and subacute high altitude diseases. High Alt Med Biol 6:147–157
27. Li JB, Sui GJ (1984) Pathological findings in high altitude heart disease. In: Applied High Altitude Medicine. Tibet Press, Lhasa, Tibet, pp 288–305
28. Li JB, Wang IY (1966) Infantile malacclimatized to high altitude. A pathologic observation. Chin J Pathol 10:98–99 (in Chinese)
29. Li YD, Ji L (1989) Clinical analysis of 500 cases of adult high altitude heart disease (in Chinese). Chin J Int Med 28:173–176
30. Lin CP, Wu TY (1974) Clinical analysis of 286 cases of pediatric high altitude heart disease. Chin Med J 54:99–100 (English supplement to No. 6)
31. Maggiorini M, Leon-Velarde F (2003) High-altitude pulmonary hypertension: a pathophysiological entity in different diseases. Eur Respir J 22:1019–1025
32. Manier G, Guénard H, Castaing Y, Varene N, Vargas E (1988) Pulmonary gas exchange in Andean natives with excessive polycythemia-effect of hemodilution. J Appl Physiol 65:2107–2117
33. McGoon M, Gutterman D, Steen V, Barst RJ, McCrory DC, Fortin TA, Lloyd JE (2004) Screening, early detection and diagnosis of pulmonary arterial hypertension. ACCP Evidence-Based Clinical Practice Guidelines. Chest 126:14S–34S
34. Miao CY, Sun SY, Tan XF, Yeng ZG, Xiao SJ (1989) Analysis of pulmonary arterial pressure in 162 subjects at high altitude. Chin J Circ 4:27–29
35. Michelli A, Villacis P, De la Mora P, Alvarez V (1960) Observaciones sobre los valores hemodinámicos y respiratorios obtenidos en sujetos normales. Arch Inst Cardiol Mex 30:507–511
36. Mirrakhimov MM (1985) Chronic high-altitude cor pulmonale. In: Transactions of the International Symposium on Pulmonary Arterial Hypertension. Kyrgyz Institute of Cardiology, Frunze, Kyrgyzstan, pp 267–287
37. Monge-MC (1928) La Enfermedad de los Andes. Síndromes eritrémicos. Anales de la Facultad de Medicina. Lima
38. Monge-MC, Monge-CC (1966) High Altitude Diseases. Charles Thomas, Springfield, pp 38–39
39. Niermeyer S (2003) Cardiopulmonary transition in the high altitude infant. High Alt Med Biol 4:225–239
40. Ordoñez JH (1969) Physiological observations in residents of Bogotá, Colombia, altitude 8700 feet. Rocky Mtn Med J 66:33–36
41. Pei SX, Chen XJ, Si Ren BZ, Liu YH, Chen XS, Harris EM, Anand IS, Harris, PC (1989) Chronic mountain sickness in Tibet. QJ Med 266:555–574
42. Penaloza D (1966) Physiological patterns: Cardiovascular characteristics of healthy man. In: Life at High Altitudes. Pan American Health Organization. Scientific Publications No. 140. Washington DC, pp 27–31

43. Penaloza D (2003) Circulación pulmonar. En: El Reto de Vivir en los Andes. Monge C, León Velarde F (eds) IFEA-UPCH, Lima, Perú pp 135–206
44. Penaloza D (2003) Mal de montaña subagudo. En: El Reto de Vivir en los Andes. Monge C, León Velarde F (eds) IFEA-UPCH, Lima, Perú pp 399–408
45. Penaloza D (2004) Chronic mountain sickness: an open debate of scoring systems used for its diagnosis. J Qinghai Med College 25:248–255
46. Penaloza D, Arias-Stella J (2007) The heart and pulmonary circulation at high altitude. Healthy highlanders and chronic mountain sickness. Circulation. In press. Lippincot Williams & Wilkins
47. Penaloza D, Gamboa R (1986) Hipertensión pulmonar. En: Cardiología Pediátrica Vol 2. Sanchez P (ed) Salvat, Barcelona, Spain, pp 1216–1238
48. Penaloza D, Sime F (1969) Circulatory dynamics during high altitude pulmonary edema. Am J Cardiol 23:369–378
49. Penaloza D, Sime F (1971) Chronic cor pulmonale due to loss of altitude acclimatization (chronic mountain sickness). Am J Med 50:728–743
50. Penaloza D, Gamboa R, Dyer J, Echevarría M, Marticorena E (1960) The influence of high altitudes on the electrical activity of the heart. Electrocardiographic and vectorcardiographic observations in the newborn, infants and children. Am Heart J 59:111–128
51. Penaloza D, Gamboa R, Marticorena E, Echevarría M, Dyer J, Gutierrez E (1961) The influence of high altitudes of the electrical activity of the heart. Electrocardiographic and vectorcardiographic observations in adolescence and adulthood. Am Heart J 61:101–115
52. Penaloza D, Sime F, Banchero N, Gamboa R, Cruz J, Marticorena E (1963) Pulmonary hypertension in healthy men born and living at high altitudes. Am J Cardiol 11:150–157
53. Penaloza D, Arias-Stella J, Sime F, Recavarren S, Marticorena E (1964) The heart and pulmonary circulation in children al high altitudes: Physiological, anatomical and clinical observations. Pediatrics 34:568–582
54. Penaloza D, Del Río C, Luy G, Cruz, J, Gamboa R, Marticorena E, Dyer J, Sime F (1965) Relationship between AQRS° and the level of altitude. Progress Report. US. PHS Research Grant HE-06910, pp 1–5
55. Penaloza D, Sime F, Ruiz L (1971) Cor pulmonale in chronic mountain sickness: present concept of Monge's disease. In: Porter R, Knight J (eds) High Altitude Physiology: Cardiac and Respiratory Aspects. Churchill Livingstone, Edinburgh and London, pp 41–60
56. Penaloza D, Ruiz L, Arias-Stella J, Scavino Y, Hurtado A (1977) Mal de montaña crónico: formas vascular y respiratoria (Resumen 95). En: Jornadas Científicas por el XV Aniversario de la Universidad Peruana Cayetano Heredia. UPCH, Lima, Perú, p 52
57. Pietra GG, Capron F, Stewart S, Levine O, Humbert M, Robbins IM, Reid LM, Tuder RM (2004) Pathologic assessment of vasculopathies in pulmonary hypertension. J Am Coll Cardiol 43:25S–32S
58. Recavarren S, Arias-Stella J (1964) Right ventricular hypertrophy in people living at high altitudes. Brit Heart J 26:806–812
59. Reeves JT, Groves BM (1984) Approach to the patient with pulmonary hypertension. In: Weir EK, Reeves JT (eds) Pulmonary Hypertension. Futura, Mt Kisco, NY, pp 1–44
60. Reeves JT, Grover RF (2005) Insights by Peruvian scientists into the pathogenesis of human chronic hypoxic pulmonary hypertension. J Appl Physiol 98:384–389
61. Rich, Dantzer DR, Ayres SM, et al. (1987) Primary pulmonary hypertension: a national prospective study. Ann Intern Med 107:108–123
62. Ri-Li Ge, Helun G (2001) Current concept of chronic mountain sickness: pulmonary hypertension-related high-altitude heart disease. Wilderness and Environmental Medicine J 12:190–194
63. Ri-Li Ge, Gaowa H, Guo-en J, Ying-Zhong Y (2003) High-altitude heart diseases in Qinghai-Tibet. In: Viscor G, Ricart A, Leal C (eds) Health & Height. Proceedings of the 5th World Congress on Mountain Medicine and High Altitude Physiology. Universitat de Barcelona Publicacions, Barcelona, pp 197–204

64. Rotta A, Cánepa A, Hurtado A, Velásquez T, Chávez R (1956) Pulmonary circulation at sea level and at high altitude. J Appl Physiol 9:328–336
65. Ru-Yan Ma, Hai-Ying Q, Peng Y, Kun S, Ri-Li Ge (2004) Comparative study of pulmonary arterial pressure in healthy children at different altitudes by Doppler echocardiography. (Abstract 197). High Alt Med Biol 5:259
66. Ru-Yan Ma, Pang Y, Ri-Li Ge (2004) Clinical study of 55 cases of high altitude heart disease in children in Qinghai. (Abstract 196). High Alt Med Biol 5:259
67. Sarybaeb A, Mirrakhimov M (1998) Prevalence and natural course of high altitude pulmonary hypertension and high altitude cor pulmonale. In: Ohno H, Kobayashi T, Masuyama S, Nakashima M (eds) Progress in Mountain Medicine and High Altitude Physiology. Matsumoto, Japan, pp 126–131
68. Sime F, Banchero N, Penaloza D, Gamboa R, Cruz J, Marticorena E (1963) Pulmonary hypertension in children born and living at high altitudes. Am J Cardiol 11:143–149
69. Simmoneau G, Galie N, Rubin LJ, Langleben D, Seeger W, Domenighetti G, Gibbs S, Lebrec D, Speich R, Begheti M, Rich S, Fishman A (2004) Clinical classification of pulmonary hypertension. J Am Coll Cardiol 43:5S–12S
70. Sui GJ, Liu YH, Cheng XS, Anand IS, Harris E, Harris P, Heath D (1988) Subacute infantile mountain sickness. J Pathol 155:161–170
71. Vargas E, Spielvogel H (2006) Chronic mountain sickness, optimal hemoglobin and heart disease. High Alt Med Biol 7:138–149
72. Vogel JHK, Weaver WF, Rose RL, Blount SG, Grover RF (1962) Pulmonary hypertension on exertion in normal man living at 10,150 feet (Leadville, Colorado). Med Thorac 19:269–285
73. Wu DC y Liu YR (1955) High altitude heart disease (in Chinese). Chin J Pediat 6:348–350
74. Wu TY (1979) Excessive polycythemia of high altitude: an analysis of 82 cases (in Chinese) Chin J Hematol 3:27–32
75. Wu TY (2005) Chronic mountain sickness on the Qinghai-Tibetan plateau. Chinese Med J 118:161–168
76. Wu TY, Miao CY (2002) High altitude heart disease in children in Tibet. High Alt Med Biol 3:323–325
77. Wu TY, Li CH, Wang ZW (1965) Adult high altitude heart disease; an analysis of 22 cases. Chin Int Med J 13:700–702
78. Wu TY, Die TF, Huo KS, Zang B, Jing YS, Liu PF (1987) An epidemiological study on high altitude disease at Qinghai-Tibetan plateau. Chin J Epidemiol 8:65–69 (Chinese with English Abstract)
79. Wu TY, Xue FD, Jing BS (1989) A study on the diagnosis of high altitude heart disease. Clin Cardiovasc Dis J 5:229–232 (Chinese with English Abstract)
80. Wu TY, Jing BS, Xu FD, Cheng QH (1990) Clinical features of adult heart diseases. An analysis of 202 cases (Chinese with English abstract). Acta Cardiovassc & Pulm Dis 9:32–35
81. Wu TY, Zhang Q, Jin B, Xu F, Cheng Q, Wang X (1992) Chronic mountain sickness (Monge's disease): An observation in Qinghai-Tibet Plateau. In: High Altitude Medicine. Ueda G, Reeves JT, Sekiguchi M (eds) Shinshu University Press, Matsumoto, Japan, pp 314–324
82. Wu TY, Li W, Li Y, Ri-Li G, Cheng Q, Wang Z, Zhao G, Wei L, Jin Y, Don G (1998) Epidemiology of chronic mountain sickness: ten years study in Qinghai-Tibet. In: Ohno H, Kobayashi T, Masuyama S, Nakashima M (eds) Progress in Mountain Medicine and High Altitude Physiology. Matsumoto, Japan, pp 120–125
83. Wu TY, Li W, Wei L, Ri-Li G, Wang S, Cheng Q, Yin Y (1998) A preliminary study on the diagnosis of chronic mountain sickness in Tibetan populations. In: Ohno H, Kobayashi T, Masuyama S, Nakashima M (eds) Progress in Mountain Medicine and High Altitude Physiology. Matsumoto, Japan, pp 337–342

84. Wu TY, Miao CY, Li WS, Cheng QH, Xu FD, Wang XZ, Wei TY, Chao GC (1999) Studies on high altitude pulmonary hypertension. Chin J High Alt Med 9:1–8
85. Wu TY, Fan M, Feng G, Gao Y, Ma J, Wang X (2004) High-Altitude Medical and Physiological Researches in China. Abstracts from the last 50 years. The Milky Way Publishing House, Hong Kong
86. Yang JS, He ZQ, Zhai HY, Yan Z, Zhang HM, Qin F (1987) A study of the pulmonary artery pressure in healthy people living at lowland and high altitude under exercise. Chin J Cardiovasc Dis 15:39–41
87. Yang Z. He ZQ, Liu XL (1985) Pulmonary hypertension and high altitude. Chin Cardiovasc Dis 13:32–34
88. Zubieta-CG, De Urioste L, Zubieta-CL (1998) High altitude residents in Bolivia. In: Ohno H, Kobayashi T, Masuyama S, Nakashima M (eds) Progress in Mountain Medicine and High Altitude Physiology. Matsumoto, Japan, pp 185–189

CHAPTER 3

THE CELLULAR EFFECTS OF HYPOXIA IN THE PULMONARY CIRCULATION

ANDREW PEACOCK, OLEG PAK,
DAVID WELSH

Scottish Pulmonary Vascular Unit, Glasgow, United Kingdom

Abstract: Hypoxia causes pulmonary hypertension in nearly all species studied. The pulmonary hypertension is accompanied and augmented by pulmonary vascular remodelling. Vascular remodelling is characterised largely by fibroblast, smooth muscle cell (SMC) and endothelial cell proliferation, which results in lumen obliteration. Chronic hypoxia elicits expression of several mitogens, growth factors and cytokines by pulmonary vascular cells and the suppression of anti-proliferative factors. Although hypoxic pulmonary vascular remodelling is associated with medial hypertrophy, in vitro hypoxia does not lead directly to an increase in smooth muscle cell proliferation. It is possible that hypoxia is sensed by fibroblasts, endothelial cells, or both, and intercellular signalling by growth factors, cytokines and other mitogens to adjacent pulmonary artery SMC is the underlying mechanism for the medial hypertrophy of pulmonary vascular remodelling.

Keywords: proliferation, remodelling, smooth muscle cells, endothelial cells, fibroblast and hypoxia

Introduction

Since 1946 it has been known that hypoxia causes constriction of the pulmonary circulation. This was first shown in the intact vascular bed of the cat but subsequently also shown in isolated vessels (small resistance vessels) and isolated smooth muscle cells. The purpose of hypoxic pulmonary vasoconstriction is thought to be twofold. Firstly, in utero, it keeps the pulmonary circulation closed during gestation and allows it to open up quickly following birth. Secondly, it preserves ventilation-perfusion matching when there is obstruction of the airways. This benign physiological response becomes malign when the lung is faced with global hypoxia such as in the context of lung disease or for residents at high altitude. In this case all areas of the lung

A. Aldashev and R. Naeije (eds.), Problems of High Altitude Medicine and Biology, 39–55.

are subjected to hypoxia and thus there is generalised vasoconstriction with a rise in pulmonary artery pressure and increased strain on the right heart. For this reason, both man and animals who have lived at high altitude for many generations have a diminished hypoxic pulmonary vasoconstrictive reflex. Perhaps surprisingly, they do not seem to miss the reflex and do just as well as their sea level counterparts. For those of us investigating pulmonary hypertension, there are few models of pulmonary hypertension and hypoxia has become one of the most important. As well as being relevant to those with lung disease and those who live at high altitude, it is also apparent that the histological changes induced by hypoxia are quite similar to those seen in patients who develop pulmonary hypertension of another cause.

When the pulmonary circulation is faced with hypoxia there is initially vasoconstriction, but shortly afterwards there is a development of remodelling of the pulmonary circulation with thickening of all three layers, endothelium (endothelial cells) the media (smooth muscle cells) and the adventitia (fibroblast). This remodelling is not seen in the systemic circulation, which tends to dilate in the face of hypoxia.

In this article we shall try to answer a number of questions:

- What is the effect of hypoxia on the proliferation of the three cellular components of the pulmonary circulation, namely the endothelial cells, smooth muscle cells and fibroblasts, and what are the cellular processes that lead to this proliferation?
- Is there cross talk between the three cell types in the development of the cellular response to hypoxia?
- Do we see similar changes in cells from the systemic circulation?

Vascular Remodelling in Response to Hypoxia

Under normal conditions, the thickness of the vascular wall is maintained at an optimal level by a fine balance between proliferation and apoptosis of the resident cell types. If this balance is disturbed in favour of proliferation, the vascular wall thickens and eventually obliterates the vessel lumen, leading to increased resistance (Figure 1). This structural change of the vascular bed is called vascular remodelling [23]. PA remodelling leads to an increase in pulmonary pressure and furthers remodelling. Proliferation of adventitial fibroblasts increases within hours of hypoxic exposure [44]. A few days after exposure (to hypoxia), thickening of the media layer begins in small resistance pulmonary arteries [22]. It is known that hypertrophy of SMC makes a greater contribution than hyperplasia in the larger, more proximal arteries, whereas hyperplasia is more prevalent in the smaller resistance arteries [31, 32]. Furthermore, fibroblasts migrate into the media layer and can transform into SMC [51]. EC also participate in hypoxic

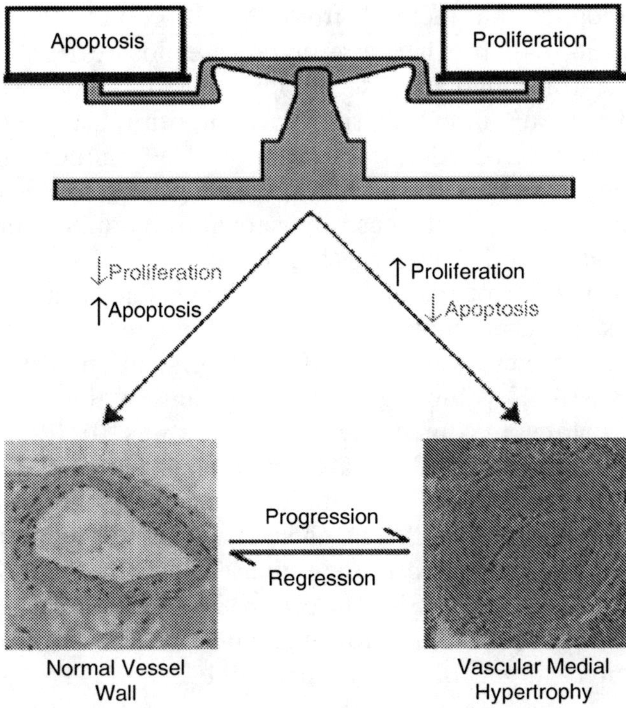

Figure 1. The balance of cell proliferation and apoptosis in pulmonary artery smooth muscle cells (PASMC) maintains the thickness and tissue mass of the arterial walls at an optimal level. If this balance is disturbed such that there is more proliferation and/or less apoptosis, the arterial wall thickens, narrowing the lumen and ultimately leading to the obliteration of the vessel and to an overall increased PVR. The histological examination of pulmonary arteries in lung tissues isolated from normotensive patients (left) and patients with pulmonary hypertension (right) shows the severe degree of medial hypertrophy in the diseased artery.

pulmonary remodelling by producing more vasoconstricting pro-proliferative factors (ET-1, angiotensin II, thromboxane A_2), and less vasodilating, antiproliferative mediators (NO, PGI_2). McLoughlin et al. [20] have shown that volume of intima and adventitia from lungs of hypoxic rats were 1.5-fold more and volume of media was 6-fold more than in control.

It is accepted that hypoxia is a cause of cell proliferation and vascular remodelling, but the mechanisms remain unclear. In vitro studies have demonstrated that hypoxia has direct effects on cell proliferation in some but not all cell preparations [61, 62, 63]. Hypoxia is able to increase cell proliferation by inhibition (production and/or release) of antimitogenic factors (e.g., NO, prostacyclin) and/or increasing the production and/or release of different mitogenic stimuli (e.g., serotonin (5-hydroxytryptamine (5-HT)), endothelin-1, PDGF, serotonin, VEGF) and inflammatory mediators (e.g., IL-6, IL-8, monocyte chemoattractant factor-1) from SMC, fibroblasts, EC and platelets [11, 21,25 ,26, 36, 64]. Furthermore, hypoxic exposure leads to increased production of extracellular matrix components [50]. Hypoxia dramatically increases the level Ca^{2+} in cytoplasm [2] of smooth muscle cells. Increased Ca^{2+} level in cytoplasm leads to activation of Ca^{2+}/calmodulin and MAP kinase II and expression of the early responsive gene, c-fos [5, 17]. Elevated Ca^{2+} level in cytoplasm of cells has been shown to modulate smooth muscle cellular proliferation and growth [5] (Figure 2).

Previous work from our laboratory has shown that acute hypoxic exposure leads to increased proliferation of pulmonary artery fibroblasts in a p38 mitogen-activated protein kinase (MAPK) dependent manner [61, 62, 63] (Figure 3). p38 MAPK is among the key mechanisms that transmit signals from the cell surface to the nucleus and belongs to Ras/ERK (Ras/extracellular-signal-regulated kinase) signalling pathway [29, 55]. p38 MAPK activation leads to cell proliferation by activating mitogen and stress-activated protein kinase 1 (MSK1), the MAP kinase-interacting kinase 1 (MNK1), the MAPK-activated protein kinase 2, 3 (MapKapK2,3), and the ribosomal protein kinase B (RSK-B). Also, p38 MAP kinase can also directly influence gene transcription, as a growing number of transcription factors are known to be direct targets of p38 (ATF-1, ATF-2, and ATF-6, the myocyte

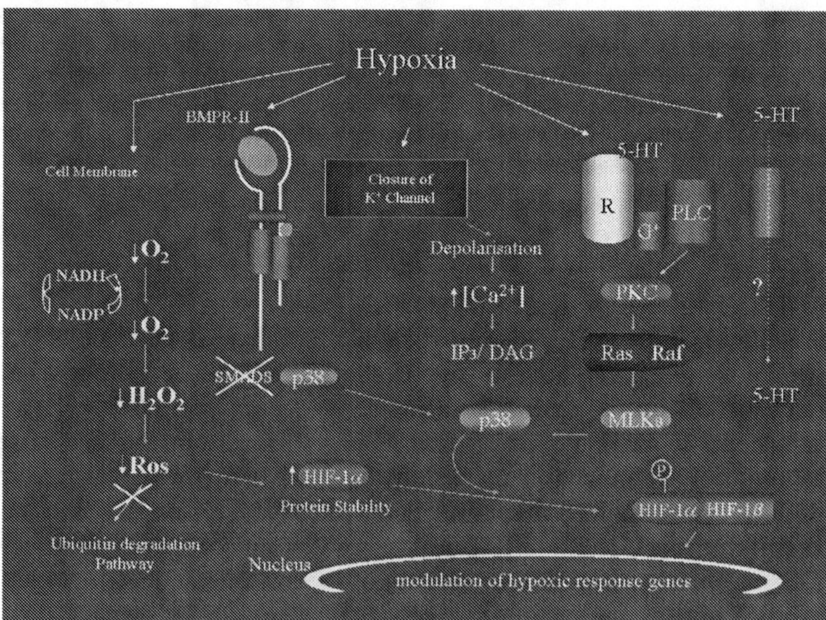

Figure 2. Possible pathways of Hypoxia induced pulmonary vascular cell proliferation.

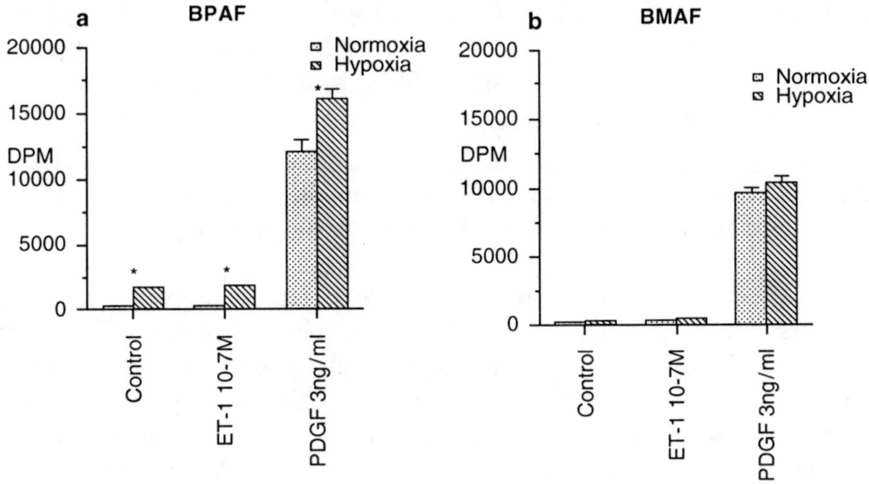

Figure 3. Effect of hypoxia on endothelin-1 and PDGF-induced stimulation of BPAF and BMAF cell proliferation. Bovine Pulmonary Artery Fibroblasts (BPAF) **(a)** and Bovine Mesenteric Artery Fibroblasts (BMAF) **(b)** cells were grown to approximately 60% confluency in 24-well plates. The cells were then allowed to grow in either normoxic or hypoxic conditions for a period of 24h in the presence or absence of ET-1 (10^{-7}M) or PDGF (3ng/ml). Cell growth was assessed by [^{3}H]thymidine uptake. Endothelin-1 did not stimulate either type of cell above control level under either normoxic or hypoxic conditions. PDGF had a marked effect on both BPAF and BMAF cells, but the effect on BPAF (though not BMAF) cells was enhanced by hypoxia ($p < 0.05$). Values shown are the mean ± SD for four replicate plates from the same animal. The experiment was repeated in four different animals and the results shown are typical of those obtained. DPM = disintegrations per minute; Norm = normoxic; Hyp = hypoxic, ET-1 = endothelin 1; PDGF = platelet-derived growth factor.

enhance factor 2C and A (MEF2 C, A), the signalling lymphocytic activation molecule associated protein 1A (SAP1A) and others [38]. Another important target of the p38 MAP kinase is the tumour suppressor protein p53 [24]. We have established a link between p38 MAPK and HIF-1α induction; our results have shown that there was a reduction of HIF-1α expression in HPAF grown in conditions of acute hypoxic preincubated with SB203580, a specific p38 MAPK inhibitor [35]. A relationship between p38 MAPK and HIF-1α is an attractive explanation for the role of p38 MAPK in hypoxia-mediated HPAF proliferation: HIF-1α is known to be responsible for the up-regulation of hypoxia-sensitive gene products assisting in cell adaptation to both acute and chronic hypoxic conditions. The mechanism of this relationship is unclear: HIF-1α may be a down-stream effector of p38 MAPK or p38 MAPK may contribute towards HIF-1α stability. Reduction of apoptosis also plays an important role in the remodelling of the pulmonary vasculature [42, 67]. A hallmark of human PAH and experimental PAH in rodents is loss of Kv (voltage-gate K^+ channel) current [48] due to decreased expression of certain Kv channels [39, 43, 66]. Chronic Kv down-regulation precipitates hypertrophy and hyperplasia of SMC and prevents removal of cells by reducing apoptosis rates [67].

Effects of Hypoxia on Vascular Cells and Pulmonary Vascular Remodelling Effects of Hypoxia on EC and PA Remodelling

The endothelial cell layer forms a permeable barrier between circulating blood cells and the underlying vascular tissue, which is composed of fibroblasts and SMC. As such, it is in a unique position to respond to circulating factors or environmental stresses and serve as a signal integrator and transducer to modulate events in the vasculature via paracrine effects. EC and SMC appear to co-operate intricately in various physiological events including the control of vascular tone and cellular growth [16].

Effect of Acute Hypoxia on EC

There is little information in the literature about the influence of acute hypoxia on pulmonary EC proliferation. During acute hypoxic exposure, EC division slows but does not arrest; progression through the G-to-S transition point and/or progression from S to G2/M of the cell cycle is altered with an increased percentage of EC in the S phase [58].

Effect of Chronic Hypoxia on EC

Endothelial cell proliferation is increased by chronic hypoxia. In the chronically hypoxic rat model of PH, there is an increase in the number of EC in the main PA and also in the small muscular arteries [20]. In hypoxic neonatal calves the endothelial proliferative index is enhanced after 14 days exposed to 8% oxygen [52].

Some of this EC proliferation appears disorganised and leads to the formation of plexiform lesions [7, 60], similar to those seen in primary PH (idiopathic PAH).

Effects of Hypoxia on SMC and PA Remodelling

SMC are a main determinant of pulmonary vascular resistance. Precapillary segments of the pulmonary vascular bed contribute to the majority of pulmonary vascular resistance. It therefore follows that small changes in tone and/or structure in this area can lead to a large elevation of pulmonary arterial pressure. These vessels are normally only partially muscularised, but hypoxic pulmonary vascular remodelling leads to enhanced muscularisation. PA smooth muscle cell proliferation is a key feature of hypoxic pulmonary vascular remodelling.

Effect of Acute Hypoxia on SMC

There is disagreement in the scientific literature about the influence of acute hypoxia on cultures of PA SMC in vitro. It is unclear whether hypoxia has direct mitogenic or comitogenic effects on human PA SMC or whether hypoxia induces human PA SMC to produce an autocrine growth factor or whether hypoxia is in fact anti-proliferative in PA SMC. Some studies have shown that acute hypoxia is not a direct stimulus for PA SMC proliferation [10, 28] and some investigators have found that acute hypoxia actually decreases the PA SMC proliferation stimulated by foetal calf serum (FCS) [11, 53]. Nevertheless, other studies have shown that acute hypoxia alone is an effective mitogenic stimulus for PA SMC [1, 4, 8, 13, 15, 30, 40, 54, 56]. There are several possible reasons for the observed conflicts in the literature.

a) Variation in the level of the pulmonary arterial tree chosen for study.

It is known that hypertrophy of PA SMC makes a greater contribution than hyperplasia in the larger, more proximal arteries, whereas hyperplasia is more important in the smaller resistance arteries [31, 32]. However, experiments using explants from the same part of the pulmonary arterial tree, gave conflicting results. For example, Dempsey [10] did not find that hypoxia stimulated proximal PA SMC proliferation, whereas Ambalavan [1] showed that proximal PA SMC proliferated at oxygen concentrations of 5–10%. Stiebellehner [53] did not find that hypoxia stimulated distal PA SMC proliferation, whereas Stotz [54] showed 5–10% increase in proliferation rates of pulmonary microvascular SMC to acute hypoxia. Thus we have not found that the source of pulmonary artery cells influences the proliferative response of PA SMC to acute hypoxia.

b) Phenotypic variations of SMC within the arterial media

Recent studies of the pulmonary circulation have demonstrated that morphologically, physiologically and immunohistochemically distinct SMC exist within the arterial media of the pulmonary artery [15]. Frid isolated four phenotypically unique cell subpopulations from inner, middle, and outer compartments of the arterial media of the PA and showed that that L1 (from inner media – subendothelial layer) and L3-"R" (from outer media) cells exhibited a highly proliferative phenotype and, unlike "traditional" SMC, proliferated under hypoxic conditions. Whereas, L2 (middle media) and L3-"S" (from the outer layer of the media) had a decreased proliferative response under hypoxic conditions when compared with normoxia.

c) Severity of hypoxia used for study

An interesting similarity between all investigators who discovered a positive correlation between acute hypoxia and a PA SMC proliferation was the use of moderate levels of acute hypoxia (1–5% Oxygen) [4, 56 – 1, 8, 13, 30, 54]. In contrast, in studies where anoxia (0 % Oxygen) was used there was a decrease in PA SMC proliferation [8, 11,18, 65] .

d) Density of seeding of SMC in cell culture plates

We found that in all studies where increased proliferation was seen to acute hypoxia, PA SMC were seeded at a density ≈ 5000 cells/cm^2 [4, 8, 30, 40, 54] but in all studies where a decrease in proliferation to hypoxia was noticed, cells were seeded at a density of more than 10000 cells/cm^2 [10, 11, 15, 53]. It is likely that contact inhibition could appear earlier in experiments where cells were seeded at higher densities. Kuehl [27] showed a correlation between the cell proliferation in response to hypoxia and seeding density.

e) Concentration of serum in the cell culture plates

In the studies showing a positive correlation between acute hypoxia and PA SMC proliferation, the serum concentration used for stimulation of proliferation was more than 2% and less than 10% [4, 56 – 1, 8, 13, 30, 54].

Effect of Chronic Hypoxia on SMC

Chronic hypoxia leads to proliferation of pulmonary artery SMC in vivo. Histological and morphological analysis of pulmonary arteries of animals exposed to chronic hypoxia and humans who died from high altitude PH showed a significant thickening of muscular layers [19]. Chronic hypoxia also causes extension of SMC into normally non-muscular arteries.

Effects of Hypoxia on Fibroblasts and PA Remodelling

An increasing volume of experimental data supports the idea that the adventitial fibroblast plays an important role in vascular remodelling of PA. The vascular adventitia can act as a biological processing centre for the production, storage and release of key regulators of vessel wall function. In response to stress or injury (e.g., hypoxia), resident adventitial cells can be activated and reprogrammed to exhibit different functional and structural behaviours, which include proliferation, differentiation, up-regulation of contractile and extracellular matrix proteins and release of factors that directly affect medial smooth muscle cell tone and growth.

Effect of Acute Hypoxia on Fibroblasts

Our laboratory and others have shown that acute hypoxia is a direct trigger for fibroblast proliferation in vitro in rat, bovine and human models. (Figure 3). Exposure to acute hypoxia leads to fibroblast proliferation and hypertrophy [61–63]. Hypoxic proliferation of fibroblasts has been shown to be more sustained and to exceed that of PA EC or PA SMC in these models [3]. Acute hypoxia acts as a direct proliferative stimulus for PA adventitial fibroblasts in the absence of exogenous mitogens [51]. In our laboratory this effect of hypoxia on proliferation of adventitial FB was seen only with pulmonary vascular cells and not in those from the systemic circulation (Figure 4).

Effect of Chronic Hypoxia on Fibroblasts

Proliferation of adventitial fibroblasts occurs before other cell types in animal models of chronic hypoxia [44]. In small pulmonary arteries, fibroblasts increase production of extracellular matrix proteins (type I collagen, elastin), that contribute to the narrowing of the vascular lumen [57]. In addition, there is early and dramatic up-regulation of collagen, fibronectin and tropoelastin mRNAs, followed by the subsequent deposition of these proteins [46]. The work in our laboratory has shown that chronic hypoxia (like acute hypoxia) causes selective proliferation of pulmonary vascular (cf systemic) FB and the process is p38 dependent. (Figure 5).

Repair of the injured tissue is an essential requirement for any living organism. PH is a haemodynamic stress leading to injury of the arterial wall. SMC, EC, and fibroblasts in the pulmonary vascular wall play specific roles in the response to this injury. Fibroblasts are in a unique position for this role, since they are less differentiated and have remarkable plasticity, allowing for a tremendous capacity for rapid migration, proliferation, synthesis of connective tissue, contraction, cytokine production, and, most importantly, transdifferentiation into other types of cells (e.g., PA SMC) [51]. Hypoxia-induced changes in fibroblast proliferative and matrix-producing phenotypes are accompanied by the appearance of smooth muscle α-actin in tissues from pulmonary hypertensive subjects, suggesting that some of the fibroblasts are being transdifferentiated into myofibroblasts [51]. This transdifferentiation involves a complex network of micro-environmental factors and pathways in which extracellular matrix components as well as growth factors, cytokines, and adhesion molecules may play a role. Therefore, in rats exposed to hypoxia, precapillary vessels of a diameter of ~25 μm, which normally do not have smooth muscle cells, begin to generate this cell type from adventitial fibroblasts within 24 h [49]. Light microscopic examination of nonmuscular arterioles after exposure to hypoxia show that smooth muscle begins to form

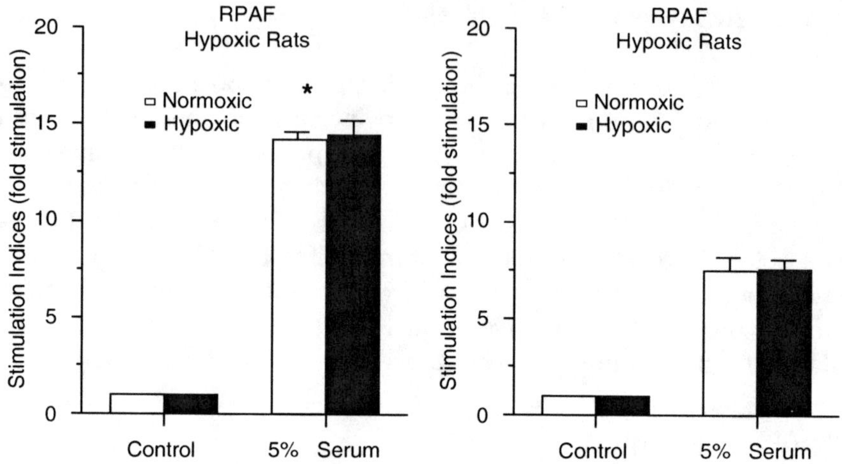

Figure 4. Chronic Hypoxia induces enhanced levels of serum-induced proliferation of RPAF but not RAF cells. Rat Pulmonary Artery Fibroblasts (RPAF) and Rat Aortic Fibroblasts (RAF) cells were explanted from animals kept under conditions of chronic hypoxia (PO_2 35 mm Hg) for 2 wk. Once explanted they were grown in normoxia and 10% serum in 24-well plates until 60% confluent and then quiesced in serum-free media (SFM) for 24 h before stimulation with 5% serum. The cells were then either kept in normoxic or subjected to acutely hypoxic conditions (PO_2 of 35 mm Hg) for a period of 24 h. Cell growth was assessed by [^{3}H]thymidine uptake. RPAF cells from chronically hypoxic rats kept in normoxic conditions showed substantially enhanced serum-stimulated DNA synthesis, which could not be further enhanced by the addition of acute hypoxia. RAF cells from chronically hypoxic rats maintained in either normoxic or hypoxic conditions showed no increase in serum-stimulated levels of DNA synthesis. Values shown are the pooled data of stimulation indices (mean ± SD) for eight different animals. *Value for hypoxia significantly greater than normoxia, $p < 0.05$.

by day 2 at simulated altitude, the proportion of muscularised arterioles increasing along with increasing PAP [41]. Interestingly, all these studies show that after return to normoxia, smooth muscle cells persist in normally nonmuscularised arterioles, suggesting that smooth muscle cells may remain for a long time after chronic exposure to hypoxia.

The pulmonary vascular adventitia of neonatal calves has been found to contain multiple and functionally distinct subpopulations of fibroblasts [46]. Proliferation under hypoxic conditions is highly variable among these subpopulations, with some exhibiting a more than 2-fold increase in DNA synthesis, while others show a decrease in DNA synthesis. These observations suggest that hypoxia specifically selects certain phenotypically and functionally distinct subpopulations of fibroblasts to act as 'stem cells' for the vascular wall to expand and proliferate. Since each subpopulation of fibroblast responds uniquely to hypoxia, they may serve special functions in response to injury. Thus, the adventitial fibroblast residing in the vessel wall may be a critical regulator of vascular remodelling under hypoxic conditions.

Interactions Between Fibroblasts, SMC and EC and Pulmonary Vascular Remodelling

Studies have shown that EC secrete mitogenic factors under hypoxic conditions that induce SMC proliferation. Bovine aortic EC have been shown to secrete several SMC growth factors, including platelet-derived growth factor (PDGF), endothelial-derived growth factor (EDGF), insulin like growth factor 1, fibroblast growth factor (FGF) and interleukin 1 [25, 26 – 6, 47]. It is known that EC produce PDGF-B in response to hypoxia [63], but SMC do not [1]. It has also been shown that increased ET-1 expression in pulmonary vascular EC appears to be transcriptionally mediated by hypoxia [25, 26]. The expression of such vasoactive agents as endothelin-l (ET-1) and platelet-derived growth factor-B (PDGF-B) is dramatically increased in EC exposed to low oxygen tension [26] and similarly, vascular endothelial growth factor is induced in SMC. In addition to increasing the release of growth factors, hypoxia stimulates the production of some extracellular matrix proteins, such as thrombospondin-1 in human EC [37]. Thrombospondin-1 modulates smooth muscle cell proliferation and migration and may be a negative regulator of angiogenesis [14]. Because of their localisation at the interface between blood and tissue, EC are responsible for the maintenance of vascular homeostasis. They fulfil a series of various functions and constantly interact with circulating leukocytes and SMC present in the media. Any disturbance of their metabolism can thus lead to alterations of blood vessel functions. It has been shown that hypoxia, resulting from venous stasis, induces the activation of EC from human umbilical vein that then release inflammatory mediators able to activate neutrophils and to induce their infiltration as well as growth factors for SMC [34].

The addition of conditioned medium, obtained from pulmonary EC exposed to hypoxia, to cultures of quiescent PA SMC has been shown to result in a significant increase in total cell number [34, 59]. However, other work has shown conversely that [18] hypoxia stimulates the release by bovine PA EC of an inhibitor of PA SMC growth isolated from the main pulmonary artery of calves.

A strong proliferative response of PA SMC to hypoxia was noted when SMC were co-incubated with adventitial fibroblasts from human and rat pulmonary artery [45]. (Figure 6). A number of pieces of experimental evidence demonstrate that fibroblasts exert significant paracrine effects on other cells. Fibroblasts are known to produce a wide array of cytokines, growth factors (TGF-β, epithelial growth factor, insulin-like growth factor,

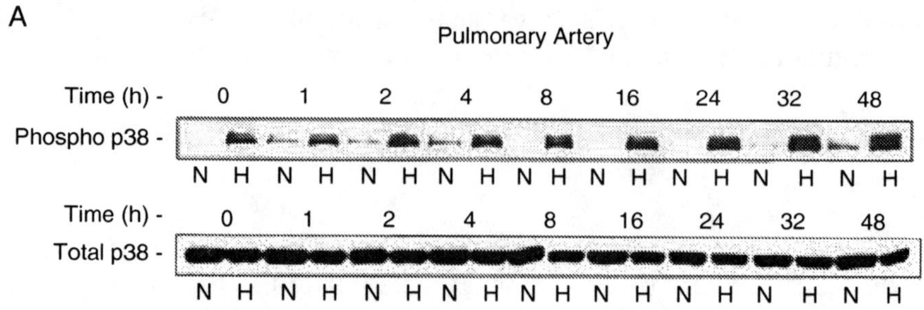

Figure 5. p38 activity in RPAF cells from normoxic and chronically hypoxic rats. Rat Pulmonary Artery Fibroblasts (RPAF) cells derived from rats kept in either normoxic or hypoxic conditions for 2 wk were grown to 90% confluency in 6-well plates and quiesced in serum-free media for 24 h under normoxic conditions. Cells were then stimulated with 5% serum for the times indicated and then prepared for Western blot analysis. RPAF cells from normoxic rats showed little or no p38 activity in unstimulated cells: serum weakly stimulated this activity in a multiphasic manner over the 48-h time period tested. In contrast, RPAF cells from chronically hypoxic animals exhibited constitutively and strongly activated p38 MAP kinase, which could be further stimulated in response to serum over the time points studied. The experiment was repeated with cells from four different animals and the results shown here from a single animal are typical of all those obtained. N, cells from normoxic rats; H, cells from chronically hypoxic animals.

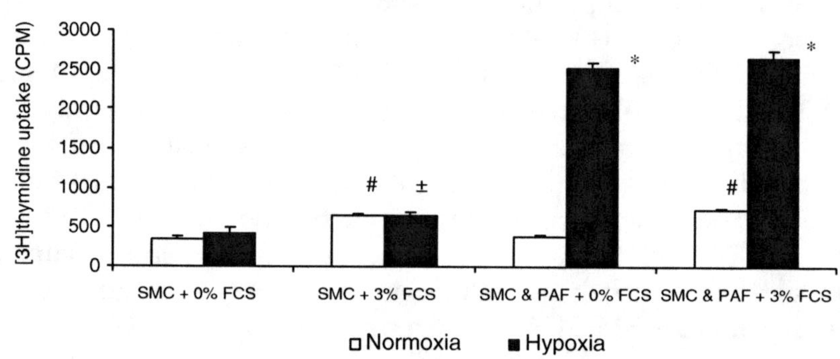

Figure 6. Effect of hypoxia on proliferation of Bovine Pulmonary Artery Smooth Muscle cells (SMC) cocultured with Bovine Pulmonary Artery Fibroblasts (PAF). Hypoxia alone or in combination with serum has no effect on SMC proliferation. However when the SMC were co-cultured with PAF under hypoxic conditions, there was a significant increase in SMC proliferation. * - hypoxic values significantly different to normoxic values ($p<0.01$) (means ± S.D.). # - 3% FCS - increase proliferation of bovine pulmonary artery smooth muscle cells ($p<0.05$) (means±S.D.).

platelet-derived growth factor) and inflammatory mediators, which function as autocrine regulators of fibroblasts and paracrine regulators of neighbouring cell (endothelial, SMC, epithelial) proliferation [9]. It has been established that matrix proteins such as collagen, fibronectin and proteoglycans play a prominent role in migration, proliferation and differentiation [50]. It is possible that hypoxia sensing by fibroblasts may lead to extracellular signalling to adjacent PA SMC, resulting in their proliferation.

Summary

Acute hypoxia has direct proliferative effects on PA fibroblasts. Hypoxia does not appear to have a direct effect on PA SMC proliferation but may increase the effect of other mitogenic factors on PA SMC. Quiescent PA SMC may require a priming step for acute hypoxia-induced proliferation. Acute hypoxia may decrease PA EC proliferation but hypoxic EC and adventitial fibroblasts can release factors that are mitogenic for SMC, and moderate acute hypoxia can enhance the proliferative effects of peptide growth factors and other growth stimulants. It is feasible that fibroblasts could be a hypoxic sensor and a key determinant of PA SMC proliferation. Chronic hypoxia leads to the proliferation all three vascular layers of pulmonary arteries.

Acknowledgments

This work is supported by grant from the European Respiratory Society and is an adaptation of an article published in the European Respiratory Journal.

References

1. Ambalavanan N, Mariani G, Bulger A, Philips JB. (1999) Role of nitric oxide in regulating neonatal porcine pulmonary artery smooth muscle cell proliferation. Biol Neonate 76:291–300.
2. Ashida T, Blaustein MP. (1987) Regulation of cell calcium and contractility in mammalian arterial smooth muscle: the role of sodium-calcium exchange. J Physiol. Nov;392:617–635
3. Belknap JK, Orton EC, Ensley B, Tucker A, Stenmark KR. (1997) Hypoxia increases bromodeoxyuridine labeling indices in bovine neonatal pulmonary arteries. Am. J. Respir. Cell Mol. Biol. 16:366–371.
4. Benitz WE, Coulson JD, Lessler DS, Bernfield M. (1986) Hypoxia inhibits proliferation of fetal pulmonary arterial smooth muscle cells in vitro. Pediatric research Vol. 20(10):966–972.
5. Berridge MJ. (1994) The biology and medicine of calcium signalling. Mol Cell Endocrinol. Jan;98:119–124.
6. Bohlen P, Esch F, Baird A, Gospodarowicz D. (1985) Acidic fibroblasts growth factor from bovine brain: amino-terminal sequence and comparison with basic FGF. EMBO J 4:1951–1956.

7. Cool CD, Stewart JS, Wehareha P, et al. (1999) Three-dimensional reconstruction of pulmonary arteries in plexiform pulmonary hypertension using cell-specific markers. Evidence for a dynamic and heterogeneous process of pulmonary endothelial cell growth. Am J Pathol 155:411–9.
8. Cooper A, Beasley D. (1999) Hypoxia stimulates proliferation and interleukin-1α production in human vascular smooth muscle cells. Am J Physiol. 277:H1326–H1337.
9. Davie N, Gerasimovskaya E, Hofmeister S, Richman A, Jones P, Reeves J. and Stenmark S. (2006) Pulmonary artery adventitial fibroblasts cooperate with vasa vasorum endothelial cells to regulate vasa vasorum neovascularization: a process mediated by hypoxia and endothelin-1. Am J Pathol. Jun;168:1793–807.
10. Dempsey E, Mcmurtry I, and O'Brien RF. (1991) Protein kinase C activation allows pulmonary artery smooth muscle cells to proliferate to hypoxia. Lung Cell. Mol. Physiol. 4: L136–L145.
11. Eddahibi S, Fabre V, Boni C, Martres MP, Raffestin B, Hamon M, Adnot S. (1999) Induction of serotonin transporter by hypoxia in pulmonary vascular smooth muscle cells relationship with the mitogenic action of serotonin. Circ Res. 84:329–336.
12. Feng J, Ito M, Ichikawa K, Isaka N, Nishikawa M, Hartshorne, DJ, Nakano, T. (1999) Inhibitory phosphorylation site for Rho-associated kinase on smooth muscle myosin phosphatase. J. Biol. Chem., 274:37385–37390.
13. Frank DB, Abtahi A, Yamaguchi DJ, Manning S, Shyr Y, Pozzi A, Baldwin HS, Johnsos JE, Caestecker PD. (2005) Bone morphogenetic protein 4 promotes pulmonary vascular remodelling in hypoxic pulmonary hypertension. Circ res. 97:496–504.
14. Frazier WA. (1991) Thrombospondins. Curr. Opin. Cell Biol. 3:792–799.
15. Frid MG, Aldashev AA, Dempsey EC, Stenmark KR. (1997) Smooth muscle cells isolated from discrete compartments of the mature vascular media exhibit unique phenotypes and distinct growth capabilities. Circulation Research. 81:940–952.
16. Furchgott RD, Zawadzki JV. (1986) The obligatory role of endothelial cells in the relaxation of smooth muscle cells by scetylcholine. Nature. 28:373–376.
17. Hardingham GE, Chawla S, Johnson CM, Bading H. (1997) Distinct functions of nuclear and cytoplasmic calcium in the control of gene expression. Nature. Jan 16;385:260–5
18. Hassoun PM, Pasricha PJ, Teufel E, Lee SL, Fanburg BL. (1989) Hypoxia stimulates the release by bovine pulmonary artery endothelial cells of an inhibitor of pulmonary artery smooth muscle cells growth. Am J Respir Cell Moll Biol Vol1:377–384.
19. Heath D, Smith P, Harris P, Yacoub M. (1988) Plexiform lesion in bronchopulmonary anastomosis. Br J Dis Chest. Jul;82:294–299.
20. Howell K, Preston RJ, Mcloughlin P. (2003) Chronic hypoxia causes angiogenesis in addition to remodelling in the adult rat pulmonary circulation. J Physiol. Feb 15;547:133–145.
21. Humar R, Kiefer FN, Berns H, Resink TJ, and Battegay EJ. (2002) Hypoxia enhances vascular cell proliferation and angiogenesis in vitro via rapamycin (mTOR)-dependent signalling. FASEB J 16:771–780.
22. Hunter C, Barer GR, Shaw JW, Clegg EJ. (1974) Growth of the heart and lungs in hypoxic rodents: a model of human hypoxic disease. Clin Sci Mol Med. Mar;46:375–91.
23. Kato M, Staub NC. (1996) Response of small pulmonary arteries to unilobar hypoxia and hypercapnia. Circ Res 19:426–440.
24. Katsoulidis E., Li Y., Mears H., Platanias LC. (2005) The p38 mitogen-activated protein kinase pathway in interferon signal transduction. J Interferon Cytokine Res. Dec;25: 749–56.
25. Kourembanas S, Hannan RL, and Faller DV. (1990) Oxygen tension regulates the expression of the platelet-derived growth factor-B chain gene in human endothelial cells. J. Clin. Invest. 86:670–674.
26. Kourembanas, S, Marsden PA, McQuillan LP, and Faller DV. (1991) Hypoxia induces endothelin gene expression and secretion in cultured human endothelium. J. Clin. Invest. 88:1054–1057.

27. Kuehl KS, Bruttig SP, Singer DV, Rubio , Berne RM. (1981) Growth of aortic vascular smooth muscle cells in lowered oxygen tension. Cell Tissue Res. 216:591–602.
28. Lanner MC, Raper M, Pratt WM, and Rhoades RA. (2005) Heterotrimeric G proteins and the platelet-derived growth factor receptor - contribute to hypoxic proliferation of smooth muscle cells. Am J Respir Cell Mol Biol Vol 33:412–419.
29. Lewis TS, Shapiro PS, Ahn NG. (1998) Signal transduction through MAP kinase cascades. Adv Cancer Res 74: 49–139.
30. Lu S, Wang D, Zhu M, Zhang Q, Hu Y, Pei J. (2005) Inhibition of hypoxia-induced proliferation and collagen synthesis by vasonatrin peptide in cultured rat pulmonary artery smooth muscle cells. Life Sciences 77:28–38.
31. McKenzie JC, Clancy J, Klein RM. (1984) Autoradiographic analysis of cell proliferation and protein synthesis in the pulmonary trunk of rats during the early development of hypoxia-induced pulmonary hypertension. Blood vessels 21:80–89.
32. Meyrick B, Reid L. (1980) Hypoxia-induced structural changes in the media and adventitia of the rat hilar pulmonary artery and their regression. Am J Pathol. Jul;100:151–78.
33. Michiels C, Bouaziz N, Remacle J. (2002) Role of the endothelium and blood stasis in the development of varicose veins. Int Angiol. Jun;21:18–25.
34. Michielis C, Leener F, Arnould T, Dieu M, Remarcle J. (1994) Hypoxia stimulates human endothelial cells to release smooth muscle cells mitogens: role of prostoglandins and bFGF. Exper Cell research 213:43–54
35. Mortimer HJ, Peacock AJ, Kirk K and Welsh DJ. (2006) p38 MAP kinase: Essential role in hypoxia-mediated human pulmonary artery fibroblast proliferation. Pulm Pharmacol Ther. Sep 8 [epub ahead of print]
36. Mukhopadhyay D, Tsiokas L, Zhou XM, Foster D, Brugge JS, Sukhatme VP. (1995) Hypoxic induction of human vascular endothelial growth factor expression through c-Src activation. Nature 375:577–581.
37. Phelan MW, Forman LW, Perrine SP, Faller DV. (1998) Hypoxia increases thrombospondin-1 transcript and protein in cultured endothelial cells. J. Lab. Clin. Med. 132:519–529.
38. Pouyssegur J, Lenormand P. (2003) Fidelity and spatio-temporal control in MAP kinase (ERKs) signalling. Eur J Biochem 270: 3291–9.
39. Pozeg ZI, Michelakis ED, McMurtry MS, Thebaud B, Wu XC, Dyck JR, Hashimoto K, Wang S, Moudgil R, Harry G, Sultanian R, Koshal A, Archer SL. (2003) In vivo gene transfer of the O2-sensitive potassium channel Kv1.5 reduces pulmonary hypertension and restores hypoxic pulmonary vasoconstriction in chronically hypoxic rats. Circulation 107:2037–2044.
40. Preston, N, Hill R, Warburton B, Fanburg. (2006) The role of 12-lipoxygenase in hypoxia-induced rat pulmonary artery smooth muscle cell proliferation. Am J Physiol Lung Cell Mol Physiol. Feb;290:L367–74.
41. Rabinovitch M, Konstam MA, Gamble WJ, et al. (1983) Changes in pulmonary blood flow affect vascular response to chronic hypoxia in rats. Circ Res 52:432–441.
42. Rabinovitch, M. (1998) Elastase and the pathobiology of unexplained pulmonary hypertension. Chest 114:213–224S.
43. Reeve HL, Michelakis E, Nelson DP,Weir EK, Archer SL. (2001) Alterations in a redox oxygen sensing mechanism in chronic hypoxia. J Appl Physiol 90:2249–2256.
44. Reid LM and Davies P in Lung Biology in Health and Disease (Lenfant C, exec.ed). (1989) Pulmonary vascular physiology and pathophysiology. (Weir E.K. eds). Marcel Decker, NY. 38:541–611
45. Rose F, Grimminger F, Appel J, Heller M, Pies V, Weisssmann N, Fink L, Schmidt S, Krick S, Camenisch G, Gassmann M, Seeger W. and Hanze J. (2002) Hypoxic pulmonary artery fibroblasts trigger proliferation of vascular smooth muscle cells – role of hypoxia-inducible transcription factors. FASEB J. Oct;16:1660–1.
46. Sartore S, Chiavegato A, Faggin E, Franch R, Puato M, Ausoni S, Pauletto P. (2001) Contribution of adventitial fibroblasts to neointima formation and vascular remodelling. Circ. Res. 89:1111–1121.

47. Shreeniwas R, Koga S, Karakurum M, Pinsky D, Kaiser E, Brett J, Wolitzky BA, Norton C, Plocinski J, Benjamin W, et al. (1992) Hypoxiamediated induction of endothelial cell interleukin-la. J. Clin. Invest. 90:2333–2339.
48. Smirnov SV, Robertson TP, Ward JP, Aaronson PI. (1994) Chronic hypoxia is associated with reduced delayed rectifier K+ current in rat pulmonary artery muscle cells. Am J Physiol 266:H365–H370.
49. Sobin SS, Tremer HM, Hardy JD, Chiodi HP. (1983)Changes inarteriole in acute and chronic hypoxic pulmonary hypertension and recovery in rat. J Appl Physiol 55:1445–1455.
50. Stenmark KR, Mecham RP. (1997) Cellular and molecular mechanisms of pulmonary vascular remodelling. Annu Rev Physiol 59:89–144
51. Stenmark KR, Gerasimovskaya EV, Nemenoff RA, Das M. (2002) Hypoxic activation of adventitial fibroblasts: role in vascular remodelling. Chest 122: 326S– 334S.
52. Stiebellehner L, Belknap JK, Ensley B et al. (1998) Lung endothelial cell proliferation in normal and pulmonary hypertensive neonatal calves. Am. J. Physiol. 275:L593–600.
53. Stiebellehner L, Frid M, Reeves J, Low R, Gnanasekharan M, and Stenmark K. (2003) Bovine distal pulmonary arterial media is composed of a uniform population of well-differentiated smooth muscle cells with low proliferative capabilities. Am J Physiol Lung Cell Mol Physiol 285:L819–828.
54. Stotz W, Li D, Johns RA. (2004) Exogenous nitric oxide upregulates p21waf1/cip1 in pulmonary microvascular smooth muscle cells. J Vasc Res 41:211–219.
55. Sturgill TW, Wu J. (1991) Recent progress in characterization of protein kinase cascades for phosphorylation of ribosomal protein S6. Biochim Biophys Acta 1092:350–7.
56. Tamm M, Bihl M, Eickelberg O, Stulz P, Perruchoud AP, and Roth M. (1998) Hypoxia-induced interleukin-6 and interleukin-8 production is mediated by platelet-activating factor and platelet-derived growth factor in primary human lung cells. Am. J. Respir. Cell Mol. Biol. 19:653–661.
57. Tozzi CA, Christiansen DL, Poiani GJ, Riley DJ. (1994) Excess collagen in hypertensive pulmonary arteries decreases vascular distensibility. Am J Respir Crit Care Med. May;149:1317–26.
58. Tucci M, Hammerman S, Furfaro S, Saukonnen J, Conca T, and Farber H. (1997) Distinct effect of hypoxia on endothelial cell proliferation and cycling. Am. J. Physiol. 272:C1700–C1708.
59. Vender RL, Clemmons DR, Kwock L, Friedman M. (1987) Reduced oxygen tension induces pulmonary endothelium to release a pulmonary smooth muscle cells mitogen(s). Am Rev Respir Dis 135:622–627.
60. Voelkel NF, Tuder RM, Weir EK. (1997) Pathophysiology of primary pulmonary hypertension. In: Rubin L, Rich S, editors. Primary Pulmonary Hypertension. New York, NY: Marcel Dekker, pp 83–129.
61. Welsh DJ, Scott PH, Plevin R, Wadsworth R, Peacock AJ. (1998) Hypoxia enhances cellular proliferation and 1,4,5 – triphosphate genetarion in fibroblasts from bovine pulmonary artery but not from mesenteric artery. Am J Respir Crit Care Med. 158:1757–1762.
62. Welsh DJ, Peacock AJ, MacLean MR, Harnett M. (2001) Chronic hypoxia induces constitutive p38 MAPK activity which correlates with enhanced cellular proliferation in fibroblasts from rat pulmonary not mesenteric artery. Am J Respir Crit Care Med. 164:282–289.
63. Welsh D, Scott P, Peacock A. (2006) p38 MAP kinase isoform activity and cell cycle regulators in the proliferative response of pulmonary and systemic artery fibroblasts to acute hypoxia. Pulm Pharmacol Ther. 19:128–38.
64. Yan SF, Tritto I, Pinsky D, Liao H, Huang J, Fuller G, Brett J, May L, Stern D. (1995) Induction of interleukin 6 (IL-6) by hypoxia in vascular cells. Central role of the binding site for nuclear factor-IL-6. J. Biol. Chem. 270:11463–11471.
65. Yang X, Sheares K, Davie N, Upton PD, Taylor GW, Horsley J, Wharton J, and Morrell NW. (2002) Hypoxic induction of cox-2 regulates proliferation of human pulmonary artery smooth muscle cells. Am. J. Respir. Cell Mol. Biol. 27:688–696.

66. Yuan XJ, Wang J, Juhaszova M, Gaine SP, Rubin LJ. (1998) Attenuated K+ channel gene transcription in primary pulmonary hypertension. Lancet 351:726–727.
67. Zhang S, Fantozzi I, Tigno DD, Yi ES, Platoshyn O, Thistlethwaite PA, Kriett JM, Yung G, Rubin LJ, Yuan JX-J. (2003) Bone morphogenetic proteins induce apoptosis in human pulmonary vascular smooth muscle cells. Am. J. Physiol.: Lung Cell. Mol. Physiol. 285: L740–754.

CHAPTER 4

ANGIOGENESIS AND CHRONIC HYPOXIC PULMONARY HYPERTENSION

SAADIA EDDAHIBI[1], BERNADETTE RAFFESTIN[2], SERGE ADNOT[1]

[1] *INSERM U 651, Département de Physiologie, CHU Henri Mondor AP-HP, 94010 Créteil, France*
[2] *Département de Physiologie, UFR Paris-Ouest, Hôpital Ambroise Paré AP-HP, 92104 Boulogne, France*

Abbreviations: PH: pulmonary hypertension; EC: human microvascular endothelial cells; PA-SMC: pulmonary arterial smooth muscle cells; VEGF: vascular endothelial growth factor; PDGF: platelet derived growth factor; FCS: fetal calf serum.

Abstract: Exposure to hypoxia leads to the development of pulmonary hypertension (PH) as a consequence of pulmonary smooth muscle hyperplasia. Hypoxia concomitantly stimulates lung expression of angiogenic factors. Increased expression of the angiogenic factor VEGF and its receptors has been found in the lungs of chronically hypoxic rats. In addition to VEGFA, VEGF C and D, other growth factors or cytokines including PDGF, acidic and basic FGF, transforming growth factor, angiogenin, and prostaglandin E2 have also been shown to increase during exposure to hypoxia, suggesting that activation of several lung angiogenic processes contribute to the lung adaptation to chronic hypoxia. Labeling studies also indicate that activation of lung angiogenic processes in response to hypoxia is associated with an increased number of peripheral pulmonary vessels. Pharmacological blockade of VEGF receptors or increased expression of antiangiogenic factors such as angiostatin, aggravate hypoxic pulmonary hypertension and structural vascular remodeling of pulmonary vessels. Concomitantly, these treatments decrease the number of peripheral pulmonary vessels. This suggests that activation of endogenous lung angiogenic processes during chronic hypoxia attenuates the severity of pulmonary hypertension by at least two mechanisms, protection against vascular remodeling and stimulation of peripheral vessel development.

Another critical aspect of vessel development is maturation, during which endothelial cells (ECs) no longer proliferate or migrate but instead

A. Aldashev and R. Naeije (eds.), Problems of High Altitude Medicine and Biology, 57–68.

promote vessel stabilization by recruiting peri-endothelial support cells, which differentiate into smooth muscle cells. Because this maturation phase is partly under the control of angiopoietin-1 (Ang1), which acts selectively on ECs via the Tie2 receptor, one theory is that EC stimulation by Ang1 contributes to pulmonary vascular remodeling via the release of signaling molecules that act on smooth muscle cells. The exact role of these mechanisms in hypoxic pulmonary hypertension is still under investigation.

In conclusion, exposure to chronic hypoxia is associated with the activation of endogenous lung angiogenic processes, which attenuate the severity of pulmonary hypertension. Angiogenic factors such as angiopoietin-1 may contribute to the process of pulmonary vascular remodeling.

Keywords: pulmonary hypertension; hypoxia; angiogenesis; vascular endothelial growth factor; platelet derived growth factor; angiopoietin-1; angiostatin

Introduction

Hypoxia is a well recognized stimulus for pulmonary blood vessel remodeling. One mechanism that may account for this effect is a direct action of hypoxia on the expression of specific genes involved in pulmonary artery smooth muscle cell proliferation, such as those encoding the serotonin transporter and endothelin [18,10]. Hypoxia is also a potent stimulus for the expression of angiogenic factors, which trigger endothelial cells [19,3]. Numerous angiogenic factors and cytokines, including VEGF and VEGF receptors, PDGF, acidic and basic FGF, transforming growth factor, angiogenin, and prostaglandin E2 have been shown to be increased in lungs of experimental hypoxic animals as well as in tissues from patients with chronic hypoxemic lung disease [33,7,30]. The physiological or pathological consequences of hypoxia-induced activation of lung angiogenic processes, however, are not completely understood.

Moreover, angiogenesis now appears as a complex process, which encompasses an activation and a resolution phase. In the activation phase, increased vascular permeability and basement membrane degradation allows endothelial cells (ECs) to proliferate and migrate into the extracellular space and form new capillary sprouts. In the resolution phase, ECs cease proliferation and migration, reconstitute the basement membrane and promote vessel maturation [14]. Mesenchymal cells are recruited and subsequently differentiate into pericytes and smooth muscle cells surrounding the newly formed vessel. While the activation phase is mainly under the control of growth factors such as VEGF, the resolution phase is mostly under the control of angiopoietin-1 (Ang1), which acts selectively on ECs via the Tie2 receptor[14]. Other molecular factors are involved in this process, such as TGF-β acting on activin-like kinase type 1 receptors (Alk-1), which are predominantly located on Ecs [16].

In this review, we will focus first on the role of VEGF in hypoxia-induced pulmonary vascular remodeling. Second, we will discuss the potential role of the Ang1/Tie 2 pathway on development of PH.

LUNG VEGF EXPRESSION DURING PULMONARY HYPERTENSION OR DURING EXPOSURE TO CHRONIC HYPOXIA

Vascular endothelial growth factor (VEGF) was first described as a potent and specific mitogen for endothelial cells and a vascular permeability factor [13]. It was then found to play an important role in normal as well as pathological angiogenesis. VEGF is a homodimeric 34- to 42-kDa heparin-binding glycoprotein, that fulfils its function on endothelial cells by binding to flt-1 and KDR/flk-1, two highly specific tyrosine kinase receptors expressed almost exclusively on endothelial cells [13]. Evidence has been provided that stimulation of angiogenesis under hypoxic and ischemic conditions involves upregulation of VEGF and its receptors. A unique feature of VEGF is its sensitivity to hypoxia [19]. Hypoxia is a strong inducer of VEGF expression in vitro [20]. The mechanism of hypoxic induction of VEGF expression has been partially elucidated. Hypoxia activates a specific transcription factor (Hypoxia Inducible Factor) that binds to identified hypoxia-sensitive elements in the promoter of the VEGF gene. Hypoxia may also increase VEGF expression by stabilizing VEGF mRNAs [20].

In recent studies, we examined the effects of exposure to chronic hypoxia (CH) and treatment with monocrotaline (MCT) on VEGF gene expression in heart and lung tissues of rats (Figure 1). The main finding of our study is that an angiogenic process is associated with right ventricular hypertrophy in hypoxia-induced pulmonary hypertension and that this process may be related to upregulation of VEGF expression in right ventricular tissue [27]. In contrast, monocrotaline-induced pulmonary hypertension caused right ventricular hypertrophy without cardiac angiogenesis, a finding consistent with down-regulation of VEGF gene expression in the right ventricular myocardium [27]. Taken together, these findings strongly suggest that VEGF plays an important role in controlling right ventricular perfusion during hypertrophy secondary to pulmonary hypertension. Moreover, lung VEGF mRNA levels were also strikingly decreased in rats given MCT, but remained unchanged after exposure to hypoxia. Since muscularization in distal vessels was also more marked in MCT than in hypoxic rats, it can be speculated that alterations in lung VEGF expression also affected pulmonary vascular remodeling.

Other studies have reported increased VEGF expression in lungs from rats exposed to chronic hypoxia [33,7]. Moreover, labeling studies in rats have suggested a burst of endothelial cell multiplication in intraacinar arteries at the end of the first week of exposure to hypoxia. In recent studies performed

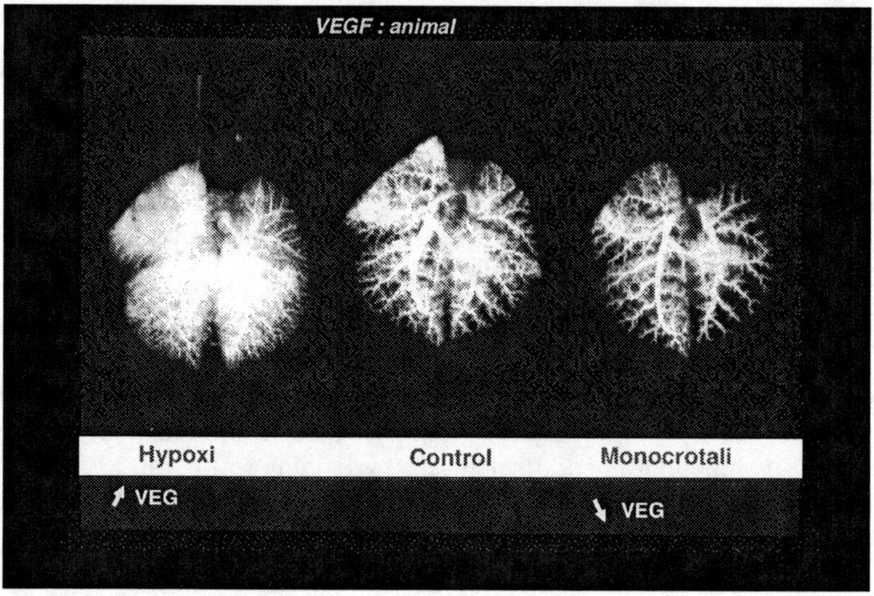

Figure 1. Lung angiograms illustrating changes in lung vascular density in rats exposed to normoxia (control), hypoxia (hypoxia) or treated with monocrotaline (monocrotaline). Lung VEGF expression is increased in lungs from animals exposed to hypoxia but decreased in animals treated with monocrotaline (Partovian C et al.).

in our laboratory, lung density of factor VIII immunostaining was increased in mice exposed to chronic hypoxia [29]. These results suggest that activation of lung angiogenic processes in response to hypoxia is associated with an increased number of peripheral pulmonary vessels.

PLATELET VEGF CONTENTS IN PATIENTS WITH PULMONARY HYPERTENSION OR WITH CHRONIC HYPOXEMIC LUNG DISEASE

It is now well established that VEGF is also synthetized by megacaryocytes and stored in circulating platelets, where it colocalizes with PDGF [23]. One speculative role for VEGF in platelets is promotion of vascular repair and wound healing in conjunction with PDGF. Platelet VEGF and PDGF are released during blood clotting or following platelet adhesion to the subendothelial basement membrane at sites of blood vessel injury. PDGF, as a potent mitogen for fibroblasts and smooth muscle cells, effectively promotes wound healing, while VEGF may initiate angiogenesis and accelerate repair of the endothelial cell lining [21]. From a physiological point of view, platelets could thus be regarded as transporters of circulating VEGF that restrict its angiogenic activity to sites of vascular injury.

VEGF released from platelets and acting specifically on endothelial cells may play a pivotal role. In systemic vessels, increasing VEGF bioavailability at sites of endothelial denudation has been shown to accelerate endothelial repair and to limit neointima formation [34]. Moreover, VEGF overexpression within the vascular wall has been shown to restore endothelium-dependent relaxation and to protect against vasoconstriction and platelet activation. The overall balance between VEGF and other platelet-derived non-specific mitogens such as PDGF may, therefore, be of importance in pulmonary vascular diseases and pulmonary hypertension.

In recent studies, we investigated serum and platelet VEGF and PDGF in a large population of patients with pulmonary arterial hypertension, either idiopathic or associated with various diseases, as well as in patients with chronic hypoxemic lung disease. We found that platelet VEGF content was markedly elevated in patients with idiopathic or associated PH, compared with normal controls, whereas platelet PDGF content was unchanged [11]. These findings imply that sustained pulmonary artery pressure elevation, regardless of its cause, may lead to an increase in platelet VEGF content and, potentially, to an increase in platelet delivery of VEGF to the pulmonary vasculature. Intrestingly, platelet VEGF content was increased by continuous prostacyclin infusion, suggesting that continuous prostacyclin therapy results in enhanced VEGF release at sites of vascular injury. In polycythemic patients with severe chronic hypoxemic lung disease, only moderate increases in platelet VEGF and PDGF contents were observed, suggesting that hypoxemia was the main factor leading to the increases in platelet VEGF and PDGF contents. We suggest that platelet VEGF elevation during PH may be a protective mechanism against pulmonary vascular injury and remodeling.

Effects of Exogenous VEGF on Development of Experimental Pulmonary Hypertension and Endothelium-dependent Relaxation

In addition to its well-known angiogenic properties, VEGF has been shown to protect against endothelial vascular injury and to improve endothelial function. Our previous finding of impaired endothelium-dependent relaxation in chronic hypoxic pulmonary hypertension [1] invited an investigation of whether lung VEGF overexpression can protect against hypoxic pulmonary hypertension and alter the development of pulmonary vascular remodeling.

Gene therapy may be a valuable therapeutic approach in pulmonary hypertension. Several studies using intratracheal administration of adenovirus vectors have shown that transgene expression is mainly located in epithelial cells [15]. Using this route of administration, previous studies demonstrated that adenoviral-mediated gene transfer of human endothelial nitric oxide synthase (eNOS) in rats was associated with a reduction in acute pulmonary vasoconstriction [17]. We therefore reasoned that overexpression of a secreted and diffusible form of VEGF ($VEGF_{165}$) in epithelial cells following adenoviral-mediated gene transfer may affect endothelial cell behavior and protect against pulmonary vascular remodeling during development of hypoxic pulmonary hypertension. To investigate this hypothesis, we used a previously described adenovirus vector containing an expression cassette with the cytomegalovirus (CMV) early/intermediate promoter/enhancer driving the human $VEGF_{165}$ cDNA (Ad.VEGF) [24].

We evaluated the efficiency of gene transfer after a single intratracheal instillation of Ad.VEGF by measuring levels of VEGF protein in bronchoalveolar fluid and serum after various doses of the adenovirus vector and at various times after the instillation [28]. We also evaluated the effect of Ad.VEGF on pulmonary vessel permeability by measuring the extravascular accumulation of radiolabeled albumin corrected for lung blood weight. In the second part of the study, we assessed pulmonary hemodynamics, right ventricular hypertrophy and pulmonary vascular remodeling in rats pretreated with intratracheal administration of Ad.VEGF two days before the start of a two-week exposure to normoxia or hypoxia. Finally, to investigate the mechanisms of the protective effect of Ad.VEGF on the development of hypoxic pulmonary hypertension, we measured eNOS activity in lung tissue and examined pulmonary vasoreactivity using isolated lungs from normoxic and chronically hypoxic rats pretreated with Ad.VEGF.

We found that adenoviral-mediated lung VEGF overexpression, which had no effect on the pulmonary circulation during normoxia, protected rats exposed to chronic hypoxia against development of pulmonary hypertension [28]. Values were lower for pulmonary arterial pressure, right ventricular hypertrophy and distal vessel muscularization in hypoxic rats pretreated with Ad.VEGF compared to rats pretreated with the control vector Ad.Null. Our results also suggest that this protective effect of VEGF on the pulmonary circulation during exposure to chronic hypoxia was, at least partially, related to an improvement in endothelial function. Indeed, Ad.VEGF pretreatment was associated with increased lung eNOS activity, partial restoration of the vasodilator response to the endothelium-dependent agent ionophore A23187 and with marked blunting of endothelin-1-induced vasoconstriction.

Effects of Inhibition of Lung Overexpression of Angiostatin on Development of Experimental Pulmonary Hypertension in Mice

As mentioned earlier, the physiological or pathological consequences of hypoxia-induced activation of lung angiogenic processes are not completely understood. Pharmacological blockade of VEGF receptors aggravates [32] whereas lung VEGF overexpression by adenovirus mediated gene transfer attenuates development of hypoxic pulmonary hypertension [28]. However, VEGF is only one among various angiogenic molecules that are upregulated during chronic hypoxia. Moreover, VEGF receptors are present not only on endothelial cells but also on lung epithelial cells and monocytes [2,4]. Finally, the regulation of angiogenesis is a complex process, which depends upon the local balance between proangiogenic and antiangiogenic molecules. In recent studies, we questioned whether changing the angiogenic set point by inducing lung overexpression of an endogenous angiogenesis inhibitor would alter development of hypoxic pulmonary hypertension. Indeed, physiological angiogenesis is a highly regulated process under the control of both angiogenic and antiangiogenic factors. A number of endogenous angiogenesis inhibitors have been identified that antagonize the effects of VEGF, FGFs and other angiogenic factors. Among those is angiostatin, a 38-kDa fragment of plasminogen, which has been shown in vitro to inhibit endothelial cell proliferation and in vivo to exhibit potent antitumor and antiangiogenic properties [25]. Although the mechanism of its action is not completely understood, numerous studies indicate that angiostatin is a highly specific angiogenesis inhibitor [6,5].

In these studies, angiostatin delivery was achieved by a defective adenovirus expressing a secretable angiostatin K3 molecule driven by the cytomegalovirus promoter (Ad.K3) [29]. We first evaluated the efficiency of gene transfer in the lungs from mice with a single intratracheal instillation of the adenovirus by detecting the protein in bronchoalveolar lavage (BAL) fluid. We found that adenoviral-mediated lung overexpression of the angiogenesis inhibitor, angiostatin, aggravated development of hypoxic pulmonary hypertension in mice. Evidence for an activation of endogenous angiogenic processes in the lung during exposure to hypoxia was highly suggested by the observation that factor VIII endothelial cell immunostaining was increased in chronically hypoxic mice (Figure 2). This change was suppressed by pretreatment with Ad-angiostatin, which also inhibited in vitro endothelial cell growth and migration [29]. Since treatment with Ad-angiostatin did not affect PA-SMCs function in vitro, but potentiated pulmonary hypertension and aggravated structural vascular remodeling in chronically hypoxic mice, the results indicate that counteracting lung angiogenic processes aggravates development of hypoxic pulmonary hypertension.

These results differ to some extent from those obtained by Taraseviciene-Stewart et al. [32]. In this study, treatment of rats with SU5416, a selective VEGF receptor tyrosine kinase inhibitor caused mild pulmonary hypertension and pulmonary vascular remodeling in normoxic rats and severe, irreversible pulmonary hypertension associated with some endothelial cell proliferation in chronically hypoxic rats [32]. It is not clear why

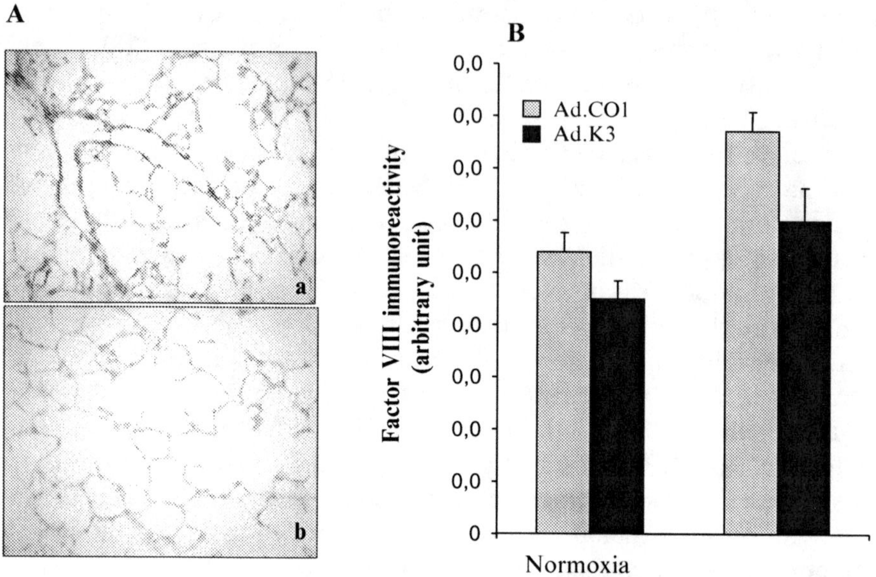

Figure 2. Von Willebrand factor immunoreactivity in lung sections from mice. Panel A shows a lung section from mice with a specific Von Willebrand factor immunoreactivity in pulmonary arterial endothelial cells (a). No immunoreactivity is detected in sections incubated with secondary antibody but no primary (b). Panel B; quantification of vascular density assessed by the ratio of Von Willebrand factor immunostaining density/ total tissue area in lung sections from mice pretreated with Ad.CO1 or Ad.K3 (10^9 pfu) and exposed to normoxia or chronic hypoxia during two weeks. Hypoxia significantly increased and pretreatment with Ad.K3 decreased vascular density. Modified from Pascaud MA et al.

pulmonary endothelial cells proliferate in response to SU5416. Because in the Taraseviciene-Stewart study, endothelial cell death occurred prior to or concomitantly with endothelial cell proliferation, the authors proposed that endothelial cell death, together with chronic hypoxia, resulted in the selection of an apoptosis-resistant, proliferating endothelial cell phenotype. No such effect of angiostatin was observed in our study, where immunostaining to factor VIII-related antigen was markedly decreased, with no evidence of a significant increase in apoptosis of lung cells. Findings obtained in the angiostatin study might therefore be interpreted as reflecting the consequence of angiogenesis inhibition. The use of VEGFR2 inhibitors likely caused additional effects, potentially related to suppression of VEGF-dependent survival of endothelial cells or to other associated effects.

Thus, exposure to chronic hypoxia is associated with the activation of endogenous lung angiogenic processes, which attenuate the severity of pulmonary hypertension. This counteracting mechanism may not be found in other models of pulmonary hypertension and may explain why hypoxic pulmonary hypertension is reversible and usually less severe than other forms of the disease. Moreover, they provide further support to the concept that stimulation of angiogenesis in the lung may be viewed as a therapeutic approach of pulmonary hypertension.

The Maturation Phase of Angiogenesis: Role of the Angiopoietin1/Tie2 Pathway on Development of Pulmonary Hypertension

A critical aspect of vessel development is maturation, during which ECs no longer proliferate or migrate but instead promote vessel stabilization by recruiting peri-endothelial support cells, which differentiate into smooth muscle cells [14]. Because this maturation phase is partly under the control of angiopoietin-1 (Ang1), which acts selectively on ECs via the Tie2 receptor [8], one theory is that EC stimulation by Ang1 leads to the release of signaling molecules that act on smooth muscle cells [26,31]. In accordance with a role for such a mechanism in the pulmonary circulation, it was recently shown that ECs stimulated with Ang1 were capable of promoting PA-SMC growth [31]. In a more recent study, we obtained evidence that serum-free medium of quiescent human ECs elicited marked PA-SMC proliferation, although the ECs were not previously stimulated by Ang1 [12]. Interestingly, this effect was greater with ECs from patients with idiopathic PH than with ECs from controls, suggesting dysregulation of this mechanism in idiopathic PH. Thus, an intriguing hypothesis is that the angiopoietin/Tie2 pathway, which seems to play a role in normal vessel wall development, may be altered in idiopathic PH, thereby leading to excessive smooth muscle proliferation.

In recent studies we investigated the angiopoietin-1/Tie2 pathway in patients with idiopathic PH [9]. For this purpose, we sampled lung tissue from patients with idiopathic PH and controls and we investigated the expression of Ang1, Ang2, and Tie2 receptor in cultured PA-SMCs and in ECs, as well as in whole lung homogenates. Second, we investigated whether treatment of cultured ECs with Ang1 increased the growth-promoting activity of culture medium from ECs of patients and controls.

We found that the angiopoietin/Tie2 pathway effectively contributed to PA-SMC proliferation by stimulating the release of growth factors by ECs. The stimulating effect of EC media on PA-SMC growth was greater with ECs from patients with iPAH than from controls and treatment with Ang1 in both cases stimulated the PA-SMC growth-promoting activity of EC media. We found that Ang1 expression in PA-SMCs did not differ between patients with iPAH and controls, whereas the Ang1 receptor Tie2 was overexpressed in ECs from patients with idiopathic PH. Consequently, stimulation by

Ang1 of ECs from patients with iPAH increased the release of the signaling molecules such as serotonin and ET-1, which was less marked in ECs from controls. Taken together, these results suggest that the Ang1/Tie2 pathway is abnormal in idiopathic PH and contributes to PA-SMC hyperplasia.

Conclusion

In conclusion, exposure to chronic hypoxia is associated with the activation of endogenous lung angiogenic processes, which attenuate the severity of pulmonary hypertension. Recent studies also provide evidence that the angiopoietin-1/Tie2 pathway is abnormal in idiopathic PAH and contributes to PA-SMC hyperplasia through excessive release of growth factors by ECs. Since Ang1 is now considered a pericyte-derived paracrine signal for the endothelium, these findings identify dysregulation of cross-talk between endothelial and smooth muscle cells as an important component of pulmonary vascular remodeling. Further studies are needed to better understand the importance of these abnormalities in the process of hypoxia-induced smooth muscle proliferation.

References

1. Adnot, S., B. Raffestin, S. Eddahibi, P. Braquet, and P. E. Chabrier. (1991). Loss of endothelium-dependent relaxant activity in the pulmonary circulation of rats exposed to chronic hypoxia. J. Clin. Invest 87: 155–162.
2. Barleon, B., S. Sozzani, D. Zhou, H. A. Weich, A. Mantovani, and D. Marme. (1996). Migration of human monocytes in response to vascular endothelial growth factor (VEGF) is mediated via the VEGF receptor flt-1. Blood 87: 3336–3343.
3. Boussat, S., S. Eddahibi, A. Coste, M. Gouge, B. Housset, S. Adnot, and B. Maitre. (2000). Expression and regulation of vascular endothelial growth factor in human pulmonary epithelial cells. Am J Physiol Lung Cell Mol Physiol 279: L371–L378.
4. Brown, K. R., K. M. England, K. L. Goss, J. M. Snyder, and M. J. Acarregui. (2001). VEGF induces airway epithelial cell proliferation in human fetal lung in vitro. Am J Physiol Lung Cell Mol Physiol 281: L1001–1010.
5. Cao, Y., A. Chen, S. S. An, R. W. Ji, D. Davidson, and M. Llinas. (1997). Kringle 5 of plasminogen is a novel inhibitor of endothelial cell growth. J Biol Chem 272: 22924–22928.
6. Cao, Y., R. W. Ji, D. Davidson, J. Schaller, D. Marti, S. Sohndel, S. G. Mccance, M. S. O'Reilly, M. Llinas, and J. Folkman. (1996). Kringle domains of human angiostatin. Characterization of the anti-proliferative activity on endothelial cells. J Biol Chem 271: 29461–29467.
7. Christou, H., A. Yoshida, V. Arthur, T. Morita, and S. Kourembanas. (1998). Increased vascular endothelial growth factor production in the lungs of rats with hypoxia-induced pulmonary hypertension. Am J Respir Cell Mol Biol 18: 768–776.
8. Davis, S., T. H. Aldrich, P. F. Jones, A. Acheson, D. L. Compton, V. Jain, T. E. Ryan, J. Bruno, C. Radziejewski, P. C. Maisonpierre, and G. D. Yancopoulos. (1996). Isolation of angiopoietin-1, a ligand for the TIE2 receptor, by secretion-trap expression cloning. Cell 87: 1161–1169.

9. Dewachter, L., S. Adnot, E. Fadel, M. Humbert, B. Maitre, A. M. Barlier-Mur, G. Simonneau, M. Hamon, R. Naeije, and S. Eddahibi. (2006). Angiopoietin/Tie2 pathway influences smooth muscle hyperplasia in idiopathic pulmonary hypertension. Am J Respir Crit Care Med 174: 1025–1033.
10. Eddahibi, S., V. Fabre, C. Boni, M. P. Martres, B. Raffestin, M. Hamon, and S. Adnot. (1999). Induction of serotonin transporter by hypoxia in pulmonary vascular smooth muscle cells. Relationship with the mitogenic action of serotonin. Circ Res 84: 329–336.
11. Eddahibi, S., M. Humbert, S. Sediame, C. Chouaïd, E. Teiger, C. Partovian, B. Maître, S. Rideau, G. Simonneau, O. Sitbon, and S. Adnot. (2000). Imbalance between platelet VEGF and PDGF in pulmonary hypertension, effects of prostacyclin infusion. Am J Respir Crit Care Med 162: 1493–1499.
12. Eddahibi, S., C. Guignabert, A. M. Barlier-Mur, L. Dewachter, E. Fadel, P. Dartevelle, M. Humbert, G. Simonneau, N. Hanoun, F. Saurini, M. Hamon, and S. Adnot. (2006). Cross talk between endothelial and smooth muscle cells in pulmonary hypertension: critical role for serotonin-induced smooth muscle hyperplasia. Circulation 113: 1857–1864.
13. Ferrara, N., K. Houck, L. Jakeman, and D. W. Leung. (1992). Molecular and biological properties of the vascular endothelial growth factor family of proteins. Endocr Rev 13: 18–32.
14. Folkman, J., and P. A. D'Amore. (1996). Blood vessel formation: what is its molecular basis? Cell 87: 1153–1155.
15. Gauldie, J., F. Graham, Z. Xing, T. Braciak, R. Foley, and P. J. Sime. (1996). Adenovirus-vector-mediated cytokine gene transfer to lung tissue. Ann N Y Acad Sci 796: 235–244.
16. Goumans, M. J., G. Valdimarsdottir, S. Itoh, A. Rosendahl, P. Sideras, and P. ten Dijke. (2002). Balancing the activation state of the endothelium via two distinct TGF-beta type I receptors. Embo J 21: 1743–1753.
17. Janssens, S. P., K. D. Bloch, Z. Nong, R. D. Gerard, P. Zoldhelyi, and D. Collen. (1996). Adenoviral-mediated transfer of the human endothelial nitric oxide synthase gene reduces acute hypoxic pulmonary vasoconstriction in rats. J Clin Invest 98: 317–324.
18. Kourembanas, S., and M. Bernfield. (1994). Hypoxia and endothelial-smooth muscle cell interactions in the lung. Am J Respir Cell Mol Biol 11: 373–374.
19. Kourembanas, S., T. Morita, Y. Liu, and H. Christou. (1997). Mechanisms by which oxygen regulates gene expression and cell-cell interaction in the vasculature. Kidney Int 51: 438–443.
20. Liu, Y. L., S. R. Cox, T. Morita, and S. Kourembanas. (1995). Hypoxia regulates vascular endothelial growth factor gene expression in endothelial cells. Identification of a 5' enhancer. Circ. Res 77: 638–643.
21. Maloney, J. P., C. C. Silliman, D. R. Ambruso, J. Wang, R. M. Tuder, and N. F. Voelkel. (1998). In vitro release of vascular endothelial growth factor during platelet aggregation. Am J Physiol 275: H1054–1061.
22. Meyrick, B., and L. Reid. (1980). Endothelial and subintimal changes in rat hilar pulmonary artery during recovery from hypoxia. A quantitative ultrastructural study. Lab Invest 42: 603–615.
23. Mohle, R., D. Green, M. A. Moore, R. L. Nachman, and S. Rafii. (1997). Constitutive production and thrombin-induced release of vascular endothelial growth factor by human megakaryocytes and platelets. Proc Natl Acad Sci U S A 94: 663–668.
24. Muhlhauser, J., M. J. Merrill, R. Pili, H. Maeda, M. Bacic, B. Bewig, A. Passaniti, N. A. Edwards, R. G. Crystal, and M. C. Capogrossi. (1995). VEGF165 expressed by a replication-deficient recombinant adenovirus vector induces angiogenesis in vivo. Circ Res 77: 1077–1086.
25. O'Reilly, M. S., L. Holmgren, Y. Shing, C. Chen, R. A. Rosenthal, M. Moses, W. S. Lane, Y. Cao, E. H. Sage, and J. Folkman. (1994). Angiostatin: a novel angiogenesis inhibitor that mediates the suppression of metastases by a Lewis lung carcinoma. Cell 79: 315–328.

26. Papapetropoulos, A., G. Garcia-Cardena, T. J. Dengler, P. C. Maisonpierre, G. D. Yancopoulos, and W. C. Sessa. (1999). Direct actions of angiopoietin-1 on human endothelium: evidence for network stabilization, cell survival, and interaction with other angiogenic growth factors. Lab Invest 79: 213–223.
27. Partovian, C., S. Adnot, S. Eddahibi, E. Teiger, M. Levame, P. Dreyfus, B. Raffestin, and C. Frelin. (1998). Heart and lung VEGF mRNA expression in rats with monocrotaline- or hypoxia-induced pulmonary hypertension. Am J Physiol 275 (Heart Circ Physiol) 275–44: H1948-H1956.
28. Partovian, C., S. Adnot, B. Raffestin, V. Louzier, M. Levame, I. M. Mavier, P. Lemarchand, and S. Eddahibi. (2000). Adenovirus-mediated lung vascular endothelial growth factor overexpression protects against hypoxic pulmonary hypertension in rats. Am J Respir Cell Mol Biol 23: 762–771.
29. Pascaud, M., S. Eddahibi, B. Raffestin, P. Yeh, F. Griscelli, P. Opolon, and S. Adnot. (2001). Lung overexpression of the anti-angiogenic factor angiostatin aggravates pulmonary hypertension in hypoxic mice. American of Journal Respiratory and Critical Care Medicine 163: A119.
30. Pfeifer, M., F. C. Blumberg, K. Wolf, P. Sandner, D. Elsner, G. A. Riegger, and A. Kurtz. (1998). Vascular remodeling and growth factor gene expression in the rat lung during hypoxia. Respir Physiol 111: 201–212.
31. Sullivan, C. C., L. Du, D. Chu, A. J. Cho, M. Kido, P. L. Wolf, S. W. Jamieson, and P. A. Thistlethwaite. (2003). Induction of pulmonary hypertension by an angiopoietin 1/TIE2/serotonin pathway. Proc Natl Acad Sci U S A 100: 12331–12336.
32. Taraseviciene-Stewart, L., Y. Kasahara, L. Alger, P. Hirth, G. Mc Mahon, J. Waltenberger, N. F. Voelkel, and R. M. Tuder. (2001). Inhibition of the VEGF receptor 2 combined with chronic hypoxia causes cell death-dependent pulmonary endothelial cell proliferation and severe pulmonary hypertension. Faseb J 15: 427–438.
33. Tuder, R. M., B. E. Flook, and N. F. Voelkel. (1995). Increased gene expression for VEGF and the VEGF receptors KDR/FIK and FIt in lungs exposed to acute or to chronic hypoxia Modulation of gene expression by nitric oxide. J. Clin. Invest. 95: 1798–1807.
34. Waltenberger, J. (1997). Modulation of growth factor action: implications for the treatment of cardiovascular diseases. Circulation 96: 4083–4094.

CHAPTER 5

TETRAHYDROBIOPTERIN AND PULMONARY HYPERTENSION

LAN ZHAO, FRANCIS BAHAA, MARTIN WILKINS

Imperial College London
Faculty of Medicine, Hammersmith Campus
Dept. of Experimental Medicine and Toxicology
Du Cane Road,
London W12 0NN
United Kingdom

Abstract: The integrity of the pulmonary vascular endothelium plays a key role in pulmonary vascular homeostasis. In particular, reduced endothelial-derived nitric oxide (NO) bioavailability is implicated in the pathogenesis of pulmonary hypertension. Recent studies in complementary murine genetic models provide clear evidence that tetrahydrobiopterin (BH4), a cofactor for endothelial nitric oxide synthase (eNOS), is a key determinant of NO production in pulmonary vasculature and that lack of BH4 leads to increased superoxide production. Congenital deficiency of BH4 in the mouse is associated with structural changes in pulmonary vessels from birth and pulmonary hypertension in the adult. Conversely, increased local production in vascular endothelium protects against hypoxia-induced pulmonary hypertension. The data suggest a possible therapeutic role for BH4 in the management of pulmonary hypertension.

Keywords: tretrahydrobiopterin; pulmonary hypertension; nitric oxide.

Tetrahydrobiopterin Biosynthesis

Tetrahydrobiopterin (BH4) is an essential cofactor for the aromatic amino acid hydroxylases and nitric acid synthase (NOS). BH4 biosynthesis proceeds along a de novo pathway from guanosine triphosphate (GTP), via 7,8-dihydroneopterin triphosphate and 6-pyruvoyl-5,6,7,8-tetrahydropterin [78] (Figure 1). The committing and rate-limiting enzyme in BH4 synthesis is guanidine triphosphate cyclohydrolase I (GTPCH). Other enzymes in the synthetic pathway include 6-pyruvoyl-tetrahydropterin synthase (PTPS) and sapiapterin reductase (SR). PTPS can become rate-limiting in macrophages when GTPCH activity is up-regulated by cytokines [86]. The intermediate

A. Aldashev and R. Naeije (eds.), Problems of High Altitude Medicine and Biology, 69–86.

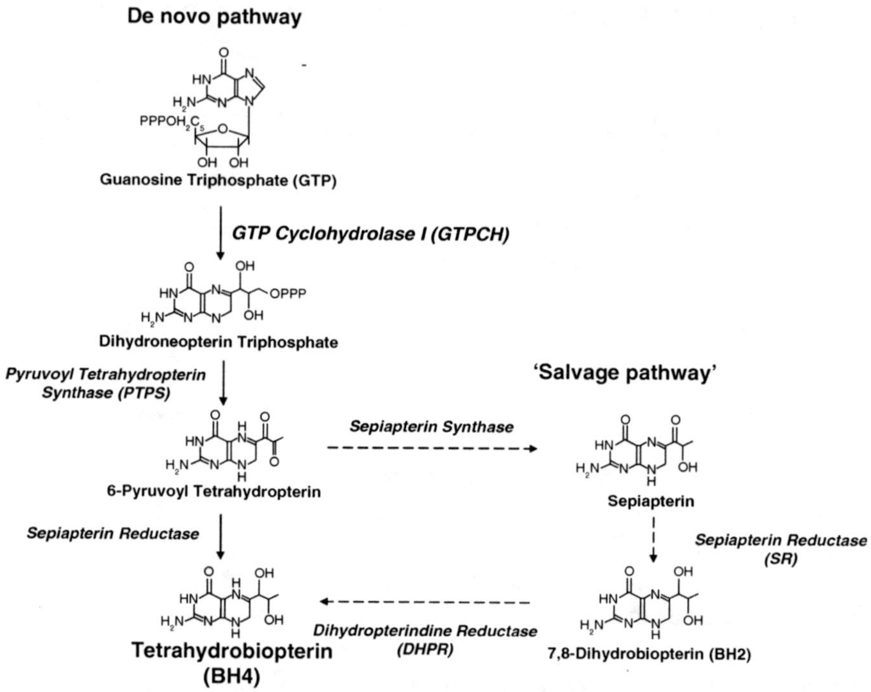

Figure 1. De novo BH4 synthesis. BH4 proceeds de novo from GTP, and GTP cyclohydrolase I (GTPCH) is a rate-limiting enzyme. A 'salvage' pathway has been described, where 6-pyruvoy-5,6,7,8-tetrahydropterin is converted to sepiapterin and then to BH4 via 7,8-Dihydrobiopterin (BH2) (adapted from Alp and Channon 2004).

7,8-dihydroneopterin triphosphate accumulates and becomes oxidized to neopterin, which is stable and detectable in plasma (Gupta et al., 1997).

GTPCH is an enzyme with 10 similar subunits, which assemble to form a 'doughnut'-shaped homodecamer of two pentamers with 10 active sites per functional unit [61]. Each 27.9 kDa subunit is encoded by the GCH gene, located on chromosome 14q22.1–q22.2 in both mice and humans, with 6 exons spanning about 30 kilobases [78]. GTPCH activity can be regulated at both the transcriptional and post-transcriptional level.

At the transcription level, cytokines are reported to increase GTPCH gene expression in endothelial cells via nuclear factor-κB, interferon-γ, tumour necrosis factor-α, interleukin-1β and Stat1/Stat3 [37]. GTPCH expression may also be up-regulated by hydrogen peroxide [71].

GTPCH is subject to post-transcriptional modification by phosphorylation in rat mesangial cells [45]. Agents that stimulate protein kinase C, such as phobol ester, platelet-derived growth factor and angiotensin II, cause an

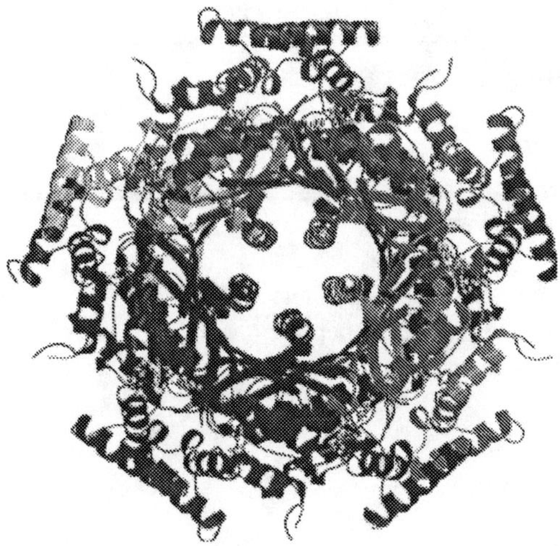

Figure 2. X-ray Crystallographic structure of GTP-Cyclohydrolase I (GTPCH, Escherichia Coli) [61]. GTPCH is the committing and rate-limiting enzyme in BH4 synthesis. Fully assembled, GTHCH is a 'doughnut'-shaped homodecamer of two staked pentamers, with 10m active sites from interactions between the subunits.

increase in GTPCH phosphorylation while specific protein kinase C inhibitors decrease phosphorylation of the enzyme. Concomitantly, phosphorylation coincides with elevated enzyme activity and an increase in cellular BH4 levels.

Recent studies suggest that GTPCH activity can also be governed by feedback regulation, mediated by GFRP, a homopentamer of 52 kDa [92]. GFRP binds to GTPCH and forms a reversible complex [53]. Through interaction with GFRP, phenylalanine stimulates GTPCH activity, while BH4 inhibits it [30]. The pattern of GPRP expression in rat tissues correlates with that of GTPCH, i.e. GFRP is highly expressed liver, heart, and brain [58,22]. Changes in BH4 levels in human endothelial cell cultures, induced by liposaccharide or hydrogen peroxide, can be mediated by GFRP [40,41]. These regulatory factors and others are summarized in Table 1.

An alternative 'salvage' pathway for BH4 synthesis has been observed in bacteria [90] and Dropsophila [44], where 6-pyruvoyl-5,6,7,8-tetrahydropterin is converted to sepiapterin by sepiapterin synthase. Endogenous sepiapterin production in humans is implied from observations of elevated sepiapterin levels in the cerebrospinal fluid of patients with sepiapterin reductase deficiency [96]. Exogenous sepiapterin can be reduced in cells by sepiapterin reductase to 7,8-dihydrobiopterin (BH2), and then by dihydropteridine reductase (DHPR), to BH4 (Nichol et al., 1983). Indeed, dietary sepiapterin administration has been used as an approach to increase BH4

TABLE 1. Regulating factors of GTPCH

Stimulating factors:
• Statins
• Ca influx
• FSH
• Epidermal growth factor
• Nerve growth factor
• Platelet-derived growth factor
• Vasoactive intestenal peptide
• TNF-α, interferon-γ, IL-1β
• Insulin
Inhibiting factors:
• NO donors
• cGMP
• BH4
• GFRP
• IL-4, TGF-β
• Glucocorticoids
• 2,4-diamino-6-hydroxypyrimidine

levels, although recent data suggested that sepiapterin itself may compete with BH4 for endothelial nitric oxide synthase (eNOS) binding to cause eNOS uncoupling (Tarpey, 2002,81)

In addition to NOS, BH4 is an essential cofactor for the aromatic amino acid hydroxylases: phenylalanine, tyrosine and tryptophan hydroxylases [78]. Phenylalanine hydroxylase is expressed in the liver, where it is involved in phenylalanine degradation. Tyrosine hydroxylase and tryptophan hydroxylase are involved in dopamine and 5–HT synthesis respectively. BH4 is oxidized to tetrahydrobiopterin-4a-carbinolamine by amino acid hydroxylases. Its regeneration requires pterin-4a-carbinolamine dehydratase (PCD) and dihydropterindine reductase (DHPR), via the quinonoid dihydrobiopterin intermediate [78]. Mutations in the PCD and DHPR genes have been associated with hyperphenylalaninaemia, but the relevance of the regeneration pathway is uncertain in endothelial cells. BH4 transiently forms the protonated trihydrobiopterin cation radical ($BH3.H^+$) during electron transfer to oxidize arginine. It reverts back to the BH4 state following the reaction [82].

BH4 deficiency arising from mutations in enzyme in BH4 synthesis can result in hyperphenylalaninaemia associated with progressive neurological deficits (Smith et al., 1975). Mutations in the GCH gene can cause DOPA-responsive dystonia (DRD), a form of BH4 deficiency syndrome without hyperphenylalaninaemia [69,39]. There are as yet no published data regarding vascular function in affected patients.

Tetrahydrobiopterin in Endothelial Nitric Oxide Synthesis

Nitric oxide synthases (NOS) are haem-containing oxidoreductases and exist as homodimers in three isoforms: endothelial (eNOS), neuronal (nNOS), and inducible (iNOS). They produce NO through a 5-step oxidation of its substrate L-arginine to L-citrulline, using molecular oxygen. The C-terminal reductase domain of NOS contains binding sites for FAD, FMN and the electron donor, NADPH (Fig 3). The N-terminal oxygenase domain contains the haem group and binding sites for the substrate, arginine and the cofactor, BH4. The reductase domain generates electron flow from NADPH through the flavins FAD and FMN and then transfers the electrons to the oxygenase domain of the other monomer, where L-arginine oxidation occurs at the haem group in the active site [4].

In the vasculature, eNOS is the main NOS isoform, constitutively expressed in normal endothelium, while iNOS expression is normally low but may be increased in certain disease states, such as atherosclerosis [88]. eNOS is localized to invaginations of the plasma membrane called caveolae. Its activity is regulated through multiple integrated pathways, including activation by calcium-camodulin, membrane localization in caveolae through lipid modifications, protein-protein interactions with caveolin and hsp90, phosphorylation at key serine and threonine residues, and subcellular trafficking between caveolae and cytosol [21].

BH4 is an essential cofactor for all 3 NOS isoforms. BH4 binds close to the haem active site at the interface between the two monomers (Fig 3). In vitro experiments have shown an important role of BH4 in maintaining and stabilizing the active dimeric form of NOS [9,68]. BH4 also participates in the transfer of electrons to L-arginine, serving as an electron donor to the haem group [67,75]. Biochemical and cellular studies have demonstrated that when BH4 levels are reduced or absent, eNOS dimerization is destabilized, leading to a reduction in the relative proportion of eNOS dimers versus monomers in the cell. eNOS catalytic activity also becomes 'uncoupled'. The stoichiometric coupling between the reductase domain and the L-arginine oxidation site is lost. The electron transfer from NADPH through flavins to molecular oxygen results in the formation of superoxide and/or hydrogen peroxide [12,80]. Besides BH4, oxidation status of the Zn 2+-thiolate centre [97] and substrate L-arginine availability are also involved in the NOS uncoupling.

Tetrahydrobiopterin and Vascular Disease

Decreased endothelial NO and increased oxidative stress are both implicated in vascular disease. The role of BH4 in contributing to endothelial dysfunction has been the subject of considerable interest in recent years.

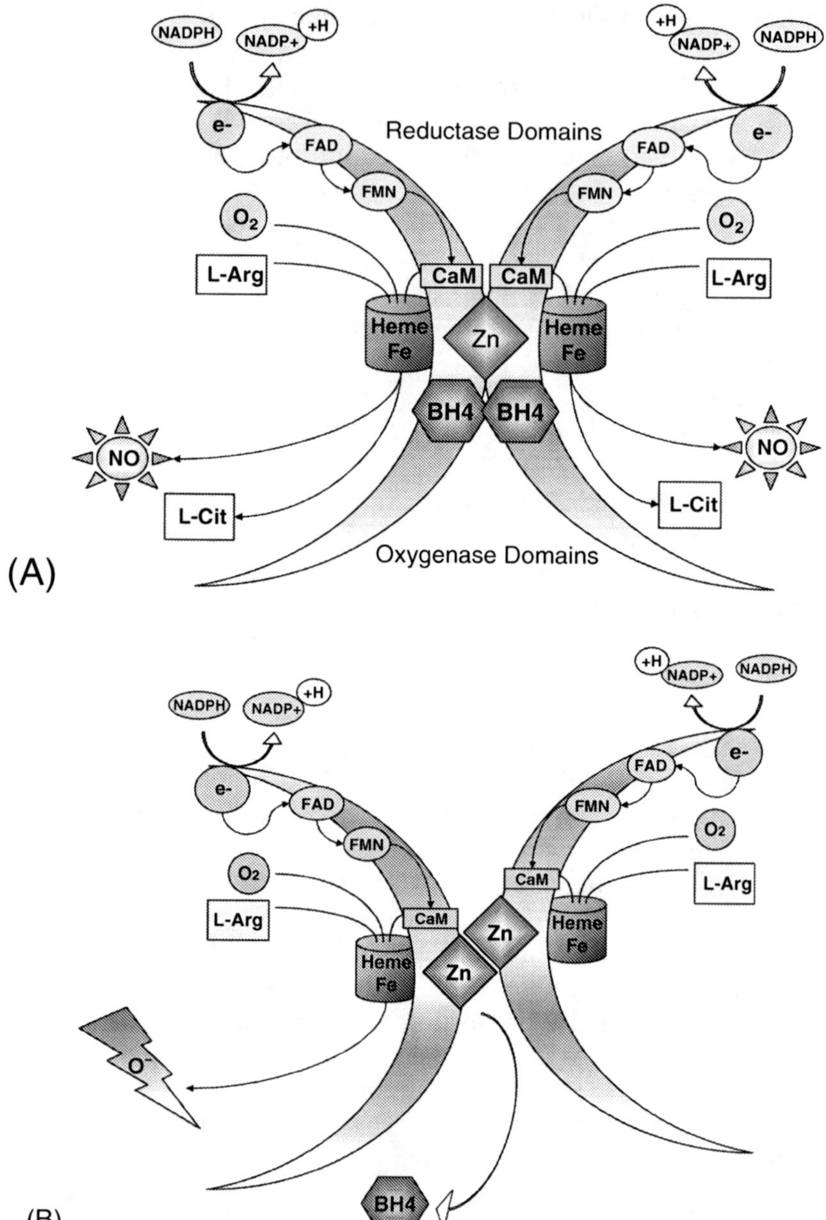

Figure 3. Schematic diagram of NOS structure and function. Active NOS is a dimmer, with each monomer consisting of a reductase domain linked to an oxigenase domain. Electron are donated by NADPH, and transferred to FAD and FMN from the reductase domain of one NOS monomer, to the heme group (Fe) in the oxygenase domain of the other monomer, resulting in NO and L-citrulline synthesis and molecular oxygen. BH4 is closely bound to the heme group, serving as an electron donor and also interacts with residues from both monomers.

Endothelial cells from the diabetic BB rat have reduced BH4 levels and reduced eNOS activity, which can be rescued by sepiapterin, a BH4 precursor [57]. NO-dependent vasodilatation is improved by sepiapterin in atherosclerotic aortas from ApoE-KO mice [47]. BH4 supplementation also improved vasodilatation in spontaneously hypertensive rats [14,36]. Verma et al (2002) showed that supplemental BH4 provides a novel cardio-protective effect on left ventricular function, endothelial-vascular reactivity, oxidative damage and cardiomyocyte injury after ischemia-reperfusion injury. NOS dimerisation and coupling is reduced in hyperglycaemic human aortic endothelial cells but can be normalized by augmenting BH4, using GTPCH gene transfer [11].

In vivo studies using disease models and gene-modified animals have also suggested an important role of BH4 in cardiovascular disease. BH4 deficiency due to increased oxidative stress appears to mediate chronic DOCA-salt induced hypertension in rodents [46,94]. Cardiac hypertrophy from pressure overload induced by aortic banding has been shown to trigger myocardial eNOS uncoupling, reversible by BH4 supplementation [77]. In eNOS transgenic/ApoE-KO mice, enhanced superoxide production and accelerated atherosclerosis were prevented by pharmacological BH4 supplementation [64]. The GTPCH deficient (hph-1) mouse has reduced levels of BH4 and appears to have impaired NOS coupling [15]. Targeted overexpression of endothelial GTPCH, augmenting BH4 levels in the endothelium, can improve eNOS function and endothelial dysfunction in diabetic mice and also reduce atherosclerosis in ApoE-KO mice [2,3].

In humans, acute BH4 administration augments NO-dependent flow-mediated vasodilatation in smokers [32], and in patients with diabetes [32], hypertension [14], hypercholesterolaemia [74] or coronary artery disease [52]. Superoxide production is increased in human diabetic vessels, which is partly inhibited by a NOS inhibitor or sepiapterin [28]. However, these studies are short-term and may be confounded by non-specific antioxidant effects, given the high doses of sepiapterin used (more than hundred-fold in excess of physiological concentration). There are few data on the long-term effects of BH4 augmentation in vascular disease.

A possible association between homocysteine, a putative risk factor for vascular disease, and BH4-dependent eNOS coupling, has also recently been suggested. Homocysteine induces oxidative stress by uncoupling

---

When heme, BH4, Zn and L-Arg are present and attach to eNOS, coupled dimmer of eNOS can produce NO (**A**). Uncoupling of eNOS as a result of loss or oxidation of BH4, eNOS produce free oxygen radicals instead of NO (**B**).

of NOS through reduction of de novo synthesis of BH4, most likely by blunting sepiapterin reductase [79,17]. BH4 supplementation attenuates homocysteine induced endothelial dysfunction. Heterozygous knockout mice for methylenetetrahydrofolate reductase, which converts homocysteine to methionine, have mildly elevated homocysteine levels and increased aortic superoxide production. These can be inhibited by sepiapterin or L-NAME [84].

Ascorbic Acid (Vitamin C) can facilitate recycling of BH4 from BH3, thus preventing formation of inactive BH2 [65]. Heller et al (2001) found that ascorbic acid plays a role in the chemical stabilization of BH4 and that saturated ascorbic acid levels in endothelial cells are necessary to protect BH4 from oxidation and to provide optimal conditions for cellular NO synthesis.

Dihydrobiopterin (BH2), the oxidation product of BH4, may also compete with BH4 for binding to eNOS [81]. Loss of BH4 to BH2 by oxidation is a feature of the increased oxidative stress that is characteristic of vascular disease states [2,46]. However, it is still uncertain whether the ratio of BH4 /BH2 is more important than absolute BH4 levels in determining eNOS activity in vascular disease.

Tetrahydrobiopterin in Pulmonary Hypertension

Nitric Oxide in Pulmonary Hypertension

All 3 NOS isoforms are expressed in the lung [62,66]. There is evidence that NO is involved in lung growth and development, in so far as eNOS knockout mice have defective lungs with a poorly developed air-blood barrier, which simulates the alveolar-capillary dysplasia [29]. Expression and activity of eNOS are developmentally regulated, with large increases in both in late gestation [62].

Loss of NO is implicated in pulmonary hypertension. Administration of NOS inhibitors, such as NG-nitro-L-arginine methyl ester (L-NAME), increases pulmonary vascular resistance and augments pulmonary vasoconstrictor responses to hypoxia [1]. Mice deficient in eNOS are more sensitive to hypoxia-induced pulmonary hypertension [19,73], whereas overexpression of eNOS in the lung is partially protective [63,13]. Patients with pulmonary hypertension have lower NO levels in their exhaled breath, a lower plasma L-citrulline/L-arginine ratio, lower urinary NO metabolites, and impaired endothelial-dependent vasorelaxation [42,50,56,26]. Furthermore, both inhaled NO and phosphodiesterase type 5 inhibitors, which act to increase NO-mediated cGMP signalling, have emerged as therapeutic options for pulmonary hypertension [23,38,89].

Reduced eNOS protein in lung tissues from patients with pulmonary hypertension has been described, which may again account for the low NO levels [24]. However, others have found normal or even increased levels of eNOS in their patients [54,91]. Indeed, mice with hypoxia-induced pulmonary hypertension have increased eNOS protein levels, without a concomitant increase in NO bioactivity [20,48]. These data suggest that eNOS may be dysfunctional rather than deficient.

Oxidative Stress in Pulmonary Hypertension

The association of oxidative stress with pulmonary hypertension is increasingly recognised. Markers of oxidative stress are increased in patients with pulmonary hypertension [6,16,59]. Superoxide mediates pulmonary smooth muscle cell proliferation after exposure to endothelin-1 [85], and pulmonary vasoconstriction after exposure to 5-HT [49]. Increased superoxide production from NADPH oxidase has been associated with pulmonary hypertension in foetal lambs after in-utero ductal ligation [8]. Superoxide produced from xanthine oxidase appears to contribute to the development of hypoxia-induced pulmonary hypertension in rodents [35].

Transgenic GTPCH Deficiency and Overexpression in Mouse

Using murine models with deficient BH4 biosynthesis, complemented by targeted transgenic animals with increased endothelial BH4 biosynthesis, we have revealed that BH4 plays a pivotal role in eNOS function and regulation of the pulmonary circulation (Figure 4).

We first demonstrate that congenital BH4 deficiency in the hph-1 mouse results in the development of pulmonary hypertension and vascular remodelling in the adult under normoxic conditions and exacerbates the response to hypoxia [43]. Conversely, augmentation of endothelial BH4 biosynthesis in the GCH transgenic mouse (in which GCH-overexpression is target to endothelial cells) protects against the development of hypoxia-induced pulmonary hypertension and vascular remodelling during 4 weeks of hypoxia (unpublished data). Selective restoration of endothelial BH4 levels in the hph1 strain by intercross with the GCH transgenic mouse rescues the effects of systemic BH4 deficiency. A striking quantitative correlation was observed between lung BH4 levels and the development of pulmonary hypertension across the 5 genetic mouse models evaluated in our studies, suggesting that BH4 bioavailability controls both pulmonary vascular tone and structural remodelling in a dose-dependent manner [43]. Significantly, our data show

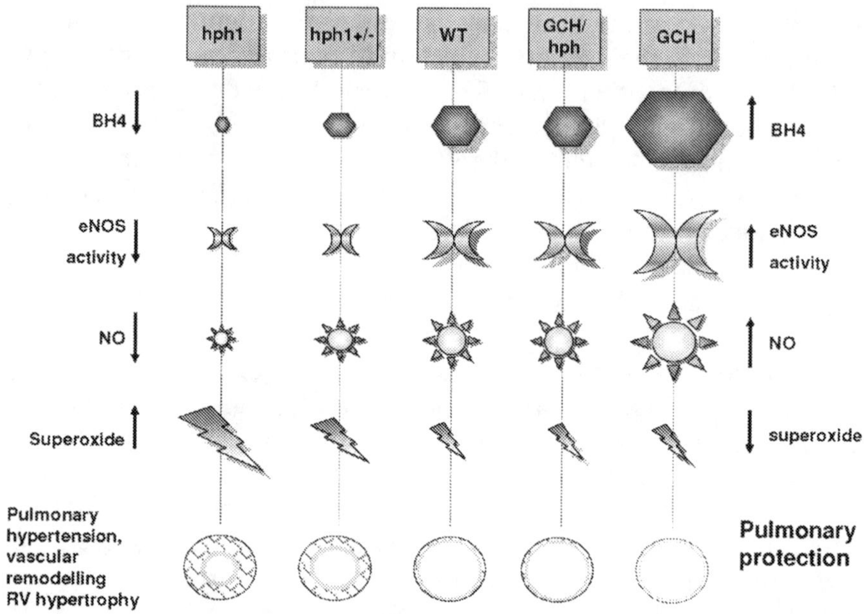

Figure 4. Schematic illustration of different parameters across the 5 genetic mouse models in our study. Gradual increase in BH4 levels, NO, eNOS activity and decrease in superoxide levels, across the genetic models, protect the pulmonary circulation (hph1 is a transgenic GTPCH deficient mice model ; hph+/− is hph1 heterozygous; GCH is a transgenic model of targeted-endothelial overexpression of GTPCH; GCH/hph1 is the cross breeding strain of hph1 and GCH.

that BH4 deficiency is associated with increased superoxide production, evidence of uncoupled NOS activity.

Our findings of pulmonary hypertension in normoxic hph-1 mice have been confirmed by independent investigators [60]. The elevated right ventricular systolic pressure in the BH4-deficient hph-1 mice is at least comparable to that previously observed in mice deficient in eNOS (eNOS- KO), with both strains showing exacerbated responses to chronic hypoxia [19,72,73]. However, vascular remodelling, a hallmark of pulmonary hypertension, was not seen in lungs from eNOS-KO mice kept in a normal oxygen atmosphere [72,93], whereas vascular remodelling was clearly evident in both hph-1 heterozygotes and homozygotes compared with wild-type littermates under normal oxygen conditions. This discordance in the severity of the phenotype between genetic eNOS deficiency and eNOS dysfunction resulting from genetic BH4 deficiency suggests that loss of NO production alone is not the sole mediator of the vascular pathology. Rather, our findings highlight the importance of increased eNOS-dependent superoxide production in playing a pathogenic role in both vascular remodelling and pulmonary hypertension.

Indeed, vascular superoxide production has a number of potentially important effects in the vascular wall, including effects on NO signalling through scavenging and peroxynitrite generation and through modulation of redox-sensitive signalling pathways [9]. Superoxide has been shown to influence proliferation and apoptosis of pulmonary vascular smooth muscle cells [85]. Our findings highlight the importance of endothelial BH4 availability as a reciprocal modulator of both NO and superoxide production by eNOS and provides a mechanistic link between previous observations of increased NOS protein levels and reduced NO bioactivity [20,48]. While chronic hypoxia increases eNOS expression in wild-type mice, BH4 levels remained unchanged, thereby leading to a relative BH4 deficiency [43]. Targeting NOS regulation and enzymatic coupling, rather than eNOS protein levels or total enzymatic activity, may be a more promising therapeutic strategy in pulmonary hypertension.

Tetrahydrobiopterin as a Therapeutic Target

Given the complex pathophysiology of pulmonary hypertension, targeting of multiple pathways with combination drug therapy may be necessary. The ability of BH4 to both augment NO synthesis and decrease superoxide production addresses two pathogenic mechanisms simultaneously. The data support evaluation of pharmacological or molecular strategies that target endothelial BH4 availability in patients with pulmonary hypertension. In this context it is interesting to note that HMG-CoA inhibitors (statins), currently generating significant interest after their reversal of experimental pulmonary hypertension in rats [25], upregulate GTPCH mRNA and BH4 levels in vascular endothelial cells [31]. A more direct approach would be to examine the clinical efficacy of oral BH4 supplementation in suitable patients.

We cannot exclude the possibility that the pulmonary changes in the hph-1 mice occur at the transition from birth to neonatal life, or that BH4 has a particularly critical role in lung development. As such, BH4 deficiency may have a more important role in the pathogenesis of persistent pulmonary hypertension of the newborn rather than adult pulmonary hypertension. As discussed earlier, eNOS is known to play a critical role in lung development, as revealed in a recent study showing alveolar capillary dysplasia in eNOS-KO mice [29]. Furthermore, mice lacking 6-pyruvoyl-tetrahydropterin synthase (PTPS), the second enzyme in the synthetic pathway for BH4, die from an undefined cause within 48 hours following birth [18,76]. A recent study in lambs has shown that the normal foetal pulmonary endothelium has high levels of BH4 and NO production but BH4 levels fall postnatally, with evidence of eNOS uncoupling and the production of reactive oxygen species in addition to NO [55]. The data suggest that BH4 availability may have an important role in regulating pulmonary eNOS function during development and the adaptation of the pulmonary vasculature to extra-uterine life.

BH4 deficiency in hph-1 mice did not reproduce the severe pulmonary hypertension with plexiform lesions seen in humans [43] even after exposure to hypoxia, and the mice appear to have a normal life expectancy. Other recently published genetic mouse models of pulmonary hypertension have also failed to recapitulate this extreme phenotype [5,51,87]. Even in mice overexpressing S100A4/Mts1, only 5% of aging mice develop plexiform arteriopathy [27]. These observations imply that additional pathways need to be invoked for the full pathogenic expression of the human disease and reinforce the idea for combination therapy in the treatment of pulmonary hypertensive patients.

References

1. Adnot S, Raffestin B, Eddahibi S, Braquet P, Chabrier PE. (1991) Loss of endothelium-dependent relaxant activity in the pulmonary circulation of rats exposed to chronic hypoxia. J Clin Invest. Jan; 87(1):155–62.
2. Alp NJ, Mussa S, Khoo J, Cai S, Guzik T, Jefferson A, Goh N, Rockett KA, Channon KM. (2003) Tetrahydrobiopterin-dependent preservation of nitric oxide-mediated endothelial function in diabetes by targeted transgenic GTP-cyclohydrolase I overexpression. J Clin Invest. Sep; 112(5):725–35.
3. Alp NJ, McAteer MA, Khoo J, Choudhury RP, Channon KM. (2004) Increased endothelial tetrahydrobiopterin synthesis by targeted transgenic GTP-cyclohydrolase I overexpression reduces endothelial dysfunction and atherosclerosis in ApoE-knockout mice. Arterioscler Thromb Vasc Biol. Mar; 24(3):445–50. Epub 2004 Jan 5.
4. Behrendt D, Ganz P. (2002) Endothelial function. From vascular biology to clinical applications. Am J Cardiol. Nov 21;90(10C):40L–48L. Review.
5. Beppu H, Ichinose F, Kawai N, Jones RC, Yu PB, Zapol WM, Miyazono K, Li E, Bloch KD. (2004) BMPR-II heterozygous mice have mild pulmonary hypertension and an impaired pulmonary vascular remodelling response to prolonged hypoxia. Am J Physiol Lung Cell Mol Physiol. Dec;287(6):L1241–7.
6. Bowers R, Cool C, Murphy RC, Tuder RM, Hopken MW, Flores SC, Voelkel NF. (2004) Oxidative stress in severe pulmonary hypertension. Am J Respir Crit Care Med. Mar 15;169(6):764–9.
7. Budhiraja, R; Rubin M. Tuder, MD; Paul M. Hassoun, MD. (2004) Endothelial dysfunction in pulmonary hypertension.Circulation. Jan 20;109(2):159–65.
8. Brennan LA, Steinhorn RH, Wedgwood S, Mata-Greenwood E, Roark EA, Russell JA, Black SM. (2003) Increased superoxide generation is associated with pulmonary hypertension in fetal lambs: a role for NADPH oxidase. Circ Res. Apr 4;92(6):683–91.
9. Cai H, Harrison DG. (2000) Endothelial dysfunction in cardiovascular diseases: the role of oxidant stress. Circ Res. Nov 10;87(10):840–4. Review.
10. Cai S, Alp NJ, McDonald D, Smith I, Kay J, Canevari L, Heales S, Channon KM. (2002) GTP cyclohydrolase I gene transfer augments intracellular tetrahydrobiopterin in human endothelial cells: effects on nitric oxide synthase activity, protein levels and dimerisation. Cardiovasc Res. Sep;55(4):838–49.

11. Cai S, Khoo J, Channon KM. (2005) Augmented BH4 by gene transfer restores nitric oxide synthase function in hyperglycemic human endothelial cells. Cardiovasc Res. Mar 1;65(4):823–31.
12. Channon KM. (2004) Tetrahydrobiopterin: regulator of endothelial nitric oxide synthase in vascular disease. Trends Cardiovasc Med. Nov;14(8):323–7. Review.
13. Champion HC, Bivalacqua TJ, Greenberg SS, Giles TD, Hyman AL, Kadowitz PJ. (2002) Adenoviral gene transfer of endothelial nitric-oxide synthase (eNOS) partially restores normal pulmonary arterial pressure in eNOS-deficient mice. Proc Natl Acad Sci U S A. Oct 1;99(20):13248–53.
14. Cosentino F, Patton S, d'Uscio LV, Werner ER, Werner-Felmayer G, Moreau P, Malinski T, Luscher TF. (1998) Tetrahydrobiopterin alters superoxide and nitric oxide release in prehypertensive rats. J Clin Invest. Apr 1;101(7):1530–7.
15. Cosentino F, Barker JE, Brand MP, Heales SJ, Werner ER, Tippins JR, West N, Channon KM, Volpe M, Luscher TF. (2001) Reactive oxygen species mediate endothelium-dependent relaxations in tetrahydrobiopterin-deficient mice. Arterioscler Thromb Vasc Biol. Apr;21(4):496–502.
16. Cracowski JL, Cracowski C, Bessard G, Pepin JL, Bessard J, Schwebel C, Stanke-Labesque F, Pison C. (2001) Increased lipid peroxidation in patients with pulmonary hypertension. Am J Respir Crit Care Med. Sep 15;164(6):1038–42.
17. Dhillon B, Badiwala MV, Maitland A, Rao V, Li SH, Verma S. (2003) Tetrahydrobiopterin attenuates homocysteine induced endothelial dysfunction. Mol Cell Biochem. May;247 (1–2):223–7.
18. Elzaouk L, Leimbacher W, Turri M, Ledermann B, Burki K, Blau N, Thony B. (2003) Dwarfism and low insulin-like growth factor-1 due to dopamine depletion in Pts –/– mice rescued by feeding neurotransmitter precursors and H4-biopterin. J Biol Chem. Jul 25;278(30):28303–11.
19. Fagan KA, Fouty BW, Tyler RC, Morris KG Jr, Hepler LK, Sato K, LeCras TD, Abman SH, Weinberger HD, Huang PL, McMurtry IF, Rodman DM. (1999) The pulmonary circulation of homozygous or heterozygous eNOS-null mice is hyperresponsive to mild hypoxia. J Clin Invest. 103: 291–299.
20. Fagan KA, Morrissey B, Fouty BW, Sato K, Harral JW, Morris KG Jr, Hoedt-Miller M, Vidmar S, McMurtry IF, Rodman DM. (2001) Upregulation of nitric oxide synthase in mice with severe hypoxia-induced pulmonary hypertension. Respir Res. 2(5):306–13.
21. Fleming I, Busse R. (2003) Molecular mechanisms involved in the regulation of the endothelial nitric oxide synthase. Am J Physiol Regul Integr Comp Physiol. Jan;284(1): R1–12. Review.
22. Gesierich A, Niroomand F, Tiefenbacher CP. (2003) Role of human GTP cyclohydrolase I and its regulatory protein in tetrahydrobiopterin metabolism. Basic Res Cardiol. 98(2):69–75.
23. Ghofrani HA, Voswinckel R, Reichenberger F, Olschewski H, Haredza P, Karadas B, Schermuly RT, Weissmann N, Seeger W, Grimminger F. (2004) Differences in hemodynamic and oxygenation responses to three different phosphodiesterase-5 inhibitors in patients with pulmonary arterial hypertension: a randomized prospective study. J Am Coll Cardiol. Oct 6;44(7):1488–96.
24. Giaid A, Saleh D. (1995) Reduced expression of endothelial nitric oxide synthase in the lungs of patients with pulmonary hypertension. N Engl J Med. Jul 27;333(4):214–21.
25. Girgis RE, Li D, Zhan X, Garcia JG, Tuder RM, Hassoun PM, Johns RA. (2003) Attenuation of chronic hypoxic pulmonary hypertension by simvastatin. Am J Physiol Heart Circ Physiol. Sep;285(3):H938–45.
26. Girgis RE, Champion HC, Diette GB, Johns RA, Permutt S, Sylvester JT. (2005) Decreased exhaled nitric oxide in pulmonary arterial hypertension: response to bosentan therapy. Am J Respir Crit Care Med. Aug 1;172(3):352–7.
27. Greenway S, van Suylen RJ, Du Marchie Sarvaas G, Kwan E, Ambartsumian N, Lukanidin E, Rabinovitch M. (2004) S100A4/Mts1 produces murine pulmonary artery changes resem-

bling plexogenic arteriopathy and is increased in human plexogenic arteriopathy. Am J Pathol. Jan;164(1):253–62.
28. Guzik TJ, Mussa S, Gastaldi D, Sadowski J, Ratnatunga C, Pillai R, Channon KM. (2002) Mechanisms of increased vascular superoxide production in human diabetes mellitus: role of NAD(P)H oxidase and endothelial nitric oxide synthase. Circulation. Apr 9;105(14):1656–62.
29. Han RN, Babaei S, Robb M, Lee T, Ridsdale R, Ackerley C, Post M, Stewart DJ. (2004) Defective lung vascular development and fatal respiratory distress in endothelial NO synthase-deficient mice: a model of alveolar capillary dysplasia? Circ Res. Apr 30;94(8):1115–23.
30. Harada T, Kagamiyama H, Hatakeyama K. (1993) Feedback regulation mechanisms for the control of GTP cyclohydrolase I activity. Science. Jun 4;260(5113):1507–10.
31. Hattori Y, Nakanishi N, Akimoto K, Yoshida M, Kasai K. (2003) HMG-CoA reductase inhibitor increases GTP cyclohydrolase I mRNA and tetrahydrobiopterin in vascular endothelial cells. Arterioscler Thromb Vasc Biol. Feb 1;23(2):176–82.
32. Heitzer T, Krohn K, Albers S, Meinertz T. (2000) Tetrahydrobiopterin improves endothelium-dependent vasodilation by increasing nitric oxide activity in patients with Type II diabetes mellitus. Diabetologia. Nov;43(11):1435–8.
33. Heitzer T, Brockhoff C, Mayer B, Warnholtz A, Mollnau H, Henne S, Meinertz T, Munzel T. (2000) Tetrahydrobiopterin improves endothelium-dependent vasodilation in chronic smokers : evidence for a dysfunctional nitric oxide synthase. Circ Res. Feb 4;86(2): E36–41.
34. Heller R, Unbehaun A, Schellenberg B, Mayer B, Werner-Felmayer G, Werner ER. (2001) L-ascorbic acid potentiates endothelial nitric oxide synthesis via a chemical stabilization of tetrahydrobiopterin. J Biol Chem. Jan 5;276(1):40–7.
35. Hoshikawa Y, Ono S, Suzuki S, Tanita T, Chida M, Song C, Noda M, Tabata T, Voelkel NF, Fujimura S. (2001) Generation of oxidative stress contributes to the development of pulmonary hypertension induced by hypoxia. J Appl Physiol. Apr;90(4):1299–306.
36. Hong HJ, Hsiao G, Cheng TH, Yen MH. (2001) Supplemention with tetrahydrobiopterin suppresses the development of hypertension in spontaneously hypertensive rats. Hypertension. Nov;38(5):1044–8.
37. Huang A, Zhang Y, Chen K, Hatakeyama K, Keaney JF Jr. (2005) Cytokine stimulated GTP cyclohydrolase I expression in endothelial cells requires coordinated activation of nuclear factor-B and Stat1/Stat3. Circ Res. 96:164 –171.
38. Ichinose F, Erana-Garcia J, Hromi J, Raveh Y, Jones R, Krim L, Clark MW, Winkler JD, Bloch KD, Zapol WM. (2001) Nebulized sildenafil is a selective pulmonary vasodilator in lambs with acute pulmonary hypertension. Crit Care Med. May;29(5):1000–5.
39. Ichinose H, Suzuki T, Inagaki H, Ohye T, Nagatsu T. (1999) Molecular genetics of dopa-responsive dystonia. Biol Chem. Dec;380(12):1355–64. Review
40. Ishii M, Shimizu S, Shiota K, Yamamoto S, Kiuchi Y, Yamamoto T. (2002) Stimulation of tetrahydrobiopterin synthesis by cyclosporin A in mouse brain microvascular endothelial cells. Int J Biochem Cell Biol. 34(9):1134–41.
41. Kalivendi S, Hatakeyama K, Whitsett J, Konorev E, Kalyanaraman B, Vasquez-Vivar J. (2005) Changes in tetrahydrobiopterin levels in endothelial cells and adult cardiomyocytes induced by LPS and hydrogen peroxide–a role for GFRP? Free Radic Biol Med. 15;38(4):481–91.
42. Kaneko FT, Arroliga AC, Dweik RA, Comhair SA, Laskowski D, Oppedisano R, Thomassen MJ, Erzurum SC. (1998) Biochemical reaction products of nitric oxide as quantitative markers of primary pulmonary hypertension. Am J Respir Crit Care Med. Sep;158(3):917–23.
43. Khoo JP, Zhao L, Alp NJ, Bendall JK, Nicoli T, Rockett K, Wilkins MR, Channon KM. (2005) Pivotal role for endothelial tetrahydrobiopterin in pulmonary hypertension. Circulation. 111:2126 –2133.

44. Krivi GG, Brown GM. (1979) Purification and properties of the enzymes from Drosophila melanogaster that catalyze the synthesis of sepiapterin from dihydroneopterin triphosphate. Biochem Genet. 17(3–4):371–90.
45. Lapize, C., Pluss, C., Werner, E. R., Huwiler, A., & Pfeilschifter, J. (1998) Protein kinase C phosphorylates and activates GTPcyclohydrolase I in rat renal mesangial cells. BiocheBiophy Res Commu 251, 802–805.
46. Landmesser U, Dikalov S, Price SR, McCann L, Fukai T, Holland SM, Mitch WE, Harrison DG. (2003) Oxidation of tetrahydrobiopterin leads to uncoupling of endothelial cell nitric oxide synthase in hypertension. J Clin Invest. Apr;111(8):1201–9.
47. Laursen JB, Boesgaard S, Trautner S, Rubin I, Poulsen HE, Aldershvile J. (2001) Endothelium-dependent vasorelaxation in inhibited by in vivo depletion of vascular thiol levels: role of endothelial nitric oxide synthase. Free Radic Res. Oct;35(4):387–94.
48. Le Cras TD, McMurtry IF. (2001) Nitric oxide production in the hypoxic lung. Am J Physiol Lung Cell Mol Physiol. Apr;280(4):L575–82.
49. Liu JQ, Folz RJ.(2004) Extracellular superoxide enhances 5-HT-induced murine pulmonary artery vasoconstriction.Am J Physiol Lung Cell Mol Physiol. Jul;287(1):L111–8.
50. Machado RF, Londhe Nerkar MV, Dweik RA, Hammel J, Janocha A, Pyle J, Laskowski D, Jennings C, Arroliga AC, Erzurum SC. (2004) Nitric oxide and pulmonary arterial pressures in pulmonary hypertension. Free Radic Biol Med. Oct 1;37(7):1010–7.
51. MacLean MR, Deuchar GA, Hicks MN, Morecroft I, Shen S, Sheward J, Colston J, Loughlin L, Nilsen M, Dempsie Y, Harmar A. (2004) Overexpression of the 5-hydroxytryptamine transporter gene: effect on pulmonary hemodynamics and hypoxia-induced pulmonary hypertension.Circulation. May 4;109(17):2150–5.
52. Maier W, Cosentino F, Lutolf RB, Fleisch M, Seiler C, Hess OM, Meier B, Luscher TF. (2000) Tetrahydrobiopterin improves endothelial function in patients with coronary artery disease. J Cardiovasc Pharmacol. Feb;35(2):173–8.
53. Maita N, Okada K, Hirotsu S, Hatakeyama K, Hakoshima T. (2001) Preparation an crystallization of the stimulatory and inhibitory complexes of GTP cyclohydrolase I and its feedback regulatory protein GFRP. Acta Crystallogr D Biol Crystallogr. 57 (Pt 8):1153–6.
54. Mason NA, Springall DR, Burke M, Pollock J, Mikhail G, Yacoub MH, Polak JM. (1998) High expression of endothelial nitric oxide synthase in plexiform lesions of pulmonary hypertension. J Pathol. Jul;185(3):313–8.
55. Mata-Greenwood E, Jenkins C, Farrow KN, Konduri GG, Russell JA, Lakshminrusimha S, Black SM, Steinhorn RH. (2006) eNOS function is developmentally regulated: uncoupling of eNOS occurs postnatally. Am J Physiol Lung Cell Mol Physiol. Feb;290(2): L232–41.
56. Mehta S, Stewart DJ, Langleben D, Levy RD. (1995) Short-term pulmonary vasodilation with L-arginine in pulmonary hypertension. Circulation. Sep 15;92(6):1539–45.
57. Meininger CJ, Marinos RS, Hatakeyama K, Martinez-Zaguilan R, Rojas JD, Kelly KA, Wu G. (2000) Impaired nitric oxide production in coronary endothelial cells of the spontaneously diabetic BB rat is due to tetrahydrobiopterin deficiency. Biochem J. Jul 1;349(Pt 1):353–6.
58. Milstien S, Jaffe H, Kowlessur D, Bonner TI. (1996) Purification and cloning of the GTP cyclohydrolase I feedback regulatory protein, GFRP. J Biol Chem. 16; 271 (33):19743–51.
59. Nagaya N, Uematsu M, Satoh T, Kyotani S, Sakamaki F, Nakanishi N, Yamagishi M, Kunieda T, Miyatake K. (1999) Serum uric acid levels correlate with the severity and the mortality of primary pulmonary hypertension. Am J Respir Crit Care Med. Aug;160(2):487–92.
60. Nandi M, Miller A, Stidwill R, Jacques TS, Lam AAJ, Haworth S, Heales S, Vallance P. (2005) Pulmonary hypertension in a GTP-cyclohydrolase1–deficient mouse. Circulation. 111:2086 –2090.

61. Nar H, Huber R, Auerbach G, Fischer M, Hosl C, Ritz H, Bracher A, Meining W, Eberhardt S, Bacher A. (1995) Active site topology and reaction mechanism of GTP cyclohydrolase I. Proc Natl Acad Sci. 19;92(26):12120–5.
62. North AJ, Star RA, Brannon TS, Ujiie K, Wells LB, Lowenstein CJ, Snyder SH, Shaul PW. (1994) Nitric oxide synthase type I and type III gene expression are developmentally regulated in rat lung.Am J Physiol. Jun;266(6 Pt 1):L635–41.
63. Ozaki M, Kawashima S, Yamashita T, Ohashi Y, Rikitake Y, Inoue N, Hirata KI, Hayashi Y, Itoh H, Yokoyama M. (2001) Reduced hypoxic pulmonary vascular remodelling by nitric oxide from the endothelium.Hypertension. Feb;37(2):322–7.
64. Ozaki M, Kawashima S, Yamashita T, Hirase T, Namiki M, Inoue N, Hirata K, Yasui H, Sakurai H, Yoshida Y, Masada M, Yokoyama M. (2002) Overexpression of endothelial nitric oxide synthase accelerates atherosclerotic lesion formation in apoE-deficient mice. J Clin Invest. Aug;110(3):331–40.
65. Patel KB, Stratford MR, Wardman P, Everett SA. (2002) Oxidation of tetrahydrobiopterin by biological radicals and scavenging of the trihydrobiopterin radical by ascorbate. Free Radic Biol Med. Feb 1;32(3):203–11.
66. Rairigh RL, Le Cras TD, Ivy DD, Kinsella JP, Richter G, Horan MP, Fan ID, Abman SH. (1998) Role of inducible nitric oxide synthase in regulation of pulmonary vascular tone in the late gestation ovine fetus. J Clin Invest. Jan 1;101(1):15–21.
67. Raman CS, Li H, Martasek P, Kral V, Masters BS, Poulos TL. (1998) Crystal structure of constitutive endothelial nitric oxide synthase: a paradigm for pterin function involving a novel metal center. Cell. Dec 23;95(7):939–50.
68. Reif A, Frohlich LG, Kotsonis P, Frey A, Bommel HM, Wink DA, Pfleiderer W, Schmidt HH. (1999) Tetrahydrobiopterin inhibits monomerization and is consumed during catalysis in neuronal NO synthase. J Biol Chem. Aug 27;274(35):24921–9.
69. Segawa M, Hosaka A, Miyagawa F, Nomura Y, Imai H. (1976) Hereditary progressive dystonia with marked diurnal fluctuation. Adv Neurol. 14:215–33.
70. Shimizu S, Ishii M, Miyasaka Y, Wajima T, Negoro T, Hagiwara T, Kiuchi Y. (2005) Possible involvement of hydroxyl radical on the stimulation of tetrahydrobiopterin synthesis by hydrogen peroxide and peroxynitrite in vascular endothelial cells.Int J Biochem Cell Biol. 37(4):864–75.
71. Shimizu, S., Shiota, K., Yamamoto, S., Miyasaka, Y., Ishii, M., Watabe, T. (2003) Hydrogen peroxide stimulates tetrahydrobiopterin synthesis through the induction of GTP cyclohydrolase I and increases nitric oxide synthase activity in vascular endothelial cells. Free Rad Bio Med 34,1343–1352.
72. Steudel W, Ichinose F, Huang PL, Hurford WE, Jones RC, Bevan JA, Fishman MC, Zapol WM. (1997) Pulmonary vasoconstriction and hypertension in mice with targeted disruption of the endothelial nitric oxide synthase (NOS 3) gene. Circ Res. Jul;81(1): 34–41.
73. Steudel W, Scherrer-Crosbie M, Bloch KD, Weimann J, Huang PL, Jones RC, Picard MH, Zapol WM. (1998) Sustained pulmonary hypertension and right ventricular hypertrophy after chronic hypoxia in mice with congenital deficiency of nitric oxide synthase 3. J Clin Invest. Jun 1;101(11):2468–77.
74. Stroes E, Kastelein J, Cosentino F, Erkelens W, Wever R, Koomans H, Luscher T, Rabelink T. (1997) Tetrahydrobiopterin restores endothelial function in hypercholesterolemia. J Clin Invest. Jan 1;99(1):41–6.
75. Stuehr DJ, Kwon NS, Nathan CF. (1990) FAD and GSH participate in macrophage synthesis of nitric oxide. Biochem Biophys Res Commun. Apr 30;168(2):558–65.
76. Sumi-Ichinose C, Urano F, Kuroda R, Ohye T, Kojima M, Tazawa M, Shiraishi H, Hagino Y, Nagatsu T, Nomura T, Ichinose H. (2001) Catecholamines and serotonin are differently regulated by tetrahydrobiopterin. A study from 6-pyruvoyltetrahydropterin synthase knockout mice. J Biol Chem. Nov 2;276(44):41150–60.
77. Takimoto E, Champion HC, Li M, Ren S, Rodriguez ER, Tavazzi B, Lazzarino G, Paolocci N, Gabrielson KL, Wang Y, Kass DA. (2005) Oxidant stress from nitric oxide

synthase-3 uncoupling stimulates cardiac pathologic remodelling from chronic pressure load. J Clin Invest. May;115(5):1221–31.

78. Thony B, Auerbach G, Blau N. (2000) Tetrahydrobiopterin biosynthesis, regeneration, and functions. Biochem J 347:1–16.
79. Topal G, Brunet A, Millanvoye E, Boucher JL, Rendu F, Devynck MA, David-Dufilho M. (2004) Homocysteine induces oxidative stress by uncoupling of NO synthase activity through reduction of tetrahydrobiopterin. Free Radic Biol Med. Jun 15;36(12):1532–41.
80. Vasquez-Vivar J, Kalyanaraman B, Martasek P, Hogg N, Masters BS, Karoui H, Tordo P, Pritchard KA Jr. (1998) Superoxide generation by endothelial nitric oxide synthase: the influence of cofactors. Proc Natl Acad Sci U S A. Aug 4;95(16):9220–5.
81. Vasquez-Vivar J, Martasek P, Whitsett J, Joseph J, Kalyanaraman B. (2002) The ratio between tetrahydrobiopterin and oxidized tetrahydrobiopterin analogues controls superoxide release from endothelial nitric oxide synthase: an EPR spin trapping study. Biochem J 362(Pt 3):733–9.
82. Vasquez-Vivar J, Whitsett J, Martasek P, Hogg N, Kalyanaraman B. (2001) Reaction of tetrahydrobiopterin with superoxide: EPR-kinetic analysis and characterization of the pteridine radical. Free Radic Biol Med 31(8):975–985.
83. Verma S, Maitland A, Weisel RD, Fedak PW, Pomroy NC, Li SH, Mickle DA, Li RK, Rao V. (2002) Novel cardioprotective effects of tetrahydrobiopterin after anoxia and reoxygenation: Identifying cellular targets for pharmacologic manipulation. J Thorac Cardiovasc Surg. Jun;123(6):1074–83.
84. Virdis A, Iglarz M, Neves MF, Amiri F, Touyz RM, Rozen R, Schiffrin EL. (2003) Effect of hyperhomocystinemia and hypertension on endothelial function in methylenetetrahydrofolate reductase-deficient mice. Arterioscler Thromb Vasc Biol. Aug 1;23(8):1352–7.
85. Wedgwood S, Black SM. (2003) Molecular mechanisms of nitric oxide-induced growth arrest and apoptosis in fetal pulmonary arterial smooth muscle cells. Nitric Oxide. Dec;9(4):201–10.
86. Werner ER, Werner-Felmayer G, Fuchs D, Hausen A, Reibnegger R, Yim JJ, Wachter H. (1991) Biochemistry and function of pteridine synthesis in human and murine macrophages. Pathobiology. 59(4):276–9. Review.
87. West J, Fagan K, Steudel W, Fouty B, Lane K, Harral J, Hoedt-Miller M, Tada Y, Ozimek J, Tuder R, Rodman DM. (2004) Pulmonary hypertension in transgenic mice expressing a dominant-negative BMPRII gene in smooth muscle. Circ Res. Apr 30;94(8):1109–14.
88. Wilcox JN, Subramanian RR, Sundell CL, Tracey WR, Pollock JS, Harrison DG, Marsden PA. (1997) Expression of multiple isoforms of nitric oxide synthase in normal and atherosclerotic vessels. Arterioscler Thromb Vasc Biol. Nov;17(11):2479–88.
89. Wilkins MR, Paul GA, Strange JW, Tunariu N, Gin-Sing W, Banya WA, Westwood MA, Stefanidis A, Ng LL, Pennell DJ, Mohiaddin RH, Nihoyannopoulos P, Gibbs JS. (2005) Sildenafil versus Endothelin Receptor Antagonist for Pulmonary Hypertension (SERAPH) study. Am J Respir Crit Care Med. Jun 1;171(11):1292–7.
90. Woo, HJ., Hwang YK, Kim YJ, Kang JY, Choi YK, Kim CG and Park YS. (2002) Escherichia coli 6-pyruvoyltetrahydropterin synthase ortholog encoded by ygcM has a new catalytic activity for conversion of sepiapterin to 7,8-dihydropterin. FEBS Lett 523(1–3): 234–8.
91. Xu W, Kaneko FT, Zheng S, Comhair SA, Janocha AJ, Goggans T, Thunnissen FB, Farver C, Hazen SL, Jennings C, Dweik RA, Arroliga AC, Erzurum SC. (2004) Increased arginase II and decreased NO synthesis in endothelial cells of patients with pulmonary arterial hypertension. FASEB J. Nov;18(14):1746–8.
92. Yoneyama T, Hatakeyama K. (1998) Decameric GTP cyclohydrolase I forms complexes with two pentameric GTP cyclohydrolase I feedback regulatory proteins in the presence of phenylalanine or of a combination of tetrahydrobiopterin and GTP. J Biol Chem. Aug 7;273(32):20102–8.

93. Zhao L, Mason NA, Morrell NW, Kojonazarov B, Sadykov A, Maripov A, Mirrakhimov MM, Aldashev A, Wilkins MR. (2001) Sildenafil inhibits hypoxia-induced pulmonary hypertension. Circulation. Jul 24;104(4):424–8.
94. Zheng JS, Yang XQ, Lookingland KJ, Fink GD, Hesslinger C, Kapatos G, Kovesdi I, Chen AF. (2003) Gene transfer of human guanosine 5`-triphosphate cyclohydrolase I restores vascular tetrahydrobiopterin level and endothelial function in low renin hypertension. Circulation. Sep 9;108(10):1238–45.
95. Zorzi G, Redweik U, Trippe H, Penzien JM, Thöny B, Blau N. (2002) Detection of sepiapterin in CSF of patients with sepiapterin reductase deficiency. Mol Genet Metab 75:174–177.
96. Zorzi G, Thöny B, Blau N. (2002) Reduced nitric oxide metabolites in CSF of patients with tetrahydrobiopterin deficiency. J Neurochem 80:362–364.
97. Zou MH, Shi C, Cohen RA. (2002) Oxidation of the zinc-thiolate complex and uncoupling of endothelial nitric oxide synthase by peroxynitrite. J Clin Invest. Mar;109(6):817–26.

CHAPTER 6

HYPOXIA-INDUCED PROLIFERATION OF HUMAN PULMONARY ARTERIAL SMOOTH MUSCLE CELLS (PASMC) IS INVOLVED IN THE SUPPRESSION OF CYCLIN-DEPENDENT KINASE INHIBITORS, p21, p27 AND p53

T. ISHIZAKI, S. MIZUNO, M. KADOWAKI, D. UESAKA, Y. UMEDA, M. MORIKAWA, M. NAKANISHI, Y. DEMURA, S. AMESHIMA, S.MATSUKAWA

Division of Pulmonary Medicine, University of Fukui Hospital, Central Laboratory, University of Fukui, Fukui Prefecture, Japan 910–1193

Abstract: It is known that hypoxia causes proliferation of pulmonary arterial smooth muscle cells (PASMC) and that hypoxia can also affect the endogenous vasodilators such as nitric oxide (NO) and Prostacyclin I2 (PGI2). Recently, it has been noted that the suppressive effect of NO on the proliferation of PASMC was partially exerted via the activation of p21, a cyclin-dependent kinase (CDK) inhibitor. We therefore decided to clarify the role of CDK inhibitors, p21, p27 and tumour suppressor p53 in PASMC in the presence/absence of exogenous NO/PGI2 during hypoxia.
HumanPASMC treated with/without NO donor or PGI2 analogue was cultured in conditions of 2% hypoxic oxygen for 24 hr. BrdU uptake for cell proliferation, flow-cytometry for cell cycle, real-time RT-PCR by Lightcycler for mRNA of CDK inhibitors and Western blot analysis for protein expression of CDK inhibitors were examined. NO donor and PGI2 suppressed the intake of BrdU and stopped the cell cycle at the G0/1 phase in humanPASMC. Concordantly, NO donor induced p21 mRNA and augmented the protein expression of p21 and p53. PGI2 analogue augmented the protein expression of p27.

These results suggest that suppression of p53, p21 and p27 are required for hypoxia-induced pulmonary vascular cell proliferation and endogenous NO and PGI2 have an anti-proliferative effect on humanPASMC via preventing the down-regulation of p53 and p21 and p27, respectively. Targeting therapy for overexpression of CDK inhibitors could be protective against the development of hypoxia-induced pulmonary arterial vascular remodelling.

Keywords: Nitric oxide, Prostacyclin, p21, p27, p53, pulmonary arterial smooth muscle cell, hypoxia

A. Aldashev and R. Naeije (eds.), Problems of High Altitude Medicine and Biology, 87–99.

Introduction

The major characteristic pathological findings of pulmonary vascular remodelling are increased wall thickening of pulmonary vessels and muscularization of small arteries. In laboratory animals, decreased ambient oxygen concentrations cause similar pathological findings, including pulmonary smooth muscle hypertrophy and proliferation [22,23]. It has been suggested that proliferation of pulmonary arterial smooth muscle cells (PASMC) is a key component of pulmonary vascular remodelling, and several in vitro studies have also addressed that exposure to hypoxia can stimulate proliferation of PASMC [13,4,1]. The proliferation of the PASMC begins when the cells enter into the cell cycle. The most important molecular event necessary for the progress of the cell cycle is phosphorylation of retinoblastoma protein by cyclin-dependent kinase (CDK)-cyclin complexes. The CDK activity can be inhibited by CDK inhibitors and the expression of CDK inhibitor is a major regulator of the transition between each phase of the cell cycle [7]. Previous studies have noted that CDK inhibitor p27 plays an important role in the inhibition of the CDK activity and proliferation in vascular smooth muscle cells [2,3]. The G1 phase in severe hypoxia is suggested to involve the CKI p27, because the expression of p27 increased in several cell-lines when they were exposed to extreme hypoxia [20,5].

Previous reports indicate that hypoxia decreases the p27 expression in the murine lung [23,24] and we found that PGI2 suppresses hypoxia-induced proliferation of PASMC and maintains p27 in PASMC [20]. We also reported that NO donors suppress thymidine incorporation and induce tumour suppressor p53 and CDK inhibitor p21 protein in human PASMC [14,15,16].

Beraprost sodium (BPS) is a stable analogue of prostacyclin (PGI2) that increases intracellular cAMP levels via activation of adenylate cyclase [17]. BPS is the first chemically stable and orally active prostacyclin analogue developed by TORAY Industries, Inc. Since 1995, BPS has been used to treat pulmonary artery hypertension in Japan, Owing to its chemical characteristics, BPS is a more stable and more long-lived molecule and has a higher affinity to the PGI2 receptor than natural PGI2 [11].

These reports indicate that CDK inhibitors can regulate proliferation of PASMC and NO or PGI2 can suppress PASMC proliferation via modulating CDK inhibitors. Furthermore, hypoxia can affect CDK inhibitors in pulmonary vessels.

Thus, our aim is to clarify the role of CDK inhibitors, p21, p27, and p53 in the presence or absence of exogenous NO/PGI2 in PASMC during hypoxia.

Materials and Methods, Chemicals

Chemicals and materials were obtained from the following sources. Humedia SG medium, recombinant human EGF and FGF, gentamycin, streptomycin, and amphotericin B came from Kurabou Ltd. (Osaka, Japan); Bromodeoxyuridine (BrdU) proliferation assay kit from OncogeneTM (Cambridge, MA); ECL system from Amersham (Buckinghamshire, UK); a QuantitechTM SYBAR Green PCR kit from Qiagen (Santa Clarita, CA); lipofectamine 2000, 4 - 12% Bis-Tris Nupage gels, and MES-SDS running buffer from Invitrogen (Carlsbad, CA); a DC protein assay kit and polyvinylidene difluoride (PVDF) membranes from Bio-Rad Laboratories (Richmond, CA); rabbit anti-p21 polyclonal antibody, rabbit anti-p27 polyclonal antibody, mouse anti-p53 monoclonal antibody, mouse anti-s-actin monoclonal antibody and horseradish peroxidase-conjugated goat anti-mouse and rabbit antibody. NO donors, S-nitroso-N-acetylpenicillamine (SNAP) and diethylenetriaminelNONOate (DETANO) were purchased from Dojindo Laboratories (Kumamoto, Japan) and BPS was kindly gifted from Toray industries Inc. (Tokyo, Japan). All other chemicals were purchased from Sigma (St. Louis, MO).

Cell Culture

HumanPASMC were supplied by Kurabou Ltd. (Osaka, Japan) and grown in Humedia SG medium containing 5% foetal bovine serum with 50 μg/ml of gentamycin, 50 ng/ml of amphotericin B, 1ng/ml of recombinant human EGF and 1ng/ml of recombinant human FGF. The cells were cultured in 75-cm2 tissue culture flasks (Corning, NY, U.S.) in a cell-culture incubator (37°C, 5% CO2, and 95% air) and used at the seventh passage after trypsinization in all of the experiments. Modifications of oxygen concentrations (0.1% ~ 10%) were performed by N2-CO2 incubators (BNR-110M, Tabai ESPEC Corp., Tokyo, Japan, and 10-0233, Ikemoto Rika Kogyo, Co., LTD., Tokyo, Japan).

Assay of BrdU Incorporation of HumanPASMC

HumanPASMC were seeded in a 96-well culture disk at a density of 6000 cells/cm^2 and incubated for 48 hours in serum-free DME, after which the medium was changed to DME with 10% FBS and antibiotics. After that, the cells were incubated for another 24 hours in various oxygen concentrations with or without NO donors or BPS. BrdU incorporations were measured by BrdU proliferation assay kit, using the manufacturer's protocol. Briefly, the cells were labelled with 10ng/ml of BrdU during the incubation. After labelling, the cells were washed three times with cold PBS and fixed. Then air dried and treated with mouse anti-BrdU monoclonal antibody (1: 1000). After aspiration the antibody, the cells were washed three times, and incubated with peroxidase goat anti-mouse IgG (1: 2000) at room temperature for 30 minutes. After incubation, the cells were washed three times and 100μM of substrate solution was added to the each well and incubated for 10 minutes in dark. After that, the absorbance of dual-wave length at 450 to 540nm was measured.

Propidium Iodide Staining

To examine whether the cell cycles were influenced by oxygen concentration, flow cytometric analysis with propidium iodide staining was performed. HumanPASMC were seeded in a 6-well culture disk at a density of 6000 cells/cm^2 and incubated for 48 hours in serum-free DME, after which the medium was changed to DME with 10% FBS and antibiotics. Next, the cells were incubated for 24 hours in normal or hypoxic oxygen concentrations with or without NO donors or BPS. To measure the DNA content, the cells were harvested by trypsin and EDTA and fixed with 70% ethanol. The ethanol was removed and the cells were incubated in PBS containing RNase (172 kunits/ml) at 37°C for 30 minutes and then stained with propidium iodide (50 μg/ml) and dissolved in PBS for 30 minutes on ice. DNA fluorescence was measured and flow cytometric analysis was performed using an EPICS XL (Beckman Coulter, CA, USA).

Real-Time RT-PCR Analysis of p27 Using LightCyclerTM

HumanPASMC were seeded in 6-cm dishes at a density of 6000 cells/cm^2 and cultured for 48 hours in serum-free DME. The cells were washed twice with PBS, then placed in DME supplemented with 10% FBS and antibiotics in normal or hypoxic oxygen concentrations for the indicated times with or without NO donors or BPS. The cells were then harvested by trypsinization, washed 3 times and pelletized by centrifugation. Total cellular RNA was obtained from the cells by a single extraction with an acid guanidinium thiocyanate-phenol-chloroform mixture [12]. RT was performed using 0.5μg of total RNA. cDNA synthesis was done with 200U of Moloney murine leukemia virus reverse transcriptase, 5μM of oligoDT, 1mM of dNTPs and 3mM of Mg^{2+} in a volume of 20 μl. The temperature profile consisted of annealing at room temperature for 5 minutes, extension at 44°C for 40 minutes and termination at 99°C for 5 minutes.

PCR was performed with the resulting RT products using specific oligonucleotide primers for p21, p27, p53, and β-actin, respectively. The sequence of the forward primer for p21 was 5-GGAAGACCATGTGGACCTGT-3 and that of the reverse primer was 5-GGCGTTTGGAGTGGTAGAAA-3, those of p27 was 5'-GCCCTCCCCAGTCTCTCTTA-3' (the forward primer) and the reverse primer 5'-TCAAAACTCCCAAGCACCTC-3' (the reverse primer), Those of p53 was 5-GTTCCGAGAGCTGAATGAGG-3 (the forward primer) and 5-TTATGGCGGGAGGTAGACTG-3 (the reverse primer) and those of β-actin was 5'-GCAAGCAGGAGTATGACGAG-3' (the forward primer) and 5'-CAAATAAAGCCATGCCAATC-3' (the reverse primer).

All PCR reactions were performed with a LightCyclerTM PCR system (Roche Diagnostics, Meylan, France) using DNA binding SYBR Green dye for the detection of PCR products. The cycling conditions were as follows: initial denaturation at 95°C for 15 minutes, followed by 50 cycles of denaturation at 94°C for 15 seconds, annealing at 55°C for 15 seconds, and extension at 72°C for 15 seconds. The β-actin gene was used as the reference. The PCR products were isolated from the LightCyclerTM glass capillaries and visualized by electrophoresis on 1.5% agarose gels with ethidium bromide staining to confirm the products. Each assay was performed in 6 independent experiments.

Western Blot Analysis

HumanPASMC were cultured in a 6-cm dish at a density of 6000 cells/cm^2 and cultured for 48 hours in serum-free DME. The cells were washed twice with PBS, and then placed in DME supplemented with 10% FBS and antibiotics. The cells were then cultured in normal or hypoxic oxygen concentrations for the indicated times with or without NO donors or BPS. After incubation, the cells were harvested and resuspended in protein lysis buffer (150mM of NaCl, 20mM of Tris-HCl, 1% NP40, 10mM of EDTA, 10% glycerol, 1mM of PMSF, 10μg/ml of aprotinin, 1μg/ml of leupeptin, 1μg/ml of gestating) and then incubated for 30 minutes on ice. After incubation, the cell lysis buffers were centrifuged at 10,000*g* for 15 minutes at 4°C to remove the cell fragments and the supernatants were analyzed for protein content using a DC protein assay kit. Each sample was quantified and then 25μg of protein was loaded onto each lane of a 4 - 12% Bis-Tris Nupage gel with MES SDS running buffer, according to the manufacturer's protocol. The gel was transferred to a PVDF membrane by electrophoresis at 100 V for 1 hour. The membrane was blocked in PBS, 0.2% Tween 20 (PBS-T), and 5% non-fat milk at room temperature for 1 hour. All antibodies were diluted in the same blocking buffer. The membrane was then probed either with rabbit anti-p21, anti-p27 or anti-p53 polyclonal antibody (1:1000 dilution) or mouse anti-s-actin monoclonal antibody (1:5000 dilution) and then incubated for 1 hour at room temperature. After incubation, the membrane was washed with PBS-T and incubated with horseradish peroxidase-conjugated goat anti-rabbit or mouse IgG (1 : 2000 dilution) for 2 hours at room temperature. After washing with PBS-T, an ECL system was used for detection of the proteins. Each assay was performed in 4 independent experiments.

Statistical Analysis

Results are expressed as the means ± SE. Statistical analysis was performed by ANOVA with Bonferroni for multiple comparisons. Comparisons were considered statistically significant at $p < 0.05$.

Results

1. NO donors suppress proliferation of humanPASMC via enhancing the expression of p21 and p53 at normoxia and at hypoxia

Both NO donors at 100μM significantly suppressed proliferation of humanPASMC at normoxia (figure 1a).

Both NO donors dose-dependently suppressed production of DNA of humanPASMC (figure 1b).

The cell cycle was significantly suppressed at the S and M phases and increased at the G0/1 phase by both NO donors at normoxia (figure 2a).

Hypoxia (2% oxygen) enhanced cell cycle at S+G2/M and G2M phase (figure 2b). NO donors significantly suppressed hypoxia-induced changes in cell cycle.

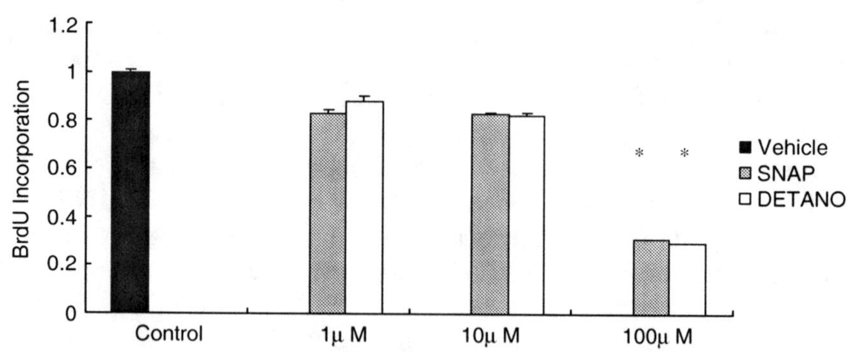

Figure 1a. HumanPASMC proliferation in the presence of NO donors at normoxia (21% oxygen). *$p < 0.05$, vs. control Data are expressed as mean ± SE (n=4).

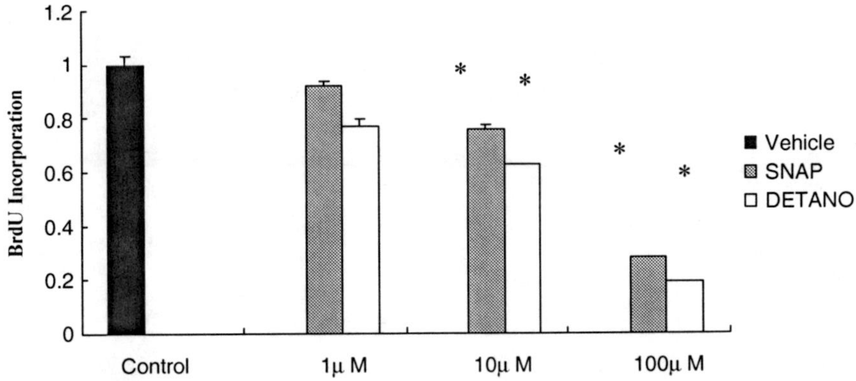

Figure 1b. HumanPASMC proliferation in the presence of NO donors at hypoxia (2% oxygen).
* $p < 0.05$, vs. control Data are expressed as mean ± SE (n=4).

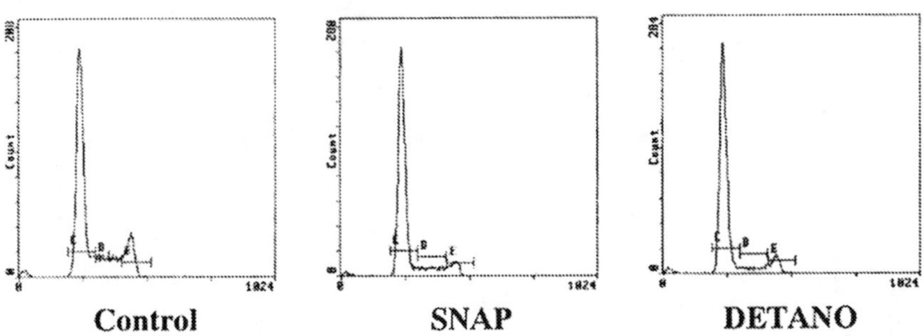

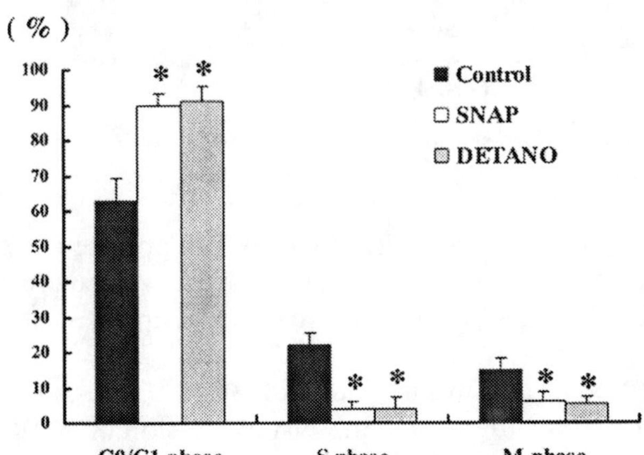

Figure 2a. Cell cycle in the presence of NO donors at normoxia.
* $p < 0.05$, vs. control Data are expressed as mean ± SE (n=6).

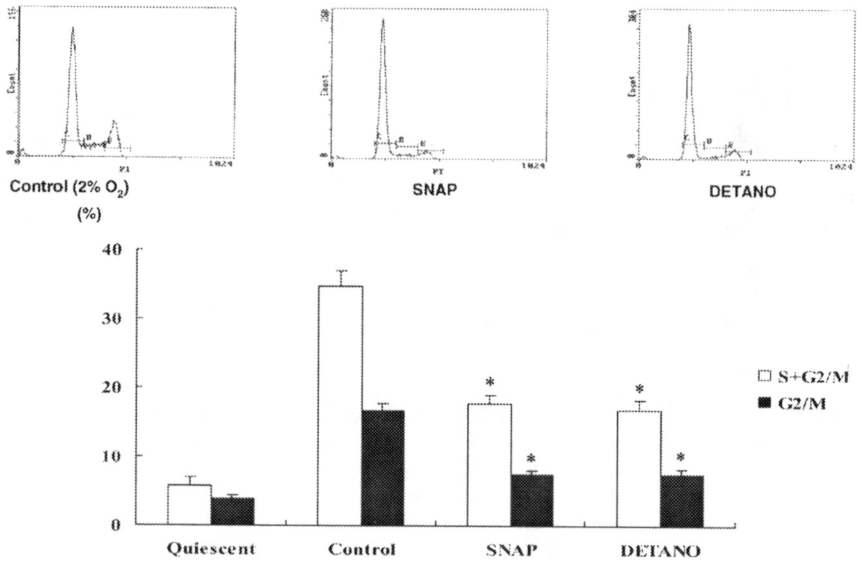

Figure 2b. Cell cycle in the presence of NO donors at hypoxia.
* $p < 0.05$ vs. control Data are expressed as mean ± SE (n=4).

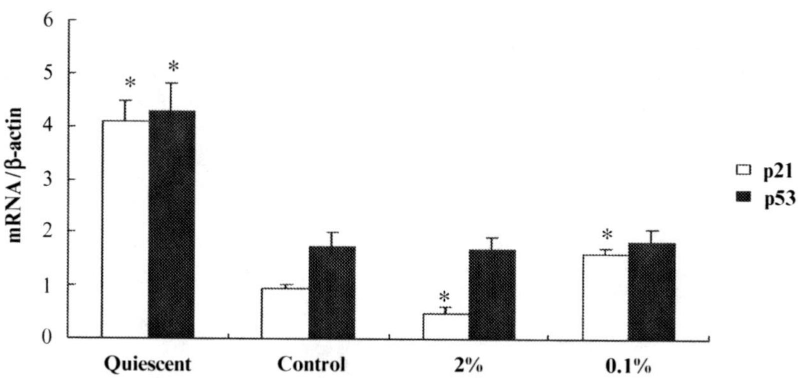

Figure 3. Hypoxia but not anoxia suppressed mRNA of p21.
* $p< 0.05$ vs. control Data are expressed as mean ± SE (n=4).

As shown in figure 3, hypoxia (2% oxygen) suppressed expression of mRNA of p21 without apparent effect on that of p53. Anoxia (0.1% oxygen) inversely enhanced that of p21 and cell cycle was suppressed at G0/1 phase (data not shown).

At normoxia, SNAP at concentrations of 30, 100 and 300μM and 100 and 300μM of DETANO augmented mRNA expression of p21 but not p53. Protein expression of p21 and p53, however, was dose-dependently strengthened by both NO donors.

When human PASMC was exposed to hypoxic air (2% oxygen)the presence of NO donors attenuated hypoxia-induced suppression of mRNA. Expression of p21(figure 5) and p53 was not affected by the NO donors. Protein expression of both p21 and p53 was elevated by SNAP at a dose of 30μM and by DATANO at a dose of 100μM, respectively (figure 6).

2. PGI2 attenuates hypoxia-induced proliferation of humanPASMC via partly preventing hypoxia-caused decrease of p27.

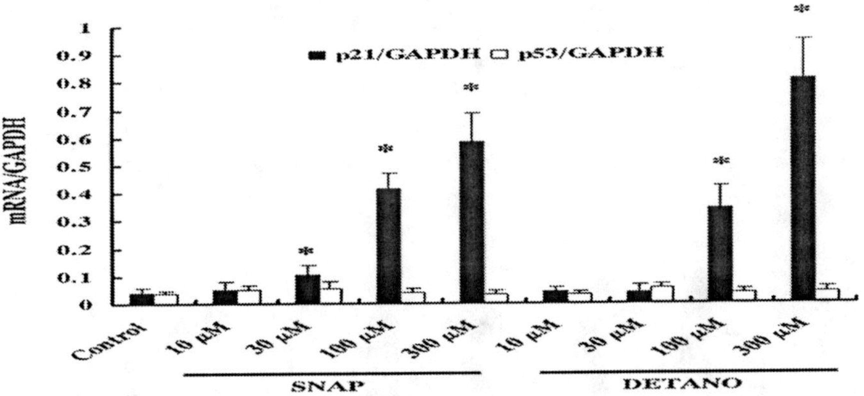

Figure 4. mRNA of p21 in the presence of NO donors at normoxia.
*p < 0.05 vs. control, Data are expressed as mean ± SE (n=4).

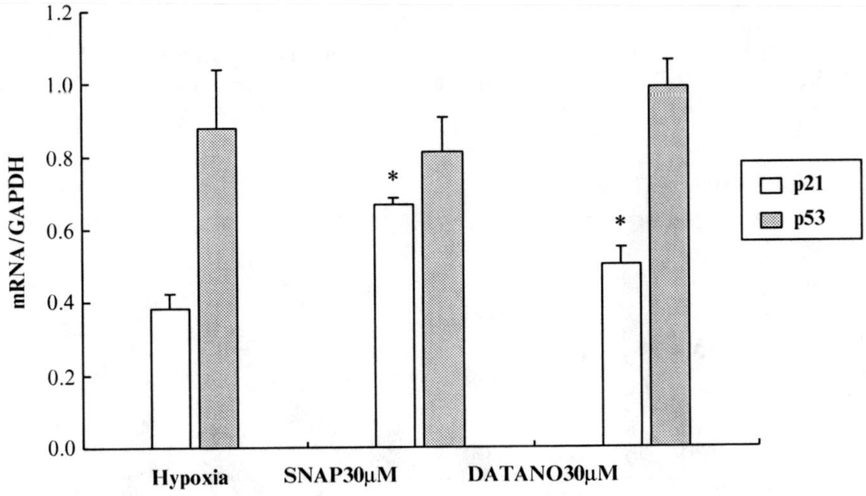

Figure 5. mRNA expression of p21 and p53 in the presence of NO donors during hypoxia.
*p< 0.05 vs. control Data are expressed as mean ± SE (n=4).

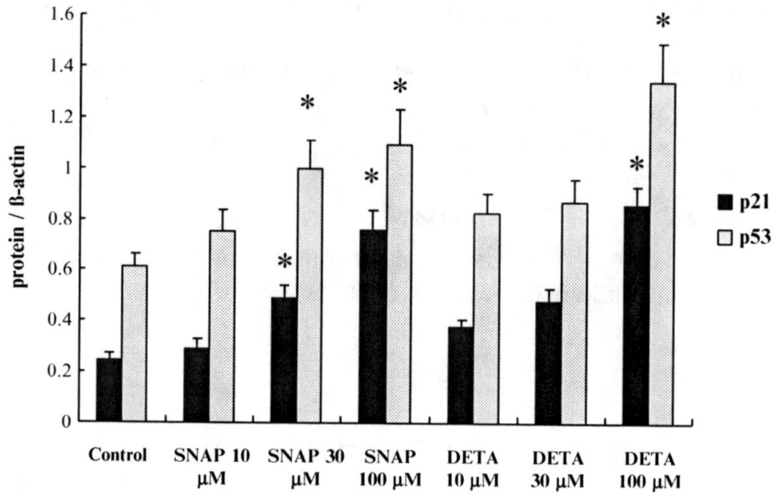

Figure 6. Protein expression of p21 and p53 in the presence of NO donors during hypoxia. *p< 0.05 vs. control DETA: DETANO Data are expressed as mean ± SE (n=4).

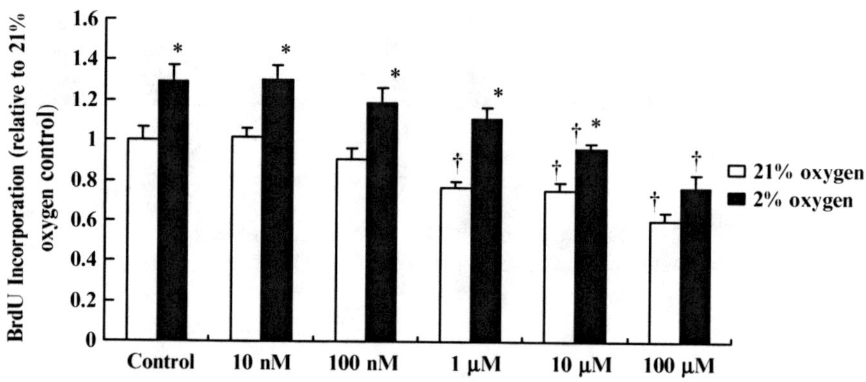

Figure 7. HumanPASMC proliferation in the presence of BPS at normoxia and hypoxia. *P < 0.05 vs. 21% oxygen. †P < 0.05 vs. without BPS Data are expressed as mean ± SE (n=4).

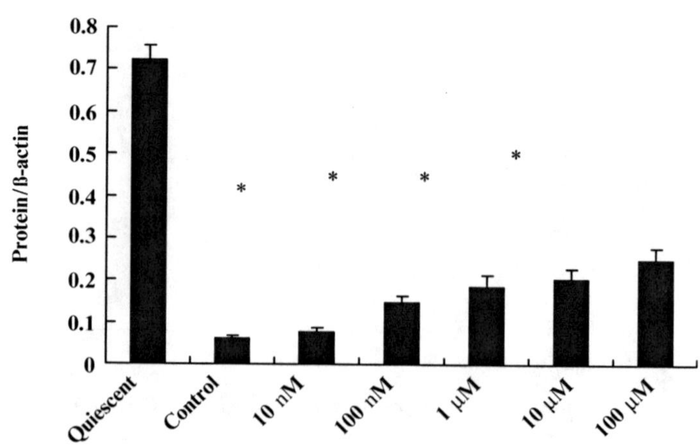

Figure 8. BPS augmented protein expression of p27.
*P < 0.05 vs. control Data are expressed as mean ± SE (n=4).

BPS at 10μM suppressed hypoxia-induced cell proliferation of humanPASMC and BPS at 1μM caused suppression of humanPASMC, even at normoxia (figure 7).

BPS dose-dependently regained protein expression of p27 in humanPASMC at hypoxia (2% oxygen) (figure 8).

Discussion

In the present study, we confirmed that exogenous NO suppresses the proliferation of humanPASMC through inhibition of the G1/S transition phases, and Exogenous NO significantly suppressed the cell cycle at G0/1 phase. We further observed that moderate hypoxia (2% oxygen) enhanced the proliferation of serum stimulated humanPASMC in accordance with the promoted degradation of p27 protein. When compared to moderate hypoxia, severe hypoxia decreased the proliferation of humanPASMC. This lower proliferation under severe hypoxia did not seem to be due to apoptosis, because the flow cytometric analyses showed only decreased S and M phases but not DNA fragmentation (data not shown) in the cells under severe hypoxia. Many other relevant papers which have noted that severe hypoxia induces a quiescent state in many cells [6,20,5], suggest that the cell cycle arrest in severe hypoxia is a common and general reaction in mammalian cells.

Our results also demonstrated that exogenous NO and BPS suppressed the humanPASMC proliferation both in the hypoxic and normoxic condition via blocking p21 and p27, and p27 protein reduction, respectively. The NO-induced preservation of p21 was compatible with the previous study using endothelial NOS gene transfer to coronary arterial SMC [18]. The finding that NO prevented hypoxia-induced suppression of p53 protein expression but not mRNA expression may indicate the post-transcription regulation of p53 protein expression [9]. CDK inhibitor p27, which blocks the cell cycle at the G0/1 phase, seemed to be regulated via multiple mechanisms, including transcription, protein degradation and translation [5,9,8]. A number of previous reports have shown that p27 levels are enhanced by hypoxia and are essential for cell cycle regulation [6,20,5]. Wang et al. reported that hypoxia-mediated loss of p27 expression correlated with enhanced entry into S phase without affecting of p27 mRNA levels [20]. These reports mean that p27 expression during hypoxia is a critical post-transcriptional regulation of hypoxia-induced proliferation. However, several reports indicate that p27 expression is also regulated at the transcriptional levels. Yu et al. reported that decreased p27 expression in the murine lung exposed to hypoxia is transcriptional regulation [23,24]. Taken together with our results, it might be that p27 expression in humanPASMC is regulated via a combination of transcriptional and post-transcriptional regulation.

Our result that humanPASMC incubated with BPS were blocked at the G0/1 phase even in the hypoxic exposure with p27 elevation, may suggest that the elevation of p27 might be the consequence of the BPS induced elevation of intracellular cAMP. Although we did not assess the cAMP in the current study, previous reports have noted that agents that increase intracellular cAMP induce the expression of p27 in an adenylate cyclase and PKA-dependent pathways and cell cycle arrest at the G0/1 phase [8, 12,19,21].

In summary, we have shown that the suppression of p53, p21 and p27 are required for hypoxia-induced pulmonary vascular cell proliferation and exogenous NO and PGI2 have an anti-proliferation effect on HPASMC via preventing the down-regulation of p53, p21 and p27, respectively. Thus, we expect targeting therapy for overexpression of CDK inhibitors could be protective against the development of hypoxia-induced pulmonary arterial vascular remodelling.

Acknowledgements

This work was supported by the Ministry of Education and Sciences of Japan (No. 16590743, No. 16406026 and No. 17790529).

References

1. Cooper AL, Beasley D (1999) Hypoxia stimulates proliferation and Interleukin-1alpha production in human vascular smooth muscle cells. Am J Physiol 277:H1326–37
2. Fasciano S, Patel RC, Handy I, Patel CV (2005) Regulation of vascular smooth muscle proliferation by heparin: inhibition of cyclin-dependent kinase 2 activity by p27 (kip1). J Biol Chem 280:15682–9
3. Fouty BW, Grimison B, Fagan KA, Le Cras TD, Harral JW, Hoedt-Miller M, Sclafani RA, Rodman DM (2001) p27(Kip1) is important in modulating pulmonary artery smooth muscle cell proliferation. Am J Respir Cell Mol Biol 25:652–8
4. Frid MG, Aldashev AA, Dempsey EC, Stenmark KR (1997) Smooth muscle cells isolated from discrete compartments of the mature vascular media exhibit unique phenotypes and distinct growth capabilities. Circ Res 81:940–52
5. Gardner LB, Li Q, Park MS, Flanagan WM, Semenza GL, Dang CV (2001) Hypoxia inhibits G1/S transition through regulation of p27 expression. J Biol Chem 276:7919–26
6. Graff P, Amellem O, Seim J, Stokke T, Pettersen EO (2005) The role of p27 in controlling the oxygen-dependent checkpoint of mammalian cells in late G1. Anticancer Res 25:2259–67
7. Hatakeyama M, Weinberg RA (1995) The role of RB in cell cycle control. Prog Cell Cycle Res 1:9–19
8. Ii M, Hoshiga M, Fukui R, Negoro N, Nakakoji T, Nishiguchi F, Kohbayashi E, Ishihara T, Hanafusa T (2001) Beraprost sodium regulates cell cycle in vascular smooth muscle cells through cAMP signalling by preventing down-regulation of p27(Kip1). Cardiovasc Res 52:500–8

9. Kabbutat MH, Jones SN, Vousden KH (1997) Regulation of p53 stability by Mdm2. Nature 387:296–299
10. Kadowaki M, Mizuno S, Uesaka D, Umeda Y, Demura Y, Ameshima S, Ishizaki T (2005) The effect of Beraprost sodium on cell proliferation of human pulmonary artery smooth muscle cell (HPASMC). Am J Respir Crit Care Med 171: A122
11. Kainoh M, Maruyama I, Nishio S, Nakadate T (1991) Enhancement by beraprost sodium, a stable analogue of prostacyclin, in thrombomodulin expression on membrane surface of cultured vascular endothelial cells via increase in cyclic AMP level. Biochem Pharmacol 41:1135– 40
12. Lee HT, Kay EP (2003) Regulatory role of cAMP on expression of Cdk4 and p27 (Kip1) by inhibiting phosphatidylinositol 3-kinase in corneal endothelial cells. Invest Ophthalmol Vis Sci. 44:3816–25
13. Lu SY, Wang DS, Zhu MZ, Zhang QH, Hu YZ, Pei JM (2005). Inhibition of hypoxia-induced proliferation and collagen synthesis by vasonatrin peptide in cultured rat pulmonary artery smooth muscle cells. Life Sci 77:28–38
14. Mizuno S, Kadowaki M, Demura Y, Ameshima S, Miyamori I, Ishizaki T (2004) P42/44 Mitogen-Activated Protein Kinase Regulated by p53 and Nitric Oxide in Human Pulmonary Arterial Smooth Muscle Cells. Am J Respir Cell Mol Biol 31:184–92
15. Mizuno S, Kadowaki M, Uesaka D, Demura Y, Ameshima S, Miyamori I, Ishizaki T (2004) Hypoxia and nitric oxide regulates the expression of p21 and VEGF in human pulmonary arterial smooth muscle cells. Am J Respir Crit Care Med 169:A166
16. Mizuno S, Uesaka D, Kadowaki M, Demura Y, Ameshima S, Miyamori I, Ishizaki T (2005) Cyclin dependent kinase inhibitor p21 and p27 regulate pulmonary arterial smooth muscle cells proliferation during hypoxia. Am J Respir Crit Care Med 171:A723
17. Nishio S, Kurumatani H (2001) Pharmacological and clinical properties of beraprost sodium, orally active prostacyclin analogue. Nippon Yakurigaku Zasshi. 117:123–30
18. Sato J, Nair K, Hiddinga J, Eberhardt NL, Fitzpatrick LA, Katusic ZS, O'Brien T (2000) eNOS gene transfer to vascular smooth muscle cells inhibits cell proliferation via upregulation of p27 and p21 and not apoptosis. Cardiovasc Res 47:697–706
19. Van Oirschot BA, Stahl M, Lens SM, Medema RH (2001). Protein kinase A regulates expression of p27 (kip1) and cyclin D3 to suppress proliferation of leukemic T cell lines. J Biol Chem 276:33854–60
20. Wang G, Reisdorph R, Clark RE Jr, Miskimins R, Lindahl R, Miskimins WK (2003) Cyclin dependent kinase inhibitor p27 (Kip1) is upregulated by hypoxia via an ARNT dependent pathway. J Cell Biochem 90:548–60
21. Xaus J, Valledor AF, Cardo M, Marques L, Beleta J, Palacios JM, Celada A (1999) Adenosine inhibits macrophage colony-stimulating factor-dependent proliferation of macrophages through the induction of p27kip-1 expression. J Immunol 163:4140–9
22. Yu AY, Shimoda LA, Iyer NV, Huso DL, Sun X, McWilliams R, Beaty T, Sham JS, Wiener CM, Sylvester JT, Semenza GL (1999) Impaired physiological responses to chronic hypoxia in mice partially deficient for hypoxia-inducible factor 1alpha. J Clin Invest 103:691–6
23. Yu L, Quinn DA, Garg HG, Hales (2005) Cyclin-dependent kinase inhibitor p27Kip1, but not p21WAF1/Cip1, is required for inhibition of hypoxia-induced pulmonary hypertension and remodelling by heparin in mice. Circ Res 97:937–45
24. Yu L, Quinn DA, Garg HG, Hales CA (2006) Gene expression of cyclin-dependent kinase inhibitors and effect of heparin on their expression in mice with hypoxia-induced pulmonary hypertension. Biochem Biophys Res Commun 345:1565–72

CHAPTER 7

PULMONARY ADAPTATION TO HIGH ALTITUDE IN WILD MAMMALS

AKIO SAKAI, ISHIZAKI TAKESHI[1], KOIZUMI TOMONOBU[2] AND MATSUMOTO TAKAYUKI[3]

Department of Sports Medicine, Shinshu University School of Medicine, Matsumoto, Japan
[1] Department of Fundamental Nursing, Fukui University, and Division of Pulmonary Medicine, University of Fukui Hospital, Fukui, Japan
[2] Department of Internal Medicine, Shinshu University School of Medicine, Matsumoto, Japan
[3] Laboratory for Exercise Physiology and Biomechanics, School of Health and Sports Sciences, Chukyo University, Toyota, Japan

Abstract: The increased pulmonary artery pressure or right ventricular hypertrophy at high altitude has been reported to vary widely among species and individuals of the same species even when they are exposed to the same altitude. Reeves et al. reported species differences in the increase in the pulmonary artery pressure resulting from chronic exposure to high altitude; although pulmonary hypertension induced by exposure to high altitudes was remarkable in the cow and horse, it was minimal in the llama, dog, sheep and rabbit. It was also shown that there are two types of cow, i.e., the susceptive type, which shows marked increases in pulmonary artery pressure when exposed to high altitude and the resistant type, which is less responsive to changes in altitude. Genetic factors have been suggested to play an important role in terms of sensitivity to exposure to high altitude. Similar differences in the responsiveness to hypoxia have also been noticed in humans; some individuals develop marked pulmonary hypertension but others do not.

When these observations are taken together, a small degree of pulmonary hypertension or right ventricular hypertrophy at high altitude indicates better adaptability to it. Pika, which is an animal completely adapted to high altitude and has relatively low hematocrite level, no pulmonary hypertension or no right ventricular hypertrophy, is a good example. Moreover, hypoxic pulmonary vasoconstriction is significantly smaller in the pika than in the rat. In conclusion, this paper reports data showing that the pika, blue-sheep and Yachi-nezumi have developed almost the same physiological adaptation

A. Aldashev and R. Naeije (eds.), Problems of High Altitude Medicine and Biology, 101–117.

mechanism, i.e., attenuated HPV and deficient hematocrite increase for a high-altitude environment as a result of the long history of habitation at high altitude, through a natural selection of better-adapted individuals. Genetic factors have been suggested to play important roles in this adaptability.

Keywords: altitude; pulmonary hypertension; hypoxic pulmonary vasoconstriction; hymatocrite

Introduction

High altitude is associated with low temperature as well as low pressure, and this has a marked effect on animal distribution. Most mammals could not live permanently at extreme altitude exceeding 5800m above sea level [4]. There are species indigenous to high altitude, such as Llama (Lama glama), Alapaca (Lama pacos), Vicuna (Lama vicugna) and Guanaco (Lama guanicoe) in the Andes. However, many species of mammal have been seen at great heights and Yak (Bos grunnins), Pika (Ochotona roylei) and Blue sheep (Pseudois nayaur) are living on the slope at 6100m in the Tibetan Himalayas [4]. Such species are well adapted biologically, physiologically and biochemically to high altitude.

When animals are exposed to a high altitude environment during a long period, the pulmonary artery pressure increases because of an increase in the hematocrit (Ht), an increase in the red blood cell count and hypoxic pulmonary vasoconstriction (HPV), resulting in pulmonary hypertension and right ventricular hypertrophy. These responses are typical responses to acclimatization to high altitude and show marked individual and species differences [9].

In the Tibetan highlands, Blue sheep, Pika, and Yak live at an altitude of 6100m and are typical of mammals adapted to high altitudes. These animals have a long history of habitation at high altitude and are considered to be "animals completely adapted to high altitude" because of their physiological and morphological traits, which are well adapted to high-altitude environments. And in Japan, small wild mammals, for example, Apodemus argenteus (the Japanese name is Hime-nezumi) and Cleterionomis andersoni (the Japanese name is Yachi-nezumi) are living in fields from the foot of the mountain to the top. Especially the Yachi-nezumi lives only at high altitude in the Japanese mountains. Thus, Yachi-nezumi is also a mammal completely adapted to high altitude like the Pika.

The purpose of this study is to make clear the physiological characteristics of pika, blue sheep and Yach-nezumi as high-altitude adapted wild mammals.

Methods

Subjects: blue sheep, pika, pig, rat, Yachi-nezumi and Hime-nezume were used in this study. The pika, Yachi-nezumi and Hime-nezumi were living in the fields as wild mammals and the blue sheep, pigs and rats were domestic mammals. The wild mammals captured by the traps at their living altitude and domestic animals were also obtained at their living altitude.

Measurements: all measurements were as follows; body weight (BW), pulmonary artery pressure (Ppa), systemic artery pressure (Psa) and the ratio of Ppa to Psa (Ppa/Psa) was calculated as an index of right ventricular workload. According to the Fulton's method [1], the ventricle was separated into the left ventricle including septum (LVW) and the right ventricle (RVW) and the weight of each was measured. The ratio of RVW to LVW (RVW/LVW) was then calculated as an index of right ventricular hypertrophy. Hematocrit (Ht) was subsequently measured by the capillary method (10,000rpm, 5min).

Experiments were started after a full recovery from the anesthetic state and all physiological measurements were made with the animals awake and standing. All measurements were carried out at each living altitude of the experimental animals because some parameters, especially Ppa or Ht, are easily affected by changes in altitude.

In this study, the following three experiments were designed; Experiment 1 is to assess cardiopulmonary differences among animals living at different altitudes and Experiment 2 is to study cardiopulmonary responses to exposure to simulated altitudes and Experiment 3 is to estimate the effect of environmental temperature to RVW/LVW and Ht at the same altitude.

Statistical analysis
Results are expressed as the mean ± SE. Statistical analysis was performed by ANOVA with Bonferroni for multiple comparisons. Comparisons were considered statistically significant at $p<0.05$.

Results

Experiment 1: Differences among living altitudes

Blue sheep, pika, pig and rat experiments were carried out in the Tibetan highlands in China and Hime-nezumi and Yachi-nezumi experiments were carried out in Japan.

Figure 1 showed the result of Ppa at the indicated altitude. As shown here, Ppa increased with elevation of living altitude in all species. The slope of the regression line of pika and blue sheep was less steep than that of rat or pig. This difference in slope angle is very clear, indicating that pika and blue

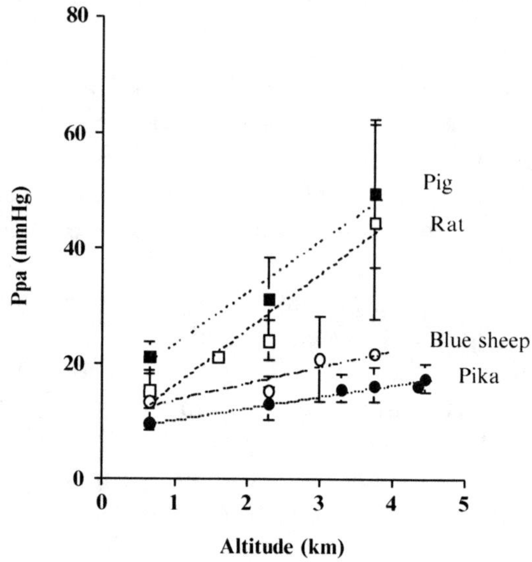

Figure 1. Pulmonary artery pressure (Ppa) in 4 species at different altitudes. X-axis shows the living altitude of each animal and the Y-axis shows the mean values for pulmonary artery pressure. The open circle means blue sheep, closed circle is pika, closed square is pig, and open square is rat, respectively. Values are mean ±SE.

sheep show significantly lower values of Ppa at high altitude compared with rat or pig. Psa did not change, despite elevation of the living altitude in all species (Figure 2). The ratio of Ppa to Psa, which means the right ventricular workload to the left or right ventricle, rose with the elevation of living altitude in all species (Figure 3). The angle of the regression line was gentle in pika and blue sheep compared with rat or pig, suggesting that pika and blue sheep show significantly lower values for Ppa/Psa at high altitude compared with rat or pig. Figure 4 shows the result of the ratio of RVW to LVW. RVW/LVW increased in accordance with living altitude in all species. However, the angles of the regression lines were gentle in pika and blue sheep compared with rat or pig. It was clear that pika and blue sheep show significantly lower values for RVW/LVW at high altitude compared with rat or pig. Figure 5 shows the result of RVW/LVW in Japanese wild mice. As shown here, both species increased with elevation of the living altitude. However, this regression line for Yachi-nezumi was shifted to the lower part and the slope of the regression line was gentler than that of Hime-nezumi. These results suggest that Yachi-nezumi has strong adaptability to high altitude, like Pika or blue sheep (see Figure 4). Figure 6 shows the result of Ht. Again, Ht rose with the elevation of living altitude in all species. However the steepness of the slopes of the regression lines were milder in pika and blue sheep than in rat or pig.

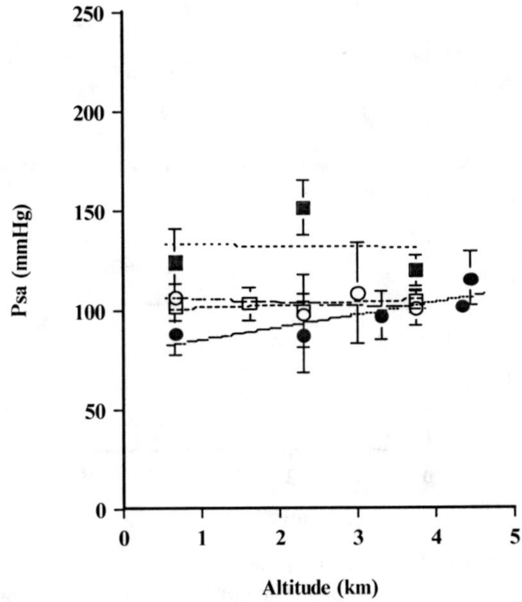

Figure 2. Systemic artery pressure (Psa) in 4 species at different altitudes. Values are mean ±SE.

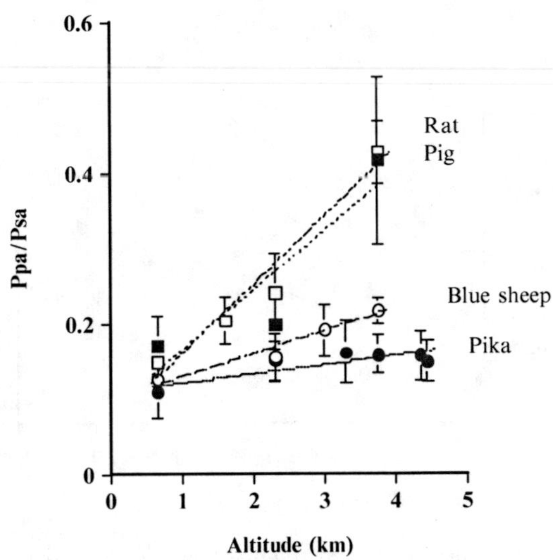

Figure 3. The ratio of systemic artery pressure to pulmonary artery pressure (Psa/Ppa) in 4 species at different altitudes. Values are mean ±SE. This ratio shows an index of right ventricular workload.

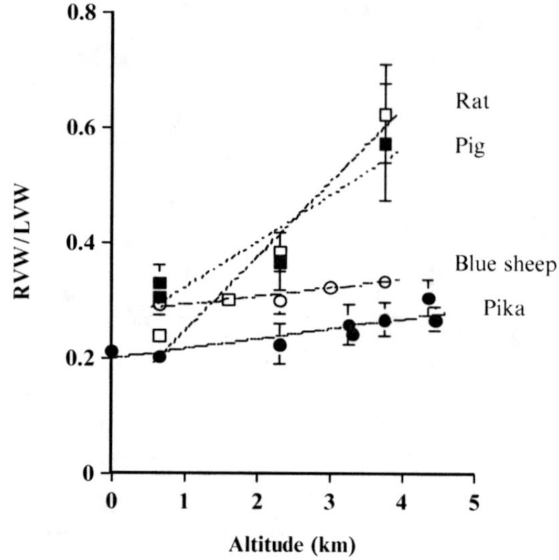

Figure 4. The ratio of the right ventricular weight to left ventricular weight (RVW/LVW) in 4 species at different altitudes. Values are mean ±SE. This ratio shows an index of right ventricular hypertrophy.

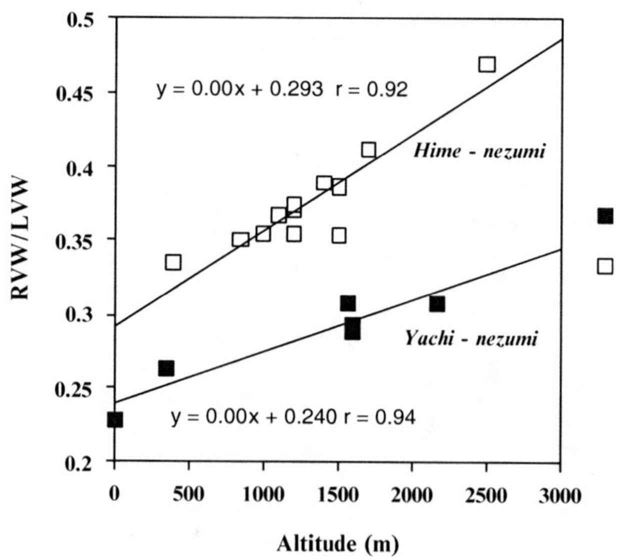

Figure 5. The ratio of the right ventricular weight to left ventricular weight (RVW/LVW) in Japanese wild mice at different altitudes. Values are mean ±SE. The open squares show Hime-nezumi and the closed squares show Yach-nezumi, respectively. This ratio shows an index of right ventricular hypertrophy.

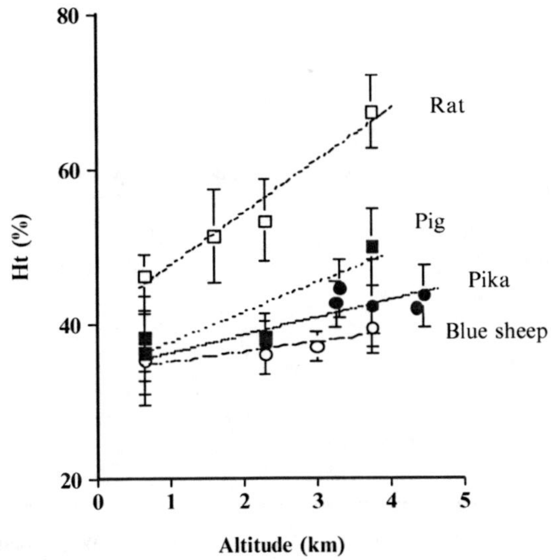

Figure 6. Hematocrit (Ht) in 4 species at different altitudes. Values are mean ±SE.

Experiment 2: Exposure to simulated altitude

Using the climatic chamber, this experiment was carried out at the Qinghai High-Altitude Medical Science Institute (2300m above sea level), Xining, China.

The animals were placed in a climatic chamber in which the atmospheric pressure could be simulated for altitudes of 0, 2300 and 4500m above sea level. Figure 7 shows changes in PPpa associated with elevations of the altitude relative to the values at 0m. As this figure clearly indicates, PPpa increased with elevations of altitude in both blue sheep and pig but the increase (slope) was milder in blue-sheep. Consequently, significant differences ($p < 0.05$) were observed in Ppa between the two species. But Psa did not change in either species, despite elevation of the altitude. Figure 8 shows the change in ΔPsa associated with an elevation of the altitude relative to the value at 0m. There was no change due to the altitude nor any differences between the species. When the altitude elevated Ppa/Psa also increased in both species, but the values of the blue sheep were lower than those of the pig at all altitudes. Moreover the angle of its increase was less steep in blue sheep (Figure 9).

Experiment 3: Effects of environmental temperature to RVW/LVW and Ht

In Japan, we studied the influence of environmental temperature on RVW/LVW and Ht using the Hime-nezumi. The Hime-nezumi is a wild wood mouse that weighs about 20g. They live on the ground surface and their physiology is greatly influenced by environmental temperature. This

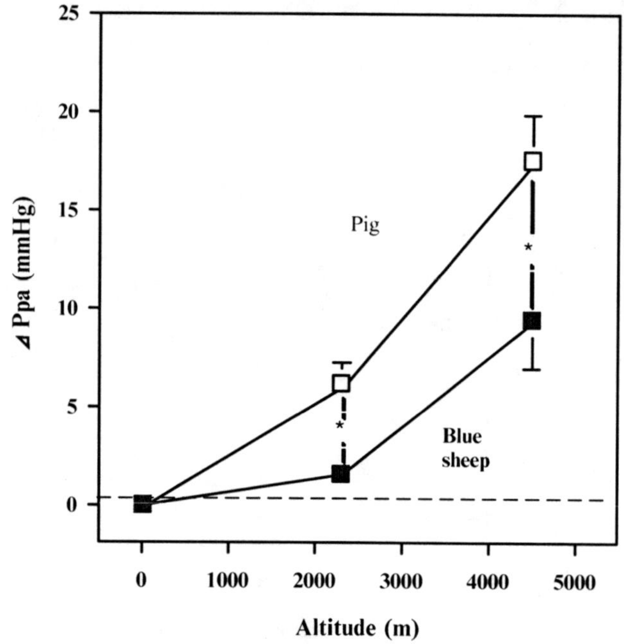

Figure 7. Changes in ΔPpa associated with elevation of altitude in blue sheep and pigs. Values are mean ±SE. ΔPpa: difference of the values at 0m. * $p < 0.05$ between the two species.

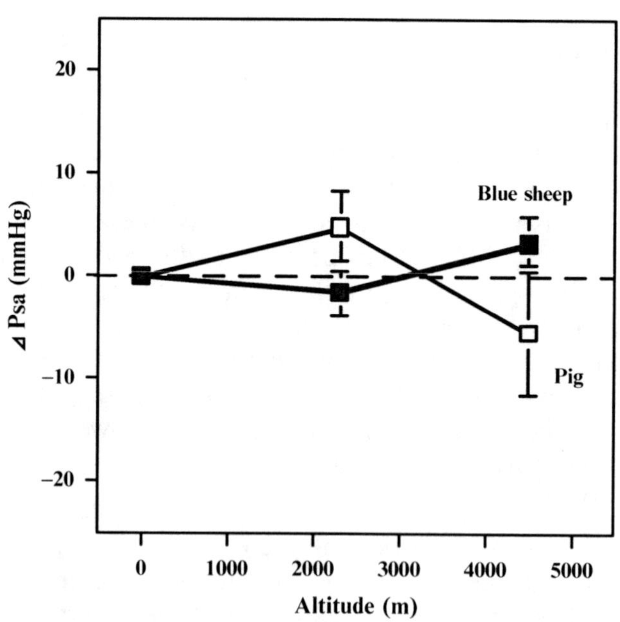

Figure 8. Changes in ΔPsa associated with an elevation of altitude in blue sheep and pigs. Values are mean ±SE. ΔPsa: difference of the values at 0m.

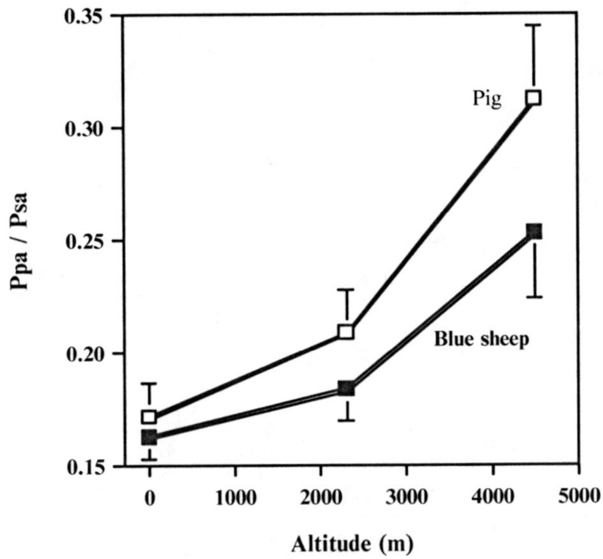

Figure 9. Changes in Ppa/Psa associated with elevation of altitude in blue sheep and pigs. Values are mean ±SE.

experiment was designed to focus on the following 3 effects, i.e., a) seasonal effects, b) latitudinal effects and c) global warming effects.

a) Seasonal effects

We captured Hime-nezumi seasonally at the same place and studied the seasonal changes of ventricular weight. Figure 10 shows the seasonal changes of ventricular weight and RVW/LVW. As shown here, all of the mean values of TVW, LVW, RVW and RVW/LVW become smaller as the season proceeds from winter to summer and then greater again towards winter. When we examined the correlation between environmental temperature and RVW/LVW, a strong negative correlation was observed between environmental temperature and RVW/LVW.

b) Latitudinal effects

This study was carried out in August at the two stations Shirakabako and Hakkouda in central Honshu island in Japan. Shirakabako is located in the southern, warm region (latitude;36° 49') and Hakkouda is located in the northern, cold region (latitude;16° 57') and the average temperature in August was 17.7°C and 16.5°C, respectively. The Hime-nezumi inhabiting warm regions (Shirakabako) had significantly lower RVW/LVW and Ht than those inhabiting cold regions (Hakkouda) (Figure 11). Also, a significant

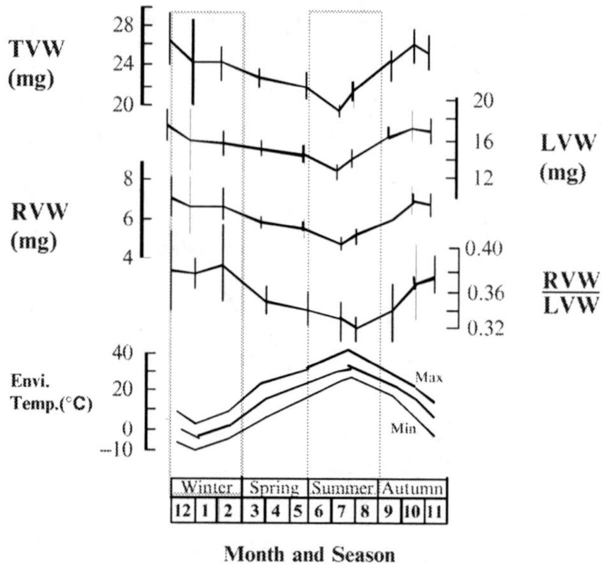

Figure 10. Seasonl changes of ventricular weights in wild mice, Hime-nezumi. TVW; total ventricular weight, LVW; left ventricular weight, RVW; right ventricular weight and RVW/LVW; the ratio of RVW to LVW, respectively.

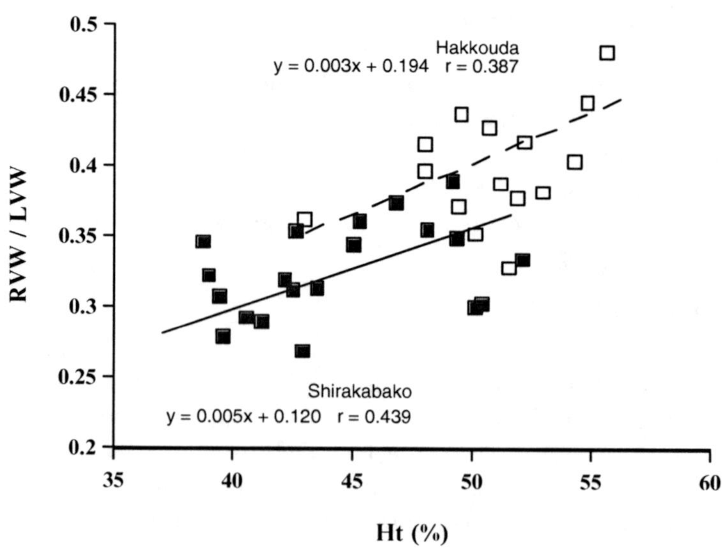

Figure 11. Relationship between hematocrit (Ht) and RVW/LVW in Shirakabako and Hakkouda.

positive correlation was observed between the level of Ht and RVW/LVW. These results suggest that hematocrit plays a role in the reduction of heart size, particularly in the right ventricle, and in the decline in RVW/LVW.

c) Global warming effects

The RVW/LVW changed comparably with the environmental temperature and this change is in accordance with the hematocrit (Ht) fluctuation. On this basis, we examined whether the decline in RVW/LVW caused by global warming is attributable to the decreases in the hematocrit. We compared the data obtained in 1971 and in 2004 at the two study sites, Shirakabako and Hakkouda. The average temperature in August was elevated 1.4°C in Shirakabako and 1.0°C in Hakkouda, respectively, probably due to global warming over the past 30 years.

We compared the ratio of RVW/LVW at the two study sites in 1971 and 2004 (Figure 12). The RVW/LVW reduced from 0.33 in 1971 to 0.29 in 2004 in Shirakabako and 0.41 in 1971 to 0.37 in Hakkouda in 2004, respectively. In both areas, the RVW/LVW in 2004 was significantly lower than that in 1971 ($p < 0.05$). Furthermore, we compared the Ht at the two study sites in 1971 and 2004 (Figure 13). Ht reduced from 44.7% in 1971 to 39.5% in 2004 in Shirakabako and 49.8% in 1971 to 46.8% in 2004 in Hakkouda, respectively. In both areas, Ht in 2004 was significantly lower than that in 1971 ($p < 0.05$). Figure 14 indicates the relation between environmental temperature and RVW/LVW. As shown here, a strong negative correlation ($r = -0.93$, $p < 0.05$) was observed. A strong negative correlation ($r = -0.99$, $p < 0.05$) between environmental temperature and Ht was observed (Figure 15). Figure 16 showed the relationship between Ht and RVW/LVW for all the

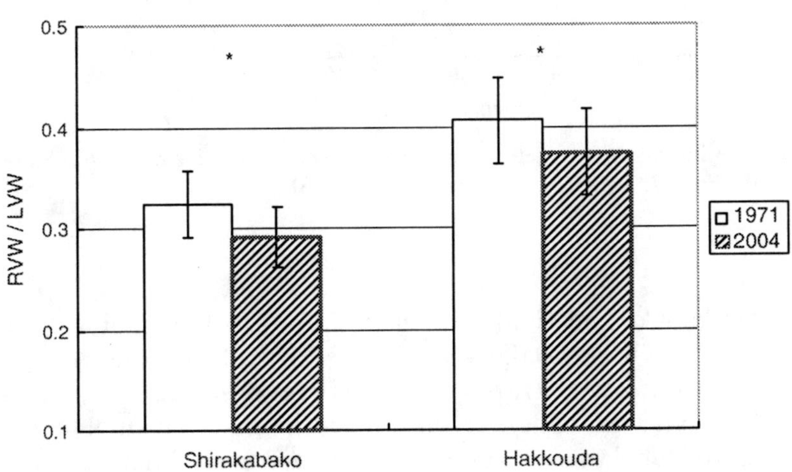

Figure 12. Comparison of RVW/LVW in Shirakabako and Hakkouda between 1971 and 2004.

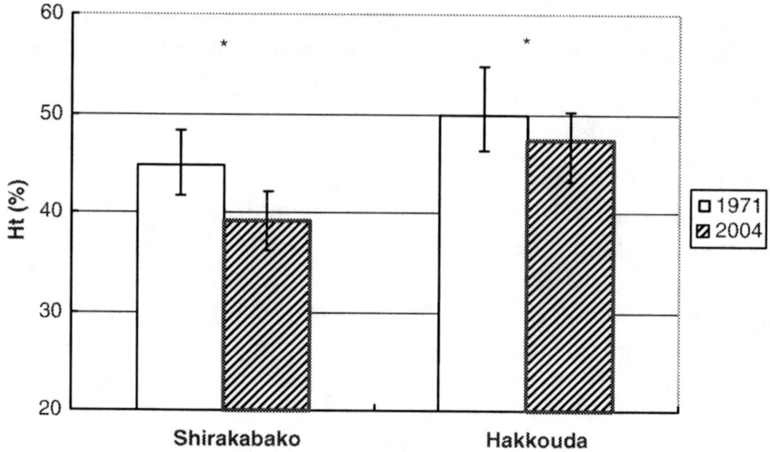

Figure 13. Comparison of hematocrit (Ht) in Shirakabako and Hakkouda between 1971 and 2004.

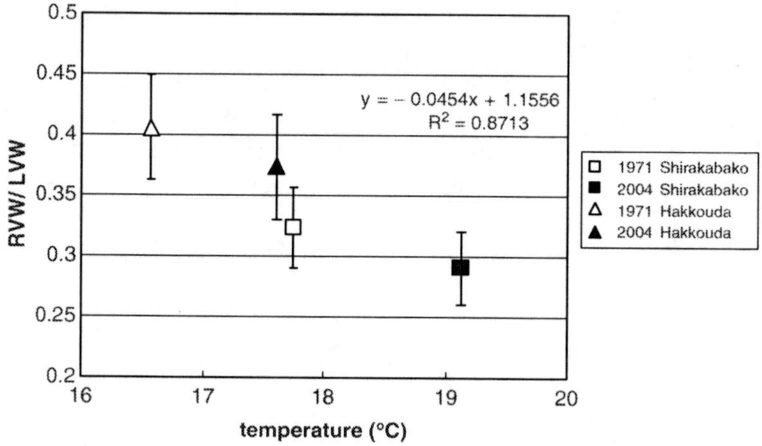

Figure 14. Relationship between environmental temperature and RVW/LVW in Shirakabako and Hakkouda in 1971 and 2004, indicated as mean ± SE.

mice at Shirakabako and Hakkouda in 1971 and 2004. A significant positive correlation ($r = 0.74$, $p < 0.05$) was observed for all the data. A significant positive correlation ($r = 0.97$, $p < 0.05$) was also observed for the data indicated in the mean ± SD. These results reflect the environmental temperature changes due to global warming and also the temperature differences according to the latitude.

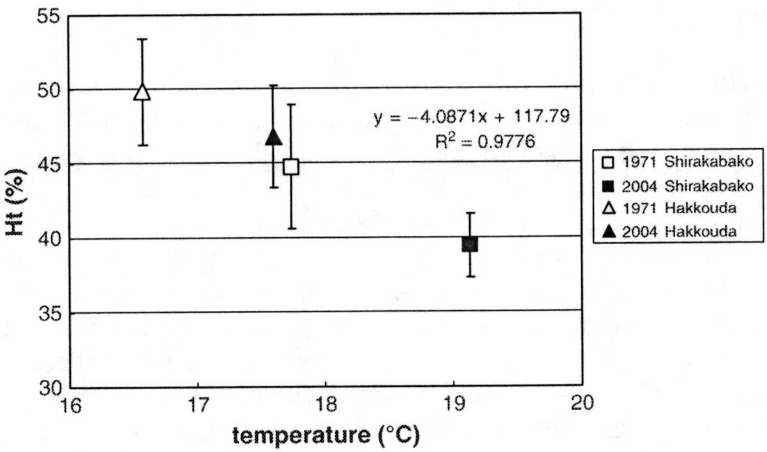

Figure 15. Relationship between environmental temperature and hematocrit in Shirakabako and Hakkouda in 1971 and 2004, indicated as mean ±SE.

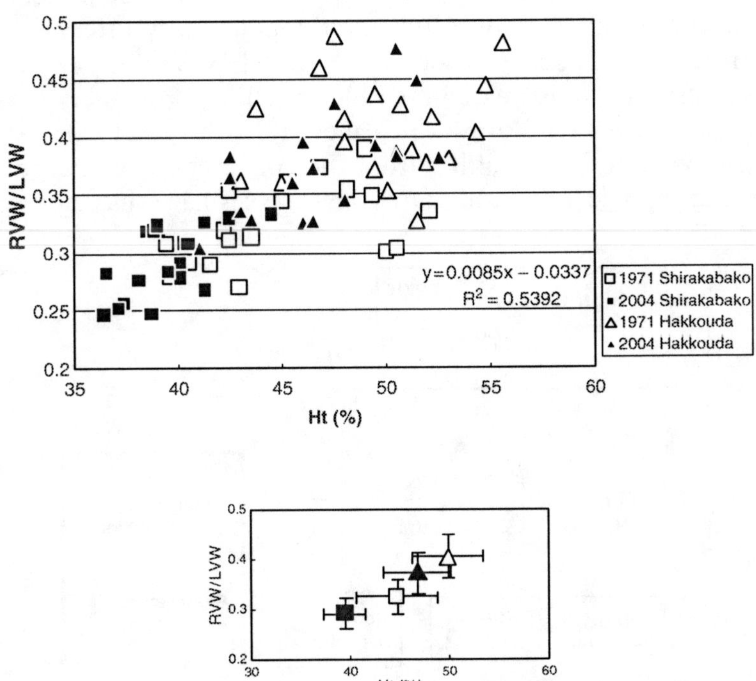

Figure 16. Relationship between RVW/LVW and hematocrit in wild mice captured in Shirakabako and Hakkouda in 1971 and 2004. The upper right box shows the relationship, indicated as mean ±SE.

Discussion

The principal findings of this study are: (a) the pulmonary artery pressure (Ppa), the ratio of right to left ventricular weight (RVW/LVW) and hematocrit (Ht) increased in accordance with the height of living altitude in all mammals, whereas in mammals well-adapted to high altitude, such as pika, blue-sheep and Yachi-nezumi, showed significantly lower values compared to other mammals; (b) when the mammals were exposed to simulated high altitude, hypoxic pulmonary vasoconstriction (HPV) in blue-sheep was significantly attenuated compared to pig; and (c) at the same altitude, a warm environment (by seasonal, latitudinal, and global warming effects) caused the decreasing RVW/LVW and Ht. These findings suggest that mammals well-adapted to high altitude such as pika, blue sheep and Yachi-nezumi have a potent adaptability to high altitude environments, having a small degree of right ventricular hypertrophy, low grade pulmonary hypertension and a small degree of Ht level at high altitude.

Generally, when animals are exposed to high altitudes, pulmonary hypertension and right ventricular hypertrophy are induced. As shown in Figure 17, the following two factors are considered to be possible causes of these phenomena: (1) constriction of the pulmonary artery because of hypoxia (hypoxic pulmonary vasoconstriction, HPV) and (2) an increase in the Ht as a result of an increase in red blood cells.

HPV, confirmed in 1946 by Von Euler [17], who used cats, is marked pulmonary hypertension resulting from the constriction of the pulmonary artery during hypoxic-air ventilation. Many reports have since appeared and

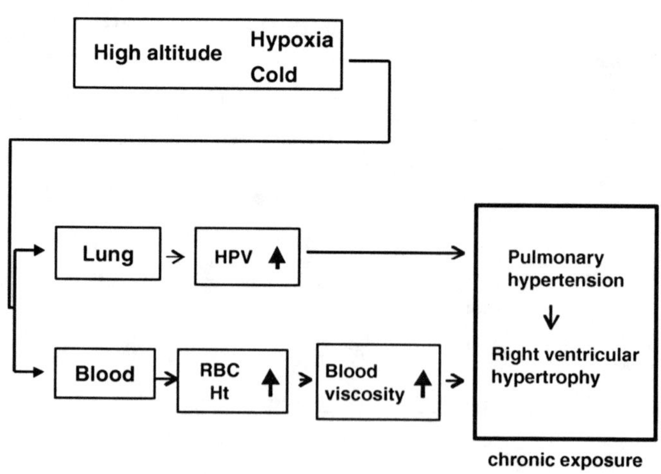

Figure 17. Diagram of pulmonary hypertension and right ventricular hypertrophy at high altitude.

HPV was shown to be observed regardless of the animal species, induced also by migration of animals to high altitude regions as well as by exposure to low atmospheric pressure. Thus, the investigation of the pathophysiological mechanism(s) of HPV has progressed, however, its precise mechanism still remains unknown.

On the other hand, the increase in Ht because of an increase in red blood cells mentioned in (2) increases the blood viscosity and this increased viscosity is considered to substantially affect the pulmonary circulation, resulting in pulmonary hypertension. Sakai (1976) examined seasonal changes in the ventricle weight and RVW/LVW of Hime-nezumi, A. argenteus [11]. Total, left, right ventricle weight and RVW/LVW decrease in summer and increase in winter, according to the seasonal temperature changes (Figure 10). A significant negative correlation is observed between these factors and the environmental temperature. It is of interest that these seasonal changes in heart characteristics are related to blood characteristics. Sealander (1962) examined seasonal changes in blood characteristics in small wild mammals and revealed that the number of red blood cells, hemoglobin concentrations and hematocrit show high values in winter and low values in summer. Swigat (1965) dosed rats and mice with cobalt chloride and artificially induced polycythemia [16]. This experiment caused enlargements of the right ventricle. In a previous study, Sakai (1974) captured Hime-nezummi (A. argenteus) in southern warm regions and northern cold regions at the same time and examined the relationship between the heart size and hematocrit [10]. The study revealed that mice inhabiting warmer regions show significantly lower ventricle weight, RVW/LVW and hematocrit than those inhabiting cold regions. Also, a significant positive relationship was observed between the level of hematocrit and RVW/LVW (Figure 11). These reports suggest that hematocrit affects heart size, particularly in the right ventricle and the decline in RVW/LVW.

Decline in pulmonary artery pressure is predicted where reduction in right ventricle size and decline in RVW/LVW occur. Sakai (1984) examined the hemo-dynamics of lung circulation when hematocrit is gradually elevated by transfusion of red blood cells to sheep. Both systemic and pulmonary artery pressure rise with the increase in hematocrit, but the rise in the pulmonary artery was more remarkable. A higher hematocrit level resulted in higher pulmonary artery pressure and caused larger load on the right ventricle [12]. Therefore, in the present study, decline in the hematocrit and pulmonary artery pressure caused by the global warming is suggested to have resulted in the reduction in heart size, right ventricle weight and RVW/LVW level, which in turn caused reduction in the right ventricle size.

As observed above, the interaction between HPV and increase in blood viscosity because of an increase in the Ht appears to be certainly involved in pulmonary hypertension and right ventricular hypertrophy observed at high altitude (Figure 17).

Therefore, we believe that analysis of these two factors is a prerequisite for the elucidation of high-altitude pulmonary hypertension and right ventricular hypertrophy.

The increased pulmonary artery pressure or right ventricular hypertrophy at high altitude has been reported to vary widely among species and individuals of the same species, even when they are exposed to the same altitude [2,3,5,6,7,9]. Reeves et al.[9] reported species differences in the increase in pulmonary artery pressure resulting from chronic exposure to high altitudes; although pulmonary hypertension induced by exposure to high altitudes was remarkable in the cow and horse, it was minimal in the llama, dog, sheep and rabbit. It was also shown that there are two types of cow, i.e., the susceptive type, which shows a marked increase in pulmonary artery pressure when exposed to high altitude and the resistant type, which is less responsive to changes in altitude [9]. Genetic factors have been suggested to play an important role in terms of sensitivity to exposure to high altitude. Similar differences in the responsiveness to hypoxia are also noticed in humans; some individuals develop marked pulmonary hypertension but others do not [3,8].

When these observations are taken into together, a small degree of pulmonary hypertension or right ventricular hypertrophy at high altitude indicates better adaptability to it. Pika, which is an animal completely adapted to high altitude and has relatively low Ht level, no pulmonary hypertension or no right ventricular hypertrophy, is a good example [13,14]. Moreover, HPV is significantly lower in the pika than in the rat [2].

In conclusion, the pika, blue-sheep and Yachi-nezumi have developed almost the same physiological adaptation mechanism, i.e., attenuated HPV and deficient Ht increase for a high-altitude environment, as a result of their long history of habitation at high altitude, through a natural selection of better-adapted individuals. Genetic factors have been suggested to play important roles in this adaptability.

References

1. Fulton RM, Hutchinson EC, Jones AM. (1952) Ventricular weight in cardiac hypertrophy. Brit Heart J 14:413–420.
2. Ge RL, Kubo K, Kobayashi T, Sekiguchi M, Honda T. (1998) Blunted hypoxic pulmonary vasoconstrictive response in the rodent Ocotona cuzoniae (pika) at high altitude. Am J Physiol 274:H1729–1799.
3. Grover RF. (1965) Pulmonary circulation in animals and man at high altitude. Ann N Y Acad Sci 127:632–639.

4. Heath D, and Williams D. (1981) In : Man at High Altitude, p14–23, Churchill Livingston., Edinburgh, London, Melbourun and New York.
5. Hultgren HN, and Miller H. (1965) Right ventricular hypertrophy high altitude. Ann N Y Acad Sci 127:627–631.
6. Hultgren HN, Kelly J, Miller H. (1965) Pulmonary circulation in acclimatized man at high altitude. J Appl Physiol 20:239–243.
7. Naeye RL. (1965) Children at high altitude: pulmonary and renal abnormalities. Circ Res 16:33–38.
8. Kawashima A, Kubo K, Kobayashi T, Sekiguchi M. (1989) Hemodynamic responses to acute hypoxia, hypobaria, and exercise in subjects susceptible to high-altitude pulmonary edema. J Appl Physiol 67:1982–1989.
9. Reeves JT, Wagner WW Jr, McMurtry IF, Grover RF. (1979) Physiological effects of high altitude on pulmonary circulation. In: International Review of Physiology, Environmental Physiology lll, ed. Robertshaw D, University Press Baltimore Vol 120, pp289–310
10. Sakai A. (1974) Hematocrit and right ventricular weight. Seasonal and latitudinal changes in hematocrit and right ventricular weights of wood mice, Apodemus argenteuse. Jpn J Physiol 36:8–16.
11. Sakai A. (1976) Seasonal changes of heart weights of wood mice, Apodemus argenteus, J Mammal Sci Jap Vol 6 : 224–230.
12. Sakai A, Ueda G, Kobayashi T, Kubo K, Fukushima M, Yoshimura K, Shibamato T, Kusama S. (1984) Effects of elevated-hematocrit levels on pulmonary circulation in conscious sheep. Jpn J Physiol 34:871–882.
13. Sakai A, Ueda G, Yanagidaira Y, Takeoka M, Tang G, Zhang Y. (1988) Physiological characteristics of pika, Ochtona, high-altitude adapted animals. In: High-Altitude Medical Science, ed. Ueda and Voelkel Shinshu Univ Press Matsumoto p99–107.
14. Sakai A, Matsumoto T, Saitoh M, Matsuzaki T, Koizumi T, Ishizaki T, Ruan ZH, Wang ZG, Chen QH, Wang XQ. (2004) Cardiopulmonary adaptation to high altitude in mammals. High Alt Med and Biol 5(2):260.
15. Sealander JA. (1962) Seasonal changes in blood values of deer mice and other small mammals. Ecology 43, 107–119.
16. Swigart RH. (1965) Polycythemia and right ventricular hypertrophy. Circulation Res. 17: 30–38.
17. Von Euler and Lijestrand (1946) Observation on pulmonary arterial blood pressure in the cat. Acta Physiol Scand 12:301–320.

CHAPTER 8

THE LUNG AT HIGH ALTITUDE: BETWEEN PHYSIOLOGY AND PATHOLOGY

ANNALISA COGO, FEDERICA CAMPIGOTTO, VALTER FASANO°, GIOVANNI GRAZZI

Sports Biomedical Studies Centre, University of Ferrara,
°Institute of Respiratory Diseases, University of Milan,
Ospedale Maggiore of Milan, IRCCS, Italy

Abstract: The lungs play a pivotal role in adaptation to high altitude. The increase in ventilation and the rise in pulmonary artery pressure are the first features of lung response to hypoxic exposure. At high altitude the lungs can also be affected by high-altitude pulmonary oedema, a severe form of acute mountain sickness. In healthy subjects the ascent to high altitude is also associated with alterations in lung function, which have been in part interpreted as an effect of extra vascular lung fluid accumulation. The patterns of respiratory function changes at high altitude are discussed, taking into account the body fluid movement and the increase in endothelial permeability induced by hypoxic exposure. As the problem of "respiratory" patients at high altitude is very important, a short summary of the guidelines for altitude exposure of asthmatic and COPD patients is reported at the end of the chapter.

Keywords: pulmonary artery pressure; high altitude; physiology.

Introduction

The lung is the first interface between environmental hypoxia and the metabolic machinery of the body, so that any factor impairing the ventilation and the lung mechanics can condition the physical performance. This is particularly true at high altitude, where the movement of large quantities of air is required, especially during exercise, and the total body function is impaired by arterial oxygen desaturation [54,55]. At altitude, many factors can affect the ability of the lung to successfully carry out its tasks, despite the facilitation induced by ongoing ventilatory acclimatization, which is secondary to carotid body sensitivity to hypoxia: as for instance, an overall greater effort for breathing,

A. Aldashev and R. Naeije (eds.), Problems of High Altitude Medicine and Biology, 119–131.

pulmonary vasoconstriction with increased pulmonary artery pressure, slightly decreased strength of respiratory muscles [17,25], ventilation/perfusion heterogeneity and oxygen diffusion limitation, essentially tied to the lower driving pressure for oxygen from the air to the blood and the shorter time for equilibration of oxygen at the alveolar-endothelial membrane site, due to the more rapid transit time [63]. Furthermore, at high altitude the lungs can also be affected by one of the two severe forms of acute mountain sickness (AMS), i.e., high altitude pulmonary oedema (HAPE), which is a well-known life-threatening complication of high altitude exposure. This illness usually develops within the first 2–5 days after acute exposure to altitudes above 2500–3000m, but is more frequent after a rapid ascent (>300m/day) to an altitude above 4000m and an overnight stay. Altitude, speed and mode of ascent and above all individual susceptibility, are the most important determinants for the occurrence of HAPE [3]. An excessive rise in pulmonary artery pressure preceding oedema formation is the crucial pathophysiological factor; decreased fluid clearance from the alveoli may also contribute to such non-cardiogenic pulmonary oedema, as well as the stress failure of pulmonary capillaries [62]. In subjects suffering from this severe and acute illness, the respiratory function and oxygenation are severely impaired [28].

Even in healthy subjects, the ascent to high altitude is associated with alterations in lung function, which have been in part interpreted as an effect of extravascular lung fluid accumulation. The mechanisms of these changes and whether they reflect early stages of high-altitude pulmonary oedema (HAPE) have been recently debated. In other words: is the HAPE the end stage of interstitial lung fluid accumulation in the same way as high-altitude cerebral oedema (HACE) is considered the end stage of AMS?

First of all, we think that the extravascular lung fluid accumulation should be seen in the wider "scenario" of the bodies fluid movement during high altitude exposure, which is a quite complex issue.

Body Fluid Movement

It is well known that exposure to high altitude is associated with changes in body fluid compartments. In particular, subjects can face both dehydration and peripheral oedema while spirometric changes, suggestive of extra vascular lung fluid accumulation, can appear [59]. Dehydration can be caused frequently by the very low absolute humidity at high and very high altitudes. This is mainly due to the fact that water loss through sweating is increased during exercise, as well as insensible water loss induced by ventilation. Increased ventilation is a common adaptation feature of high altitude and the level of ventilation may be very high, especially during exercise; furthermore, the hyperventilation of dry and cold air increases the water loss. As to peripheral oedema, it is common in newcomers at high altitude, is most frequently localized in the fingers and the face, and is tied to an increase in extra-cellular fluid [59].

An increase in endothelial permeability can be a hypothesis to explain this increase in extra-cellular fluid.

Hypoxia-induced Endothelial Permeability

A growing number of papers have shown the effects of hypoxia, both in vivo and in vitro, on capillary endothelial permeability.

The in vitro studies have shown that endothelial cell monolayers grown in culture and then exposed to low oxygen concentrations become larger, and small intercellular gaps between contiguous cells appear; permeability of monolayers to solutes increases at a dose-dependent rate. These phenomena are reversible [47,48,66]. Endothelium subjected to oxygen deprivation maintains cell viability and basic biosynthetic mechanisms but displays multiple changes in properties, including a decreased barrier function. According to these authors, hypoxia-mediated suppression of endothelial barrier function, resulting in increased vascular leakage, is likely to contribute to high-altitude pulmonary and cerebral oedema.

In vivo studies, performed in animal models, confirmed that prolonged exposure to hypoxia can result in increased vascular permeability. In fact, in rats exposed to a simulated altitude of approximately 4400m, the protein leak index increased significantly after at least 24 hours, as compared with normoxic controls. Histologic examination showed perivascular oedema cuffs in the altitude-exposed groups. The increased vascular permeability may be ameliorated and prevented by administration of glucocorticoids [57,64,27]. Extreme hypoxia has also been reported to cause an increase in microvascular permeability in isolated dog lungs [49], while hypoxic exposure in rabbits leads to an increase in interstitial fluid content (increased pulmonary interstitial pressure) [45].

Some authors suggested that the increased endothelial permeability may be at least in part mediated by the effect of vascular endothelial growth factor (VEGF), a potent mediator of capillary leak if it gains access to its receptors on the capillary endothelium [38,37].

In any case, all these data might support the hypothesis that increased endothelial permeability might be a cofactor of extravascular lung fluid accumulation at high altitude.

Lung Function at High Altitude

In the next part of the paper we discus the topic of lung function changes at high altitude, which could be related to extravascular lung fluid accumulation (i.e., interstitial lung oedema).

Exposure to high altitude is well known to induce changes in spirometry, including an increase in flow rates, a fall in vital capacity (VC) and forced vital capacity (FVC). After the observations of Paul Bert, reporting a significant reduction in vital capacity in a hypobaric chamber at a simulated altitude of 4500m [4], the first measurement of lung function testing at high altitude was provided by Angelo Mosso in 1897 [46] who observed a mean 11% decrease in VC at 4559m, as compared to sea level: he explained these changes with the increase in central blood volume due to the hypoxia-induced vasodilation of pulmonary circulation. In the early 50s Rahn and Hammond and other authors [52,58] found a reduction in lung volumes during the first week of acclimatization on Mt Evans (4347m). Similar results were reported by Cerretelli at around 5000m [7] and by Kronenberg at 4350m [39], after a variable time of acclimatization. Jaeger and co-workers were the first to attribute the altitude-induced lung function changes to an abrupt increase in thoracic intravascular fluid volume upon arrival at high altitude, followed by a more gradual increase in extravascular fluid volume in the peribronchial spaces of dependent lung regions [34]. After these observations, many other papers reported that, with increasing altitude, FVC and FEV1 as well as MEF25 (i.e., FEF75) were significantly, if variably, reduced [11,42,14,26]. After descent to below 2000m, all values normalized within one day. Some authors described a weak negative correlation between AMS and the reduction of respiratory parameters [26,14], with changes proportional to the magnitude of altitude [31], while other authors reported the absence of a correlation between the spirometric changes and SpO2 or AMS [42]. Chest radiographs on subjects immediately after a prolonged graded altitude exposure to as high as 8848m above sea level in a hypobaric chamber, showed a pattern of pulmonary artery enlargement and interstitial oedema, which could be the causes of the restricted pulmonary function pattern, together with an increase in pulmonary blood volume and respiratory muscle weakness [61]. Moreover, it has been shown in some cyclists that after prolonged high-intensity exercise at moderate altitude, there is radiographic evidence of early pulmonary oedema [2].

Beside the spirometric data, a few data regarding impedance at high altitude also support this hypothesis. In fact, Hoon and co-workers measured mean transthoracic electrical impedance, which is known to be inversely related to intrathoracic extravascular fluid volume, in 121 normal healthy volunteers at sea-level and at 3658m altitude attained with different climbing profiles, and found an overall decrease in impedance, more evident in the subjects who developed symptoms of high-altitude sickness [32]. Similar results were obtained in a group of lowlanders during a prolonged stay at 3800m. In these subjects, serial and simultaneous measurement of FVC, electrical impedance tomography (EIT) and nasal potential difference (NPD) were measured. A statistically significant relationship between the decrease in FVC and in EIT was found, as well as between NPD and both EIT changes and FVC. These changes suggest that altered respiratory epithelial ion transport might play a role in the development of subclinical pulmonary oedema at high altitude in normal subjects [43].

In 2002, Cremona was the first to study a very large number of subjects at altitude showing an increase in closing volume, indicating small airways compression by extra vascular lung fluid accumulation, in 74% of about 250 recreational climbers at 4559m [15]. According to these authors, increased pulmonary extra vascular lung fluid would track centrally along major pulmonary vessels and airways. Peribronchial fluid accumulating in this way would be expected to compress airways, thus increasing the volume at which airways close. After the appearance of this paper, many questions have arisen and are being debated in the scientific community, first of all whether these alterations of lung function consistent with interstitial fluid accumulation could indicate a subsequent progression to clinical HAPE.

We recently performed two different studies aimed at answering the following questions: at what altitude does the lung interstitial oedema appear? Does it also appear in elite climbers? Is endothelial permeability a co-factor? These data are not yet published and have only been presented as abstracts; the following summary should be therefore considered a preliminary report, pending the publication of the complete data [23,13,24].

We examined 18 subjects: 9 recreational climbers (Nepal 2003) and 9 elite climbers (Everest 2004) in two different studies with similar study designs and similar ascent profiles. None suffered from severe AMS. We tested the presence of abnormalities in the small airways in two different ways: assessing oscillatory resistances and reactance, in the first study and maximal and partial expiration flow volume curves in the second study. In fact, the effects of deep inhalation on airway calibre are considered to reflect the distensibility of intraparenchimal airways [51]. Urinary microalbumin has been measured as an indirect marker of systemic transvascular albumin leakiness and endothelial permeability [35].

The significant reduction in reactance already at 3500m [33], its further decrease at 5500m, together with a lack of reduction in oscillatory resistance (as expected on the basis of reduced density of the air), suggest that early changes in lung function (indicating an increase in lung tissue fluid) are already present at 3500m and become more evident at higher altitudes. The significant increase in urinary microalbumin already at 3500m suggests that increased endothelial permeability can play a role.

On the other hand, the significant reduction of flows, at the last part of FVC after the first night spent above 5000m, with no difference between maximal and partial expiration, can be interpreted as the narrowing of the "small airways" [41,65], which might be due to the compressing effect of extra-vascular lung fluid accumulation. Increased endothelial permeability can contribute to this phenomenon. All these changes are reduced, even if not normalized, after seven days above 5000m. Noteworthy is that all climbers reached altitudes above 7000m and four out of nine reached the summit of Mt Everest.

From these preliminary results of our research, we can summarize that the indirect signs of extravascular lung fluid accumulation seem to affect both elite and recreational climbers; they are evident starting from 3500m; more pronounced at 5000m; decrease after 7 days but in any case do not preclude successful climbing at extreme altitudes.

Further studies are needed to make clearer the link between interstitial lung oedema and HAPE, but from the data available up to now, it seems that extravascular lung fluid accumulation neither definitely evolves into HAPE nor heralds impending HAPE. These conclusions are also reported in a paper that was published after the conference at which we presented this lecture [56].

Respiratory Diseases and High Altitude

As the problem of "respiratory" patients at high altitude is very important, we add a short summary of the guidelines for asthmatic patients and for patients suffering from chronic obstructive pulmonary disease published on HAM&B [12] and discussed during the meeting. Exposure to high altitude does affect patients with chronic lung disease. Patients with obstructive disease (asthma and chronic obstructive pulmonary disease (COPD)) can have specific problems when exposed to altitude [53]. In fact, in these cases not only hypoxia but also other climatic aspects of high altitude play a potential role in the patient's wellbeing. At high altitude, in fact, there is a decrease in barometric pressure, inspired oxygen pressure, temperature, humidity, density of air but, and at the same time, an increase in solar radiation and wind. The effect is reported in Table 1.

Bronchial Asthma

Asthma is one of the most widespread diseases in the world, even if its prevalence and severity differ widely among countries and individuals. At altitude, the main problems which emerge are hypoxia and environmental and trigger factors such as exercise, hyperventilation in dry and cold air (the severity of bronchospasm induced by exercise is enhanced by hyperventilation in cold and dry air [5,22], while there is a reduction in aeroallergens and atmospheric pollution.

TABLE 1. Effect of different climatic conditions at high altitude

↓ Density of the air	→	Flows ↑ Airway resistence ↓
↓ Temperature ↓ Humidity ↑ Wind ↑ Exercise	→	Hyperventilation of dry and cold air → Asthma attack
↓ Inhaled allergens ↓ Pollution	→	Positive for "respiratory" patients

At 1500–2000m hypoxia is not severe, and the main environmental feature is the reduction in, or absence of, pollen, house dust mite and environmental pollution [8], which can play a key role in reducing the bronchial inflammation underlying airways hyper-responsiveness [60]. Avoidance of allergen exposure (especially to mite allergens) is often recommended in asthma management and a considerable reduction in exposure to allergens exists in mountain environments, a fact which reduces the bronchial inflammation and results in a dramatic clinical improvement. All the data published on this topic confirm that exposure to moderate altitude is beneficial for asthmatics.

At higher altitudes (>2500m), the effects of hypoxia and of cold and low humidity become more and more evident, so that asthmatics might be expected to worsen in this environment. Unfortunately, very limited information is available about the exposure of asthmatic subjects to high altitude and about the suitability of mountain climbing as an appropriate form of sport for asthmatics. The only two independent risk factors for asthma attacks at altitude identified in a paper by Golan [29] are: frequent use (≥ 3 times weekly) of inhaled bronchodilators before travel and participation in intensive physical exertion in the course of the treks.

At very high altitude the positive factors seem to prevail over the negative ones and the bronchial hyper responsiveness to both methacholine and hyposmolar aerosol is significantly reduced [1,11].

Recommendations for Asthmatic Patients in the Mountains

The exposure of asthmatic patients to high altitudes must be carefully evaluated in advance, keeping in mind the following recommendations [12]:

1. Asthma must be under control and in a stable state.
2. Patients should not discontinue their regular antiasthmatic prophylaxis and should always keep rescue drugs with them. At high altitude, the use of a spacer for a metered dose inhaler is more important than at sea level,

as high altitude environment might affect the delivery of the drugs, since it brings about more significant evaporation, especially if the patient does not correctly position the mouthpiece between the lips.

3. As at sea level, the patients should always be pre-medicated with short-acting beta2agonists and/or steroids before any intense physical effort, especially those who have already shown bronchospasm induced by exercise (the use of leukotriene inhibitors should also be considered).
4. As at sea level, during very cold and windy days, patients should remember to protect their mouth, e.g., with a scarf.
5. Trekking to high altitudes in remote areas would be better done in the presence of a physician. It is very important that the patient has adequate supplies of drugs, possibly packed in two different places, to avoid risks in the event of loss. In any case, patients must know how to manage asthma attacks personally, as medical care is generally poor in most high altitude areas; a check list of what to do in case of worsening asthma should be included with the medication [50].
6. Patients with moderate-severe asthma should not ascend from low altitude to above 3000m by mechanical means of transportation, as acute exposure to moderate hypoxia seems to worsen bronchial hyperresponsiveness [18,16]. A gradual ascent is recommended, so that, in case of symptoms, it is possible to stop and descend.

Chronic Bronchitis and Chronic Obstructive Pulmonary Diseases

Chronic obstructive pulmonary disease (COPD) is a leading cause of morbidity worldwide and is currently the fourth cause of death in the world.

At altitude, the most important change for patients with COPD is the reduction in atmospheric pressure, which leads to a reduction in the partial pressure of arterial oxygen and to a reduction in oxygen saturation. On the other hand, there is a slight reduction in the effort of breathing, thanks to the lower air density.

Patients who show symptoms of mild airway obstruction can take advantage of the lower density and the lower humidity of the inhaled air and of the reduction in air pollutants.

Patients with moderate to severe and very severe obstruction, with values of arterial oxygen at sea level and at rest below normal range, need a careful assessment to predict the value of arterial oxygen at altitude.

Many studies reporting recommendations for the management of respiratory patients planning an exposure to altitude (especially air travel) measured arterial blood gases and oxygen saturation at sea level and at altitudes between 1500m and 3000m either in a hypobaric chamber, or while inhaling hypoxic mixtures or during flights in non-pressurized airplanes. All studies demonstrated that both types of hypoxic exposure (hypobaric chamber and hypoxia inhalation test) are safe and can predict PaO_2 at altitude and that accuracy increases with the inclusion of spirometric variables.

General Recommendation [12]

In conclusion, hypoxic tests with the addition of spirometric testing are useful to the physician for the prediction of a patient's condition at altitudes different from the habitual residence [36,19,20,21,9,10]. The British Thoracic Society recommendations for respiratory patients planning air travel state that a minimum PaO_2 of 70 mmHg (9.3 kPa) at sea level is required in order to obtain an arterial oxygen tension not lower than 55 mmHg (7.3 kPa) at an altitude of 2,438 m (8,000 ft) (BTS 2002).

In addition to the collection of clinical information and functional data, the physician should always ask patients about:

1. the altitude of their home residence
2. the altitude they are planning to reach
3. the length of their stay at altitude
4. the altitude at which they are going to sleep
5. the level of exertion that they anticipate during recreation

Each patient should be assessed individually. In the case where exposure to hypoxia is absolutely unavoidable (e.g., if someone has to travel by air) and a PaO2 below 60mmHg is predicted, supplemental oxygen must be considered. Furthermore, it could be useful to suggest that patients measure their pulse oximetry during altitude exposure, in order to avoid activities that result in severe desaturation [44].

When planning a trip to high altitude, patients must take into account the possibility of poor medical support, additional travel diseases and problems concerning emergency rescue. It is mandatory that patients should be in a stable phase of their disease and medical treatment should be optimised. Carrying supplemental oxygen devices can be logistically difficult, time-consuming and expensive; therefore, the pre-travel assessment indicating the need of supplemental oxygen should be performed carefully (details of air travel with supplemental oxygen are described in BTS 2002).

References

1. Allegra L, Cogo A, Legnani D, Diano PL, Fasano V, Negretto GG (1995). High altitude exposure reduces bronchial responsiveness to hypoosmolar aerosol in lowland asthmatics. Eur Resp. J 8:1842–1846.
2. Anholm JD, Milne EN, Stark P, Bourne JC, Friedman P (1999). Radiographic evidence of interstitial pulmonary oedema after exercise at altitude. J Appl Physiol. Feb;86(2):503–9.
3. Bartsch P, Mairbaurl H, Maggiorini M, Swenson ER (2005). Physiological aspects of high-altitude pulmonary edema. J Appl Physiol. Mar;98(3):1101–10.
4. Bert Paul (1875) La pression barometrique. Masson
5. Boulet LP, Turcotte H. (1991). Influence of water content of inspired air during and after exercise on induced bronchoconstriction. Eur. Respir. J. 4; 979–984.
6. BTS.(2002). Managing passengers with respiratory disease planning air travel: British Thoracic Society recommendations. Thorax 57: 289–304.
7. Cerretelli P (1961) Some aspects of the respiratory function in man acclimatized to high altitude. Int Z Angew Physiol;18:386–392.
8. Charpin D, Birnbaum J, Haddi H, Genard G, Lanteaume A, Toumi M, Farai F, Van der Brembt X, Vervolet D. (1991). Altitude and allergy to house dust mite. Am. Rev. Respir. Dis.143; 983–986.
9. Chi-Lem G, Perez-Padilla R. (1998). Gas exchange at rest during simulated altitude in patients with chronic lung disease. Arch. Med. Res. Spring;29(1):57–62.
10. Christensen CC, Ryg M, Refvem OK, Skjonsberg OH. (2000). Development of severe hypoxaemia in chronic obstructive pulmonary disease patients at 2,438 m (8,000 ft) altitude. Eur. Respir. J. Apr;15(4):635–9.
11. Cogo A, Legnani D, Allegra L. (1997) Respiratory function at different altitudes. Respiration 64(6):416–21.
12. Cogo A, Fischer R, Schoene R (2004) Respiratory diseases and high altitude. High Alt Med Biol 5(4):435–44.
13. Cogo A, Paolucci E, Pomidori L, Schneider A, Bernardi L (2005) Extravascular lung fluid accumulation in èlite climbers at high altitude is a transient event and does not preclude a successful climb. ATS 2005 San Diego International Conference, May 20–25, 2005. Abstract 952886, Volume 2, p A779 (abstract).
14. Compte-Torrero L, Botella de Maglia J, de Diego-Damia A, Gomez-Perez L, Ramirez-Galleymore P, Perpina-Tordera M (2005) Changes in spirometric parameters and arterial oxygen saturation during a mountain ascent to over 3000 metres. Arch Bronconeumol. 41(10):547–52.
15. Cremona G, Asnaghi R, Baderna P, Brunetto A, Brutsaert T, Cavallaro C, Clark TM, Cogo A, Donis R, Lanfranchi P, Luks A, Novello N, Panzetta S, Perini L, Putnam M, Spagnolatti L, Wagner H, and Wagner PD (2002) Pulmonary extravascular fluid accumulation in recreational climbers: a prospective study. Lancet 359: 303–309.
16. Dagg KD, Thomson LJ, Clayton RA, Ramsay SG, Thomson NC. (1997). Effect of acute alterations in inspired oxygen tension on methacholine induced bronchoconstriction in patients with asthma. Thorax 52(5):453–7.
17. Deboeck G, Moraine JJ, Naeije R (2005) Respiratory muscle strength may explain hypoxia-induced decrease in vital capacity. Med Sci Sports Exerc 37(5):754–8.
18. Denjean A, Roux C, Herve P, Bonniot J-P, Comoy E, Duroux P, Gaultier C. (1988). Mild isocapnic hypoxia enhances the bronchial response to methacholine in asthmatic subjects. Am. Rev. Respir. Dis. 138: 789–793.
19. Dillard TA, Rosenberg AP, Berg BW. (1993). Hypoxemia during altitude exposure. A meta-analysis of chronic obstructive pulmonary disease. Chest Feb;103(2):422–5
20. Dillard TA, Moores LK, Bilello KL, Phillips YY. (1995). The preflight evaluation. A comparison of the hypoxia inhalation test with hypobaric exposure. Chest Feb;107(2):352–7.

21. Dillard TA, Rajagopal KR, Slivka WA, Berg BW, Mehm WJ, Lawless NP. (1998). Lung function during moderate hypobaric hypoxia in normal subjects and patients with chronic obstructive pulmonary disease. Aviat. Space Environ. Med. Oct;69(10):979–85.
22. Dosman JA, Hodgson WC, Cockcroft DW. (1991). Effect of cold air on the bronchial response to inhaled histamine in patients with asthma. Am. Rev. Respir. Dis. 144 45–50.
23. Fasano V, Bonardi D, Campigotto F, Donnaloja A, Farinatti M, Fioretti A, Gennari A, Pomidori L, Palange P, Cogo A (2004) Extravascular lung fluid accumulation does not immediately follow the increased capillary permeability during exposure to high altitude (HA). European Respiratory Journal (abstract).
24. Fasano V, Bonardi D, Campigotto F, Gennari A, Pomidori L, Valli G, Taccagni L, Gualdi Russo E, Cogo A (2005) Free fat mass and spirometric changes during high altitude exposure(HA) indicate a body fluid shift. Fundaments of Human Movement and Sport Practice 64–68.
25. Fasano V, Paolucci E, Pomidori L, Cogo A (2006) High-altitude exposure reduces inspiratory muscle strength. Int J Sports Med Oct 6 (e pub ahead of print).
26. Fischer R, Lang SM, Bergner A, Huber RM (2005) Monitoring of expiratory flow rates and lung volumes during a high altitude expedition. Eur J Med Res 16;10(11):469–74.
27. Fischer S., Renz D., Schaper W., Karliczek G.F. (2001). In vitro effects of dexamethasone on hypoxia-induced hyperpermeability and expression of vascular endothelial growth factor. Eur J Pharmacol 12;411(3):231–43).
28. Ge R.L., Matsuzawa Y., Takeoka M., Kubo K., Sekiguchi M., Kobayashi T. (1997). Low pulmonary diffusing capacity in subjects with acute mountain sickness. Chest 111(1):58–64.
29. Golan Y., Onn A., Villa Y., Avidor Y., Kivity S., Berger S.A., Shapira I., Levo Y., Giladi M. (2002). Asthma in adventure travellers: a prospective study evaluating the occurrence and risk factors for acute exacerbations. Arch. Intern. Med. Nov 25;162(21):2421–6.
30. Hansen J.M., Olsen N.V., Feldt-Rasmussen B., Kanstrup I.L., Dechaux M., Dubray C., Richalet J.P. (1994). Albuminuria and overall capillary permeability of albumin in acute altitude hypoxia. J Appl Physiol;76(5):1922–7.
31. Hashimoto F., McWilliams B., Qualls C. (1997). Pulmonary ventilatory function decreases in proportion to increasing altitude. Wilderness Environ Med 8(4):214–7.
32. Hoon R.S., Balasubramanian V., Tiwari S.C., Mathew O.P., Behl A., Sharma S.C., Chadha K.S. (1997). Changes in transthoracic electrical impedance at high altitude. Br Heart J 39(1):61–6.
33. Johnson M.K., Birch M., Carter R., Kinsella J., Stevenson R.D. (2005). Use of reactance to estimate transpulmonary resistance. Eur Respir J, 25, 1061–1069.
34. Jaeger J.J., Sylvester J.T., Cymerman A., Berberich J.J., Denniston J.C., Maher J.T. (1979). Evidence for increased intrathoracic fluid volume in man at high altitude. J Appl Physiol 47(4):670–6.
35. Jensen J.S., Borch-Johnsen K., Jensen G., Feldt-Rasmussen B. (1995). Microalbuminuria reflects a generalized transvascular albumin leakiness in clinically healthy subjects Clin. Sci.88(6):629–33.
36. Karrer W., Schmid T., Wuthrich O., Baldi W., Gall E., Portmann H.R.(1990). Respiration of patients with chronic lung disease at 500 and 1500 meter above sea level Schweiz Med. Wochenschr. Oct 27;120(43):1584–9.
37. Kaner RJ, Crystal RG (2004) Pathogenesis of high altitude pulmonary edema: Does alveolar epithelial lining fluid vascular endothelial growth factor exacerbate capillary leak? High Alt. Med. Biol. 5:399–409.
38. Klekamp JG, Jarzecka K, Hoover RL, Summar ML, Redmond N, Perkett EA (1997) Vascular endothelial growth factor is expressed in ovine pulmonary vascular smooth muscle cells in vitro and regulated by hypoxia and dexamethasone. Pediatr Res 42(6):744–9.
39. Kronenberg R, Safar P, Lee J, Wright F, Noble W, Wahrenbrock E, Hickeyy R, Nemoto E, Severinghaus JW (1971) Pulmonary artery pressure and alveolar gas exchanges in man during acclimatization to 12470 ft. J Clin Inves 50:827–837.

40. Lewis DM, Bradwell AR, Shore AC, Beaman M, Tooke JE (1997) Capillary filtration coefficient and urinary albumin leak at altitude. Eur J Clin Invest 27(1):64–8.
41. Macklem PT (1998) The physiology of small airways. Am J Respir Crit Care Med 157, S181–S183.
42. Mason NP, Barry PW, Pollard AJ, Collier DJ, Taub NA, Miller MR, and Milledge JS. (2002) Serial changes in spirometry during an ascent to 5,300m in the Nepalese Himalayas. High Alt Med Biol 1: 185–195.
43. Mason NP, Petersen M, Melot C, Imanow B, Matveykine O, Gautier MT, Sarybaev A, Aldashev A, Mirrakhimov MM, Brown BH, Leathard AD, Naeije R (2003) Serial changes in nasal potential difference and lung electrical impedance tomography at high altitude. J Appl Physiol 94(5):2043–50.
44. Mehm WJ, Dillard TA, Berg BW, Dooley JW, Rajagopal KR. (1991). Accuracy of oxy-hemoglobin saturation monitors during simulated altitude exposure of men with chronic obstructive pulmonary disease. Aviat. Space Environ. Med. May;62(5):418–21.
45. Miserocchi G, Passi A, Negrini D, Del Fabbro M, De Luca G (2001) Pulmonary interstitial pressure and tissue matrix structure in acute hypoxia. Am J Physiol Lung Cell Mol Physiol 280(5):L881–7.
46. Mosso A (1897) Fisiologia dell'uomo sulle Alpi. Treves, Torino.
47. Ogawa S, Gerlach H, Esposito C, Pasagian-Macaulay A, Brett J, Stern D (1990) Hypoxia modulates the barrier and coagulant function of cultured bovine endothelium. Increased monolayer permeability and induction of procoagulant properties. J Clin Invest 85(4):1090–8.
48. Ogawa S, Shreeniwas R, Brett J, Clauss M, Furie M, Stern DM (1990) The effect of hypoxia on capillary endothelial cell function: modulation of barrier and coagulant function. Br J Haematol 75(4):517–24.
49. Parker JC, Parker RE, Granger DN, Taylor AE (1981) Vascular permeability and transvascular fluid and protein transport in the dog lung. Circ Res 48(4):549–61.
50. Peacock AJ (1998). Asthma at altitude: the effect on asthma of the mountain environment and precautions for the traveller. The Asthma Journal september, 117–119.
51. Pellegrino R, Sterk PJ, Sont JK, Brusasco V (1998) Assessing the effect of deep inhalation on airway calibre: a novel approach to lung function in bronchial asthma and COPD. Eur Respir J 12(5):1219–27.
52. Rahn H, Hammond D (1951) Vital capacity at reduced barometric pressure. J Appl Physiol 4:715–724.
53. Schoene RB.(1999). Lung Disease at High Altitude. In Hypoxia into the next millennium. edited by R.R. Roach, P.D. Wagner and P.H. Hackett. Advances in Experimental Medicine and Biology vol. 474, Kluwer Academic, New York pp 47–56.
54. Schoene RB (2001) Limits of human lung function at high altitude. J Exp Biol 204(Pt 18):3121–7.
55. Schoene RB (2005) Limits of respiration at high altitude. Clin Chest Med 26(3):405–14.
56. Senn O, Clarenbach CF, Fischler M, Thalmann R, Brunner-La Rocca H, Egger P., Maggiorini M, Bloch KE (2006). Do changes in lung function predict high-altitude pulmonary edema at an early stage? Med Sci Sports Exerc. 38(9):1565–70.
57. Stelzner TJ, O'Brien RF, Sato K, Weil JV (1988) Hypoxia-induced increases in pulmonary transvascular protein escape in rats. Modulation by glucocorticoids. J Clin Invest 82(6):1840–7.
58. Tenney SM, Rahn H, Stound RC, Mithofer JC (1953) Adaptation to high altitude: changes in lung volumes during the first seven days at Mt Evans, Colorado.J Appl Physiol 5:607–613.
59. Ward MP, Milledge JS, West JB (2001) High Altitude Medicine and Physiology Chapman and Hall, London.
60. Wardlaw AJ. (1993). The role of air pollution in asthma. Clin Exp Allergy 23: 81–96.

61. Welsh CH, Wagner PD, Reeves JT, Lynch D, Cink TM, Armstrong J, Malconian MK, Rock PB, Houston CS (1993) Operation Everest. II: Spirometric and radiographic changes in acclimatized humans at simulated high altitudes. Am Rev Respir Dis 147(5):1239–44.
62. West JB, Colice GL, Lee YJ, Namba Y, Kurdak SS, Fu Z, Ou LC, Mathieu-Costello O. (1995). Pathogenesis of high-altitude pulmonary oedema: direct evidence of stress failure of pulmonary capillaries. Eur Respir J 8(4):523–9.
63. West JB (1990). Limiting factors for exercise at extreme altitudes. Clin Physiol 10(3):265–72.
64. Wood JG, Johnson JS, Mattioli LF, Gonzalez NC (2000). Systemic hypoxia increases leukocyte emigration and vascular permeability in conscious rats. J Appl Physiol 89(4):1561–8.
65. Woolcock AJ (1998). Effect of drugs on small airways. Am J Respir Crit Care Med 157, S203–S207.
66. Yan SF, Ogawa S, Stern DM, Pinsky DJ (1997) Hypoxia-induced modulation of endothelial cell properties: regulation of barrier-function and expression of interleukin-6. Kidney Int; 51(2):419–25.

CHAPTER 9

SILDENAFIL AND HYPOXIC PULMONARY HYPERTENSION

BAKTYBEK K. KOJONAZAROV[1], MIRSAID M. MIRRAKHIMOV[2], NICHOLAS W. MORRELL[3], MARTIN R. WILKINS[4], ALMAZ A. ALDASHEV[1]

[1] Institute of Molecular Biology and Medicine, Bishkek, Kyrgyzstan
[2] National centre of Cardiology and Internal Medicine, Bishkek, Kyrgyzstan
[3] Cambridge University, Cambridge, United Kingdom
[4] Imperial College of Medicine, London, United Kingdom

Abstract: We have previously demonstrated that sildenafil inhibits hypoxia-induced pulmonary vasoconstriction in healthy subjects. The aim of this study was to investigate the effects of the PDE5 inhibitor sildenafil on pulmonary hemodynamics in patients with high altitude pulmonary hypertension (HAPH). Twenty-two patients with HAPH were randomized by age and level of mean pulmonary arterial pressure (PAP) in 3 groups: a first group (n=9) treated with 25 mg of sildenafil 3 times a day; a second group (n=5) – received 100 mg of sildenafil 3 times a day; a third group (n=8) – treated with placebo. Pulmonary hemodynamics was measured by right heart catheterization at baseline and after 12 weeks of sildenafil therapy at, before and 1 hour after taking sildenafil or placebo.

In the first group the mean PAP decreased after 12 weeks of sildenafil treatment from 36±8 to 30±8 mm Hg and to 25±7 mm Hg ($p<0.007$) 1 hour after 25 mg of sildenafil, in the second group, mean PAP decreased after 12 weeks from 32±3 to 26±3 mm Hg ($p<0.01$) and to 21±2 mm Hg ($P<0.001$) 1 hour after 100 mg of sildenafil, in the third group the mean PAP did not significantly change. Both doses improved the 6-minute walk distance, in the first group of patients by 45.4 m ($p<0.01$) and in the second group by 40.0 m ($p<0.049$). No side effects were observed.

We conclude that sildenafil therapy decreases PAP and could be recommended for treatment of HAPH.

Keywords: altitude; pulmonary hypertension; sildenafil; exercise; right heart failure.

A. Aldashev and R. Naeije (eds.), Problems of High Altitude Medicine and Biology, 133–143.

Introduction

HAPH is a public health problem in the mountainous areas of the world, including Kyrgyzstan, where it is common among the highland population [2]. It is estimated that more than 140 million people reside above 2500m [3] and the number of temporary visitors to the mountains is close to 40 million [4].

HAPH is characterised by increased pulmonary vascular resistance secondary to hypoxia induced pulmonary vasoconstriction and vascular remodelling of pulmonary arterioles [2, 5, 6]. The vascular remodelling involves all cellular elements of the vessel wall with endothelial dysfunction, extension of smooth muscle into previously non-muscularised vessels and adventitial thickening [2,.5, 6]. The result is an increased pressure load on the right ventricle, reduced exercise capacity and premature death from right ventricular failure [7]. The structural changes in the pulmonary vasculature are due, at least in part, to hypoxia associated smooth muscle cell proliferation and—together with increased pulmonary vascular tone—represent targets for therapeutic intervention [7].

The biochemical pathways underlying this pathophysiology are poorly understood, but a reduction in nitric oxide (NO) production is thought to have a role. In animal studies the absence of endothelial nitric oxide synthase increases susceptibility to this condition [8]. Interestingly, indigenous Tibetans who are acclimatised to life at 3600m have twofold higher NO concentrations in exhaled breath than lowlanders [9] and inhaled NO has been shown to have beneficial effects on pulmonary haemodynamics in HAPH [10].

NO has vasorelaxant and antiproliferative effects, which are mediated by cyclic GMP [11] Cyclic GMP is hydrolysed by phosphodiesterases (PDE). PDE5 is the major PDE subtype present in pulmonary vasculature and is more abundant in the lung than in other tissues [11]. This offers the possibility of relatively selective pulmonary vasodilatation with little systemic hypotension. Agents with PDE5 inhibitory activity reduce pulmonary artery pressure (PAP) in animal models [13–16]. In an earlier study we showed that the selective PDE5 inhibitor, sildenafil, has a significant inhibitory effect on the acute pressor response to hypoxia in healthy subjects [1]. The aim of this study was to investigate the effects of PDE5 inhibitor sildenafil on pulmonary hemodynamics in patients with HAPH.

Methods

ACUTE HYPOXIA STUDY (EARLIER STUDY)

The effects of sildenafil 100mg and placebo on the pulmonary vascular response to an acute hypoxic challenge were compared in 10 male volunteers aged 18 to 27 years in a randomized, double blind study. The volunteers attended the catheterization laboratory at the National Center of Cardiology in Bishkek (760 meters above sea level), Kyrgyz Republic, on 2 occasions, 1 week apart. All gave written, informed consent and were judged to be healthy on the basis of medical examination and routine hematology and biochemistry. The study was approved by the local hospital ethics committee in Bishkek and followed international guidelines for medical research on human subjects. On each occasion, a Swan-Ganz thermodilution catheter (Baxter Healthcare Ltd) was sited in the pulmonary artery via a jugular vein. Baseline measurements were made after 30 minutes rest, and then sildenafil or placebo (lactose) was given orally in a gelatin capsule with 100 mL of water. One hour later, the volunteers breathed via a mouthpiece connected to a Douglas bag containing 11% O2. Measurements of PAP, systemic blood pressure, and heart rate were repeated after 30 minutes of hypoxia. Blood samples were taken in 1% 0.5 mmol/L EDTA on ice just before and at the end of 30 minutes of hypoxia and stored for cGMP analysis. Arterial oxygen saturation was measured by pulse oximeter (PROPAQ 102, Protocol Systems Inc).

HIGH ALTITUDE PULMONARY HYPERTENSION STUDY DESIGN OF STUDY

Suitable patients were randomised to receive sildenafil, 25 mg or 100 mg, or matching placebo every 8 hours for 12 weeks. The study was double blind. The primary end point was the change in mean PAP from baseline (week 0) after 12 weeks of treatment. Other measures of efficacy were the change in PVR (mean PAP (mm Hg) – pulmonary capillary wedge pressure (mm Hg)/cardiac output (CO, l/min) × 80 dynes.s/cm^{-5}), cardiac output (l/min), and 6-minute walk (6MW) distance from week 0 after 12 weeks of treatment. The physical limitation domain of the Kansas City Cardiomyopathy Questionnaire[16] was used to assess activity.

Both the baseline (week 0) and 12-week measurements were made at 760 m in the period 7–10 days after arrival at the hospital. Patients returned to their villages between assessments. Compliance with the protocol was assessed by tablet counts. The 6-minute walk and blood tests were made 24 hours before cardiac catheterisation. Baseline cardiopulmonary haemodynamic measurements were made following standard operating procedures after 30 minutes rest. At 12 weeks, these measurements were made 8–10 hours after administration of the study medication (trough measurements) and repeated 60 minutes after a dose of study medication was given by mouth (1 hour post-dose measurements).

STATISTICAL ANALYSIS

The data are presented as mean (SD). Differences in the response of healthy subjects to hypoxia were analyzed by repeated-measures ANOVA, with drug as a within-subject factor and order as a between-subject factor.

Changes from baseline to week 12 in the primary end point (mean PAP) and the secondary end points (PVR, CO, physical symptom score, and 6MW) were compared between the sildenafil and placebo groups using analysis of variance (ANOVA). The differences among all three treatment groups were compared using ANOVA. If a significant difference was observed among the three treatment groups, comparisons of each treatment group with placebo were conducted. In addition, the combined sildenafil dose groups (sildenafil 25 mg 8 hourly and 100 mg 8 hourly) were compared with placebo by ANOVA.

Results

Acute Hypoxia Study

The volunteers had normal PAP at rest. Inspiration of 11% O2 for 30 minutes led to a pronounced fall in arterial oxygen saturation and a 56% rise in mean PAP, from 16.0 ± 2.1 to 25.0 ± 4.8 mm Hg, on the placebo day (Table 1). The fall in arterial oxygen saturation was the same but the pressor response was almost abolished by pre-treatment with sildenafil (increase from 16.0 ± 2.1 to 18.0 ± 3.6 mm Hg). The small fall in systemic blood pressure on exposure to hypoxia was not affected by sildenafil. The rise in heart rate on the placebo day was significantly greater than on the sildenafil day.

TABLE 1. Response to breathing 11% O2 for 30 minutes after treatment with placebo or sildenafil 100 mg

	Baseline	Sildenafil	Baseline	Placebo
SaO2, %	99.0 ± 1.0	65.0 ± 11.3	99.0 ± 1.0	62.0 ± 11.2
PAP mean, mm Hg	16.0 ± 2.1	18.0 ± 3.6 *	16.0 ± 2.1	25.0 ± 4.8
PAP systolic, mm Hg	27.0 ± 3.7	30 ± 4.0 *	25.0 ± 3.5	39.0 ± 8.9
BP systolic, mm Hg	27.0 ± 3.7	30 ± 4.0 *	25.0 ± 3.5	39.0 ± 8.9
BP dyast, mm Hg	27.0 ± 3.7	30 ± 4.0 *	25.0 ± 3.5	39.0 ± 8.9
WP, mm Hg	12.2 ± 2.1	12.3 ± 1.3	10.4 ± 1.6	10.1 ± 1.5
HR, bpm	62.0 ± 6.7	82.0 ± 12.7†	67.0 ± 8.5	95.0 ± 4.5

SaO_2, systemic arterial oxygen saturation; PAP, pulmonary blood pressure; BP, blood pressure; WP, wedge pressure; HR, heart rate.

*P,0.05, †P,0.01 change from baseline on sildenafil vs change from baseline on placebo.

HIGH ALTITUDE PULMONARY HYPERTENSION STUDY SUBJECTS CHARACTERISTICS

Twenty-five patients with an elevated PAP (>25 mm Hg) volunteered for randomization of treatment. Three declined further follow-up after randomization (family commitments prevented them from travelling to Bishkek). Twenty-two patients completed the study; their ages and lung function data are shown in table 2 and baseline haemodynamic data in table 3. All subjects reported dyspnoea on moderate exertion at entry and most were judged to be in NYHA/WHO functional class II/III (table 1). There were no clinically significant baseline differences among the treatment groups.

RESPONSE TO TREATMENT
MEAN PAP

There was a statistically significant difference among the three groups in changes from baseline to week 12 in mean PAP measured 8–10 hours post-dose (trough) (p=0.039). Sildenafil 25 mg 8-hourly reduced mean PAP by −6.9 mm Hg (95% CI −12.4 to −1.3; p=0.018) compared with placebo. The treatment effect for the higher dose of sildenafil compared with placebo

TABLE 2. Mean (SD) baseline characteristics of subjects randomised to receive sildenafil or placebo treatment

	Sildenafil 25 mg tds (n = 9)	Sildenafil 100 mg tds (n = 5)	Placebo (n = 8)
Age (year)			
Mean	61 ± 8	60 ± 8	59 ± 8
Range	44 – 67	54 – 72	49 – 65
Weight (kg)	75 ± 10.6	82 ± 19.2	70 ± 10.6
BMI (kg/m^2)	30 ± 4.8	29.5 ± 4.1	26.1 ± 5.2
FEV1 (l)	2.4 ± 0.7	2.5 ± 1.0	1.9 ± 0.7
FVC (l)	2.9 ± 0.9	3.3 ± 1.1	2.6 ± 0.8
P_{O2} (kPa)	8.6 ± 0.6	9.1 ± 1.2	8.4 ± 1.8
P_{CO2} (kPa)	4.9 ± 0.5	4.8 ± 0.4	5.5 ± 1.0
Hb (g/dl)	16.4 ± 2.4	15.7 ± 1.5	16.3 ± 1.7
Haematocrit (%)	51.0 ± 6.7	48.0 ± 5.0	52.0 ± 7.3
NYHA/WHO functional class (I/II/III)	2/2/5	1/2/2	1/2/5
6 minute walk (m)	420.0 ± 85.0	449.0 ± 84.0	422.0 ± 69.0

BMI, body mass index; FEV1, forced expiratory volume in 1 second; FVC, forced vital capacity; P_{O2}, P_{CO2}, oxygen and carbon dioxide tension; Hb, haemoglobin.

TABLE 3. Response to treatment

	Sildenafil 25 mg (n = 9)			Sildenafil 100 mg (n = 5)			Placebo (n = 8)		
	Pre-treatment	Week 12		Pre-treatment	Week 12		Pre-treatment	Week 12	
Measurements	Baseline	Baseline	1 h post-dose	Baseline	Baseline	1 h post-dose	Baseline	Baseline	1 h post-dose
PAPmean (mm Hg)	36±8	30±8	25±7	32±3	26±3	21±2	34±6	35±12	35±11
PAP systolic (mm Hg)	53 ± 11	47±13	39±10	46±5	41±6	33±4	51±7	55±19	55±18
CO (l/min)	5.3±1.1	5.0±1.4	5.4±1.7	5.5±1.2	6.6±0.6	6.4±0.8	4.6±1.2	5.3±1.7	5.3±1.6
PVR (dyne.s/cm5)	441±242	391±243	284±204	328±58	185±49	130±39	457±146	390±205	388±208
WP (mm Hg)	9±1	9±2	9±2	9.6±2.1	11±2.8	11±2.8	9±2	10±3	10±3
HR (beats/min)	66±8	63±10	62±9	74±12	70±14	69±14	61±5	63±8	62±8
BPsystolic (mm Hg)	127±22	125±19	124±17	132±20	127±8	125±7	118±8	123±13	123±13
BPdiastolic (mm Hg)	77±10	78±7	78±7	80±7	81±2	81±2	75±5	75±6	76±6
SaO_2 (%)	94±3	95±2	95±2	94±2	95±1	95±1	94±5	94±5	94±5

CO, cardiac output; PVR, pulmonary vascular resistance.

was −6.4 mm Hg (95% CI −12.9 to 0.1). When patients receiving sildenafil were combined into a single treatment group, mean PAP at trough was significantly reduced by 26.7 mm Hg (95% CI −11.6 to −1.8) compared with placebo ($p=0.010$).

A statistically significant difference was also observed among the three groups in changes from baseline to week 12 in mean PAP measured 1 hour post-dose ($p = 0.001$). Sildenafil 25 mg and 100 mg reduced mean PAP by −11.4 mm Hg (95% CI −16.7 to −6.1) and −11.8 mm Hg (95% CI −18.0 to −5.6), respectively, compared with placebo. When patients receiving sildenafil were combined into a single treatment group, mean PAP at 1 hour post-dose was significantly reduced by 211.6 mm Hg (95% CI −16.3 to −6.9) compared with placebo ($p<0.001$).

PVR

There was no statistically significant difference among the three groups in changes from baseline to week 12 in PVR measured at trough levels and at 1 hour post-dose. The treatment effects of sildenafil 25 mg and 100 mg 8-hourly compared with placebo at trough levels were 16.2 dyne s/cm^{-5} (95% CI −137.3 to 169.7) and 276.9 dyne.s/cm^{-5} (95% CI −257.0 to 103.2). The treatment effect for the lower dose of sildenafil compared with placebo at 1 hour post-dose was 289.1 dyne.s/cm5 (95% CI 2214.7 to 36.5) and for the higher dose −129.9 dyne.s/cm^{-5} (95% CI −277.2 to 17.4). For the combined sildenafil treatments the effect size was −17.1 dyne.s/cm^{-5} (95% CI −157.4 to 123.2) and −103.7 dyne.s/cm^{-5} (95% CI −215.9 to 8.6) for trough and 1 hour post-dose measurements, respectively.

CARDIAC OUTPUT

There was no statistically significant difference among the three groups in changes from baseline to week 12 in cardiac output measured at trough levels ($p=0.051$), so no further statistical comparisons were carried out. The treatment effects at trough levels were −1.0 l/min (95% CI −2.1 to 0.1) and 0.5 l/min (95% CI −0.8 to 1.9) for the lower and higher doses of sildenafil compared with placebo. When patients receiving sildenafil were combined into a single treatment group, cardiac output at trough levels was reduced by was −0.4 l/min (95% CI −1.6 to 0.7) but was not significantly different from placebo. No statistically significant difference was observed among the three groups in changes from baseline to week 12 in cardiac output measured at 1 hour post-dose. The respective treatment effects for the lower and higher doses of sildenafil compared with placebo at 1 hour post-dose were −0.6

l/min (95% CI −1.8 to 0.6) and −0.2 l/min (95% CI −1.2 to 1.6). For the combined sildenafil treatments the effect size was −0.3 l/min (95% CI −1.4 to 0.8) for 1 hour post-dose.

6MW DISTANCE

There was a statistically significant difference among the three groups in changes from baseline to week 12 in 6MW distance (p=0.028). The increase on sildenafil 25 mg 8-hourly was 45.4 m (95% CI 11.5 to 79.4; p=0.011) and on sildenafil 100 mg 8-hourly it was 40.0 m (95% CI 0.2 to 79.8; p=0.049) compared with placebo. For the combined sildenafil treatment groups there was a statistically significant treatment effect size (p=0.007) of 43.5 m, compared with placebo (95% CI 13.4 to 72.6).

OTHER PARAMETERS

There was a statistically significant difference among the three groups in changes from baseline to week 12 in physical symptom score (p=0.024). The treatment effect for the lower and higher doses of sildenafil compared with placebo were 8.4 (95% CI 20.2 to 17.0) and 14.0 (95% CI 4.0 to 24.1; p=0.009), respectively. For the combined sildenafil treatments the statistically significant treatment effect size (p=0.012) was 10.4 compared with placebo (95% CI 2.5 to 18.3). There was no significant treatment effect on systemic blood pressure. Sildenafil was well tolerated. All subjects reported some improvement in wellbeing and no adverse effects were reported.

Discussion

In an earlier study we have demonstrated that exposure to hypoxia produces a rapid and sustained rise in PAP in humans. Oral treatment with sildenafil 100 mg, a PDE5 inhibitor, markedly inhibits this rise in healthy volunteers without significantly affecting systemic blood pressure [1].

Chronic treatment with the PDE5 inhibitor sildenafil was associated with a reduction in mean PAP and an improvement in exercise capacity and physical symptom score [17]. The small number of patients per treatment group resulted in a low power to detect statistically significant differences in other parameters.

Previous studies have provided evidence of therapeutic benefit from sildenafil in patients with pulmonary arterial hypertension, idiopathic or associated with collagen lung disease [18,20] and in chronic thromboembolic disease [21]. One study of five patients (four with idiopathic pulmonary arterial hypertension) in which haemodynamic measurements were made by cardiac catheterisation, reported a fall in mean PAP and PVR of 18 mm Hg and 706 dyne s cm^{-5}, respectively, with sildenafil 50 mg three times daily for 3 months [19]. Another study of nine patients (seven with pulmonary arterial hypertension) reported a 5 mm Hg fall in mean PAP with sildenafil 50 mg taken every 8 hours for 3 months [20]. In 12 patients with chronic thromboembolic disease, sildenafil 50 mg given 8-hourly reduced mean PAP by 7.7 mm Hg and PVR by 574 dyne s cm^{-5} [21]. A recent double blind, placebo controlled, crossover study of sildenafil 25–100 mg 8-hourly (dose according to body weight) for 6 weeks in 22 patients with idiopathic pulmonary arterial hypertension reported a 7 mm Hg decrease in mean PAP calculated from Doppler echocardiography derived measurements [20]. In this context, a fall in mean PAP from untreated levels in our study of around 6 mm Hg at the end of a dosing interval and 11 mm Hg 1 hour after dosing is consistent with these reports.

By comparison, the increase in exercise capacity in our study was modest compared with the effect reported in idiopathic and collagen disease related pulmonary arterial hypertension, where the 6MW distance increased by 112–225 m. It is recognised that the natural history of HAPH differs from that of idiopathic pulmonary arterial hypertension and pulmonary hypertension associated with collagen lung disease. It is evident, for example, that life expectancy is substantially better in HAPH. In keeping with this, our study population was older and the baseline 6MW distance was greater (418–456 m) than in reports of sildenafil use in other forms of pulmonary arterial hypertension studied to date (226–376 m). Nonetheless, physical activity was limited in our patient group, as demonstrated by the questionnaire, and baseline PAP and PVR were raised, even at 760 m. Patients from the same region who died of HAPH had remodelled pulmonary arterioles. The increase in exercise distance and improvement in physical activity score, together with a reduction in PAP, is consistent with a beneficial response to sildenafil.

This study extends our finding in an earlier report that sildenafil attenuates the acute pressor response to hypoxia in healthy Kyrgyz volunteers [1] and a recent study in mountaineers and trekkers [22]. The latter, using echocardiography, reported that sildenafil reduced systolic PAP during exercise and increased maximum exercise performance. The effects of PDE5 inhibition on pulmonary vessels are thought to be mediated by cyclic GMP-dependent factors, particularly NO and natriuretic factors.

Nonetheless, sildenafil is a promising treatment for the management of HAPH, a condition for which there are few treatment options. Calcium antagonists are used but have to be given in relatively high doses, lack specificity for the pulmonary vascular bed and side effects such as ankle oedema are frequent [23, 24]. Sildenafil had little effect on systemic blood pressure and was well tolerated. It is relatively expensive for a country with poor health resources and a larger study of the long-term effects of PDE5 inhibition in HAPH is warranted before sildenafil can be widely recommended.

References

1. Zhao L, Mason NA, Morrell NW, Kojonazarov B.K., et al. Sildenafil inhibits hypoxia-induced pulmonary hypertension. Circulation 2001;104:424–8.
2. Aldashev AA, Sarybaev AS, Sydykov AS, et al. Characterization of high altitude pulmonary hypertension in the Kyrgyz: association with angiotensin-converting enzyme genotype. Am J Respir Crit Care Med. 2002;166:1396–402.
3. Moore LG, Niermeyer S, Zamudio S. Human adaptation to high altitude: regional and life-cycle perspectives. Am J Phys Anthropol 1998;27:25–64.
4. Ward MP, Milledge JS, West J. High altitude medicine and physiology. New York: Oxford University Press, 2000:434.
5. Heath D. Missing link from Tibet. Thorax 1989;44:981–3.
6. Heath D, Williams D, Rios-Dalenz J, et al. Small pulmonary arterial vessels of Aymara Indians from the Bolivian Andes. Histopathology 1990;16:565–71.
7. Maggiorini M, Leon-Velarde F. High-altitude pulmonary hypertension: a pathophysiological entity to different diseases. Eur Respir J. 2003;22:1019–25.
8. Fagan KA, McMurtry I, Rodman DM. Nitric oxide synthase in pulmonary hypertension: lessons from knockout mice. Physiol Res 2000;49:539–48.
9. Beall CM, Laskowski D, Strohl KP, et al. Pulmonary nitric oxide in mountain dwellers. Nature 2001;414:411–2.
10. Anand IS, Prasad BA, Chugh SS, et al. Effects of inhaled nitric oxide and oxygen in high-altitude pulmonary edema. Circulation 1998;98:2441–5.
11. Ignarro LJ, Cirino G, Casini A, et al. Nitric oxide as a signaling molecule in the vascular system: an overview. J Cardiovasc Pharmacol 1999;34:879–86.
12. Thomas MK, Francis SH, Corbin JD. Characterisation of a purified bovine lung cGMP-binding cGMP phosphodiesterase. J Biol Chem. 1990;265:14964–70.
13. Schermuly RT, Kreisselmeier KP, Ghofrani HA, et al. Chronic sildenafil treatment inhibits monocrotaline-induced pulmonary hypertension in rats. Am J Respir Crit Care Med 2004;169:39–45.
14. Itoh T, Nagaya N, Fujii T, et al. A combination of oral sildenafil and beraprost ameliorates pulmonary hypertension in rats. Am J Respir Crit Care Med 2004;169:34–8.
15. Sebkhi A, Strange JW, Phillips SC, et al. Phosphodiesterase type 5 as a target for the treatment of hypoxia-induced pulmonary hypertension. Circulation 2003;107:3230–5.
16. Green CP, Porter CB, Bresnahan DR, et al. Development and evaluation of the Kansas City Cardiomyopathy Questionnaire: a new health status measure for heart failure. J Am Coll Cardiol 2000;35:1245–55.
17. Aldashev A.A., Kojonazarov B.K., Amatov T.A., Sooronbaev T.M., Mirrakhimov M.M., Morrell N.W., Wharton J, Wilkins M.R. Phosphodiesterase type 5 and high altitude pulmonary hypertension. Thorax. 2005; 60 (8):683-687.
18. Mikhail GW, Prasad SK, Li W, et al. Clinical and haemodynamic effects of sildenafil in pulmonary hypertension: acute and mid-term effects. Eur Heart J 2004;25:431–6.
19. Michelakis ED, Tymchak W, Noga M, et al. Long-term treatment with oral sildenafil is safe and improves functional capacity and hemodynamics in patients with pulmonary arterial hypertension. Circulation 2003;108:2066–9.
20. Sastry BK, Narasimhan C, Reddy NK, et al. A study of clinical efficacy of sildenafil in patients with primary pulmonary hypertension. Indian Heart J 2002;54:410–4.

21. Ghofrani HA, Schermuly RT, Rose F, et al. Sildenafil for long-term treatment of non-operable chronic thromboembolic pulmonary hypertension. Am J Respir Crit Care Med 2003;167:1139–41.
22. Ghofrani HA, Reichenberger F, Kohstall MG, et al. Sildenafil increased exercise capacity during hypoxia at low altitudes and at Mount Everest base camp: a randomized, double-blind, placebo-controlled crossover trial. Ann Intern Med 2004;141:169–77.
23. Hackett PH, Roach RC. High-altitude illness. N Engl J Med 2001;345:107–14.
24. Rich S, Kaufmann E, Levy PS. The effect of high doses of calcium-channel blockers on survival in primary pulmomary hypertension. N Engl J Med 1992;327:76–81.

CHAPTER 10

THE ROLE OF ANTIOXIDANTS IN MODULATION OF ACCLIMATIZATION PROCESSES

ASHYRALY Z. ZURDINOV

Clinical and Basic Pharmacology Department, Kyrgyz Medical Academy, Bishkek, Kyrgyzstan

Abstract: The purpose of this paper is to present pulmonary results of research on the pharmacological optimization of adaptation processes and a capacity for work in conditions of high-altitude hypoxia with the use of some actoprotectors and antihypoxants (bemitil, sodium oxybutyrate, and others).

Keywords: Altitude; acclimatization; antioxidant

Introduction

Research into mechanisms of human and animal adaptation to extreme environmental conditions, including high-altitude hypoxia, is very important, especially for our country. At the same time, a necessity for optimization of the processes of acclimatization and capacity for work has a topical significance because of further intensification of the industrial development of inaccessible regions. It is obvious that along with other (technical, physiological, etc.) ways of improving adaptation processes and maintaining capacity for work in extreme conditions, in particular in high-altitude conditions, an extreme necessity for the application of pharmacological drugs with protective properties exists. On this point, groups of drugs with antihypoxic, antioxidative and actoprotective properties are certainly of interest.

Based on this, the purpose of the present research was an investigation of the possibility of pharmacological optimization of adaptation processes and the capacity for work in conditions of high-altitude hypoxia, with the use of some actoprotectors and antihypoxants (bemitil, sodium oxybutyrate and others).

A. Aldashev and R. Naeije (eds.), Problems of High Altitude Medicine and Biology, 145–150.

Materials and Research Methods

The research was carried out with the participation of 54 volunteers (aged 18–21). Investigations were carried out in summer (July-August) in Bishkek (foothills, 760 m above sea level, base data) and in various periods of stay of the people tested in high-altitude conditions, during the execution of building and assembly works (at 3,200 m above sea level). The tested subjects arrived at the indicated place after a 2-day journey from Bishkek (by aircraft and then by bus) with an overnight stop at an intermediate altitude. Research using psychophysiological methods was done on the 2nd and 3rd day, and then every week of their stay in the mountains for 1 month. The lability of the visual analyzer was investigated by testing the critical frequency of flicker fusion (CFFF). Flashing lights with an on/off time ratio of 2 Hz were reproduced on red light-emitting diodes. The speed of sensory and motor response was investigated by timing the simple motor reaction (TSMR) to light (releasing the button in response to a lit red, light-emitting diode). Sensor and motor coordination was investigated by their reaction to a moving object (RMO). The speed of elementary decision making in a task of problem of choice ("reaction of choice") was estimated by the timing of correct answers to a lit red, light-emitting diode at the accidental showing of a green signal. Three indices of attention were used: volume (according to Shulte's monochrome table), stability (according to test of entangled lines) and distribution by a modified test of rest.

Tested preparations – bemitil, sodium oxybutyrate and their combinations – were prescribed by courses of 5 days with 2-day intervals from the 3rd day of their stay in the mountains after measurement of the main indices of the research parameters. Preparations were prescribed as follows: bemitil tablets in 0.25 twice a day (in the morning and in the afternoon), sodium oxybutyrate in sugary syrup in 0.5 twice a day (in the afternoon and at night), and a combination at an indicated time in the cited doses during a meal under our control. People included in the control group received "placebo" (tablets and sugary syrup). The inspected persons were divided into four randomized groups, which received preparations or a "placebo." the research was carried out using the controllable blind method. Further research was done after finishing each course, on the intervening days when no preparations were taken, during 1 month. Altogether, in conditions of high altitude, five investigations were carried out: 2nd–3rd days of stay (basic indices in mountains); after finishing the first course of preparations (8th–9th days); after the second course (15th–16th days); after the third course (22nd–23rd days); and after the fourth course (29th–30th days).

Results of Research

The results of the psychophysiological investigations conducted are shown in Tables 1–4, where it can be seen that during the first 2–3 days of adaptation to high altitude, the level of wakefulness of the examined persons had notably decreased, and the functional condition of their sensor and motor response and coordination systems, as well as attentiveness, had worsened. It may be a reason for a decreasing in the ability to reproduce sensory and operant components of an activity.

Later, on the whole, positive dynamics of research indices were noticed in the case of people who took "placebos." This may attest to the gradual adaptation of these systems to high-altitude conditions. However, on the 1st–2nd week of working in the mountains, additional peaks of worsening

TABLE 1. A dynamics of lability of visual analyzer (according to CFFF test) and speed of sensor and motor response (according to TSMR test) when taking preparations in different periods of a 30-day adaptation to high-altitude conditions

Conditions of research	CFFF	TSMR (m/s)
Low altitude (760 m above sea level)	30.82 ± 0.086	229.96 ± 7.64
3,200 m above sea level		
2nd–3rd days of stay (before taking preparations)	28.1 ± 0.095*	232.3 ± 6.12
8th–9th days of stay		
"Placebo"	29.7 ± 0.123	279.3 ± 8.4*
Bemitil	29.2 ± 0.102	295.7 ± 9.8*
Sodium oxybutyrate	29.7 ± 0.141	263.2 ± 10.8*
Bemitil + sodium oxybutyrate	28.9 ± 0.36	278.5 ± 7.7*
15th–16th days of stay		
"Placebo"	28.8 ± 0.265	272.6 ± 5.34*
Bemitil	28.6 ± 0.22	277.2 ± 8.85*
Sodium oxybutyrate	29.6 ± 0.412	256.7 ± 6.06*
Bemitil + sodium oxybutyrate	29.5 ± 0.241	270.0 ± 15.3*
22nd–23rd days of stay		
"Placebo"	29.1 ± 0.088	268.5 ± 8.36*
Bemitil	28.8 ± 0.077	275.6 ± 14.9*
Sodium oxybutyrate	29.4 ± 0.20	246.2 ± 5.5
Bemitil + sodium oxybutyrate	29.22 ± 0.20	260.3 ± 18.2
29th–30th days of stay		
"Placebo"	29.12 ± 0.142	261.39 ± 7.639
Bemitil	29.3 ± 0.153	254.0 ± 8.3
Sodium oxybutyrate	28.9 ± 1.63	252.4 ± 7.13
Bemitil + sodium oxybutyrate	29.24 ± 0.126	241.7 ± 13.31

*Statistically significant difference ($p < 0.05$) from base level (low-altitude conditions).

TABLE 2. A dynamics of index of sensor and motor coordination (according to reaction to moving object) and time of reaction of choosing during taking preparations in process of monthly adaptation to high-altitude conditions

Conditions of research	Deviations in positions	Hits the mark in %	m/s	Error in %
Low altitude (760 m above sea level)	1.54 ± 0.25	22.73 ± 3.76	364.5 ± 11.71	2.71 ± 1.47
3,200 m above sea level				
2nd–3rd days of stay (before taking preparations)	3.6 ± 0.19*	6 ± 1.23	497.7 ± 23.5*	23.3 ± 3.85*
8th–9th days of stay "placebo"	3.11 ± 0.55*	8.0 ± 2.91*	503 ± 31.3*	14 ± 4.27*
Bemitil	2.45 ± 1.15*	20 ± 10	492.1 ± 27*	17.5 ± 5.9
Sodium oxybutyrate	2.8 ± 0.33	13.3 ± 2.11	425.7 ± 34.1*	30 ± 6.83*
Bemitil + sodium oxybutyrate	2.35 ± 0.35*	15 ± 4.28	417.96 ± 14.33	13.33 ± 6.66*
15th–16th days of stay "placebo"	2.57 ± 0.35*	18 ± 2.49	456 ± 22.5*	16 ± 4.99*
Bemitil	2.96 ± 0.46*	12.5 ± 4.91	486.6 ± 27.9*	12.5 ± 5.26*
Sodium oxybutyrate	2.88 ± 0.38*	4 ± 4*	473.2 ± 31.7*	24 ± 7.48*
Bemitil + sodium oxybutyrate	2.43 ± 0.50*	11.7 ± 4.01*	456.3 ± 28.3*	10 ± 6.83*
22nd–23rd days of stay				
"Placebo"	2.67 ± 0.33*	12 ± 2.91*	475.2 ± 15.2*	4 ± 4.0
Bemitil	2.23 ± 0.27*	16.2 ± 3.75	456 ± 23.9*	7.5 ± 5.26
Sodium oxybutyrate	2.25 ± 0.30*	16.7 ± 5.6	400.8 ± 17.85	18.3 ± 9.1
Bemitil + sodium oxybutyrate	1.85 ± 0.20	18.3 ± 3.1	443.1 ± 24.8	3.3 ± 3.3
29th–30th days of stay "placebo"	1.33 ± 0.17	20 ± 5.77	437.82 ± 11.61*	7 ± 4.22
Bemitil	1.55 ± 0.23	26.2 ± 4.19	429.7 ± 32.42	5 ± 3.27
Sodium oxybutyrate			397.4 ± 17.02	16.7 ± 6.14
Bemitil + sodium oxybutyrate			415.8 ± 11.54	4 ± 2

*Statistically significant difference ($p < 0.05$) from base level (low-altitude conditions)

psychophysiological condition according to several indices were revealed: the TSMR to light, reaction of choice, etc.

From the 3rd and 4th weeks of staying in the mountains a recovery in some psychophysiological indices was noticed. RMO, reaction of choice and stability of attentiveness were recovered to the level that was noted in the foothills. The other indices remained modified in comparison with values obtained in low-altitude conditions.

As for the effects of the investigated preparations on the psychophysiological condition of the tested persons during their adaptation to conditions of high altitude, they were ambiguous and not of the same kind. In accordance with the lability of the visual analyzer (TSMR test) the most optimal effect was observed with the use of sodium oxybutyrate, especially during the initial period staying in the mountains and a tendency to worsen was noticed with the use of bemitil and its combination with sodium oxybutyrate.

TABLE 3. A dynamics of index of distribution (ID) and volume of attentiveness (VA) when taking preparations in different periods of a 30-day adaptation to high-altitude conditions

Conditions of research	ID	VA
Low altitude (760 m above sea level)	331.1 ± 14.53	35.19 ± 1.56
3,200 m above sea level		
2nd–3rd days of stay (before taking preparations)	449.6 ± 17.9*	46.4 ± 2.83*
8th–9th days of stay "placebo"	454.39 ± 30.67*	39.4 ± 2.89
Bemitil	460.9 ± 45.6*	38.2 ± 2.15
Sodium oxybutyrate	418.2 ± 33.0*	41.9 ± 4.12*
Bemitil + sodium oxybutyrate	376.9 ± 22.12	41.1 ± 2.57*
15th–16th days of stay "placebo"	435.3 ± 22.0*	40.2 ± 2.23
Bemitil	472.3 ± 50.1*	37.2 ± 2.37
Sodium oxybutyrate	431.5 ± 33.2*	40.4 ± 4.50
Bemitil + sodium oxybutyrate	457.3 ± 44.2*	38.9 ± 2.15
22nd–23rd days of stay		
"Placebo"	436.4 ± 27.9*	36.7 ± 1.77
Bemitil	435.4 ± 31.6*	33.9 ± 1.67
Sodium oxybutyrate	410.3 ± 19.7*	38.8 ± 4.15
Bemitil + sodium oxybutyrate	424.7 ± 35.7*	37.63 ± 3.2
29th–30th days of stay "placebo"	377.81 ± 14.49	38.49 ± 1.97
Bemitil	356.6 ± 19.2	36.7 ± 1.70
Sodium oxybutyrate	404.5 ± 24.19*	38.2 ± 3.47
Bemitil + sodium oxybutyrate	386.0 ± 29.56	36.5 ± 2.12

*Statistically significant difference ($p < 0.05$) from base level (low-altitude conditions)

According to the level of sensor and motor response (TSMR) the most optimal effect was detected for sodium oxybutyrate and also for a combination of this preparation with bemitil.

Recovery of functional condition of sensor and motor coordination systems was most rapid and exceeded the level of the "placebo" during the intake of bemitil, and a smaller effect was noticed in the cases of a combination of bemitil and sodium oxybutyrate and sodium oxybutyrate alone.

The results obtained attested that on the whole, taking sodium oxybutyrate in the doses used and the approved scheme has a more optimal influence than "placebos," bemitil, and its combination with sodium oxybutyrate increase some indices of psychophysiological condition in the initial period of staying in the mountains. However, in conditions of high altitude, this preparation may show no significant or a negative, effect on indices of volume and stability of attentiveness.

In conditions of high altitude, the functional state of sensor and motor coordination systems and attentiveness took a turn for the better with the dose used and the scheme for bemitil intake. But it should be pointed out

TABLE 4. Changes in index of stability of attentiveness (ISA) when taking preparations in different periods of a30-day adaptation to high-altitude conditions

Condition of research	ISA	
	s	Errors in %
Low altitude (760 m above sea level)	2.13 ± 0.084	2.73 ± 1.47
3,200 m above sea level		
2nd–3rd days of stay (before taking preparations)	2.75 ± 0.162*	7.93 ± 1.6*
8th–9th days of stay "placebo"	3.03 ± 0.141*	4 ± 1.63*
Bemitil	3.67 ± 0.262*	7.5 ± 2.5*
Sodium oxybutyrate	3.07 ± 0.117*	8.33 ± 3.07*
Bemitil + sodium oxybutyrate	3.16 ± 0.145*	6.66 ± 2.1087*
15th–16th days of stay "placebo"	2.37 ± 0.17	4 ± 1.63*
Bemitil	2.24 ± 0.113	2.5 ± 1.64
Sodium oxybutyrate	2.23 ± 0.069	10 ± 4.17
Bemitil + sodium oxybutyrate	2.38 ± 0.175	1.67 ± 1.67
22nd–23rd days of stay		
"Placebo"	2.34 ± 0.13	7 ± 2.13*
Bemitil	2.38 ± 0.056	3.75 ± 1.83
Sodium oxybutyrate	2.5 ± 0.23*	8.3 ± 4.01
Bemitil + sodium oxybutyrate	2.2 ± 0.17	8.3 ± 3.1
29th–30th days of stay		
"Placebo"	2.27 ± 0.143	3 ± 1.33
Bemitil	2.14 ± 0.129	6.25 ± 1.83*
Sodium oxybutyrate	2.18 ± 0.37	8.33 ± 1.66*
Bemitil + sodium oxybutyrate	1.92 ± 0.28	8 ± 2*

*Statistically significant difference ($p < 0.05$) from base level (low-altitude conditions)

that this preparation did not have an optimizing influence on some other psychophysiological indices.

The psychophysiological effects of a combination of bemitil with sodium oxybutyrate were not very marked.

Thus, it may be considered that for the correction of psychopshysiological conditions during the initial period of adaptation to high altitude, the prescription of sodium oxybutyrate at night is more acceptable. However, at the same time, it should be considered that this preparation may slightly worsen some indices of attentiveness. As for bemitil and its combination with sodium oxybutyrate, it is obvious that they do not correct operator activity in acute periods of adaptation to high-altitude conditions. Bemitil, in the tested dose and scheme of intake, may be most useful of all to human activity, which requires the mobilization of sensor and motor coordination and the volume of attentiveness.

CHAPTER 11

GENE POLYMORPHISMS AND HIGH ALTITUDE PULMONARY HYPERTENSION

ALMAZ A. ALDASHEV

Institute of Molecular Biology and Medicine, Bishkek, Kyrgyzstan

Abstract: High altitude pulmonary hypertension (HAPH) is a genetically determined trait, associated with the diminished oxygen content at high altitudes and it usually affects native or long-term highlanders and may reflect a loss of adaptation. This paper reviews the epidemiological evidence for a genetic trait of the altitude-related illnesses, mainly HAPH, as well as the molecular evidence for the contribution of the specific candidate genes or pathways involved. We focus on our own data and experience in the research of genetics of HAPH done on the indigenous population of Pamir and Tien-Shan mountains. These data include the existence or lack of association of polymorphisms of ACE gene, β_2–adrenoreceptor gene, C677T polymorphism of MTHFR gene, 838 C>A polymorphism of p27kip1, polymorphisms of eNOS gene and S/L polymorphism of 5-HTT gene.

The paper closes with a discussion on what could be the future of the expansion of the existing database of the genetic risk factors and polymorphisms involved in the development of HAPH.

Keywords: HAPH; hypoxic pulmonary hypertension; altitude sickness; genetic epidemiology; gene polymorphism

Introduction

High-altitude pulmonary hypertension (HAPH) is a public health problem in the mountainous areas of the world, including Kyrgyzstan. In Kyrgyzstan the Tien-Shan and Pamir mountains occupy about 90% of the territory and a significant part of the population live at an altitude higher than 2400 m above sea level.

The normal adult pulmonary circulation is a low-pressure, high-flow vascular bed with a great capacity for vascular recruitment. A unique feature of the pulmonary, as opposed to the systemic, circulation is vasoconstriction, observed at decreased levels of alveolar oxygen [64].

A. Aldashev and R. Naeije (eds.), Problems of High Altitude Medicine and Biology, 151–168.

HAPH is characterized by increased pulmonary arterial pressure (PAP) and vascular wall remodelling of the pulmonary artery compromising intimal lesions, hypertrophy of tunica media and adventitial thickening of pulmonary arteries [50,2,21,3,6]. HAPH is complicated by right ventricular hypertrophy, which could be the cause of right ventricular failure [43]. A number of factors are known to influence the development of HAPH, including the ventilatory response to hypoxia [43]. Genetic susceptibility to hypoxia-induced pulmonary hypertension in some individuals is suggested by a number of observations. The propensity to develop HAPH varies substantially among individuals, with some people seemingly resistant and while others appear to be susceptible. It is due to large interindividual differences in the magnitude of the pulmonary pressure response to hypoxia, with some subjects demonstrating exaggerated increases in pulmonary arterial pressure [6]. It was shown that susceptibility to hypoxic pulmonary hypertension in cattle ("brisket disease") is an inherited trait [66]. Moreover, strains of rat have been described with differing susceptibilities to hypoxia-induced pulmonary hypertension [4,54].

The patterns of inheritance are modulated by penetrance and gene–environment interactions (the condition is genetic, but manifests only under certain conditions), this is especially true in altitude-related diseases, which are by definition environment-dependent conditions. There is familial evidence for a genetic contribution to HAPH. Lin et al. (1984) described 13 first-degree relatives of patients with HAPH living at altitudes between 3200 and 3500 m in Qinghai, China. One patient had both siblings and children who also developed the condition, while two other patients had affected siblings [39].

HAPH occurs in both native Tibetans and Han Chinese (recent migrants to the Tibetan plateau) [49,71]. But the frequency is much lower in indigenous Tibetans than in indigenous Andeans, an observation sometimes cited as evidence that the former population is differentially [8] and perhaps better, adapted [45], which would suggest that there is some genetic basis to susceptibility that has been under either longer, greater, or more rapid selection in the Tibetans than in the Andeans. Most researchers assume that Tibetans have been at altitude for many more generations than Andeans and therefore have had more time to adapt; however, analysis of Y-chromosome haplotypes [58] indicates that the antecedents of the extant Tibetan populations migrated from the much lower Yellow River Basin about 6000 years ago, which is several thousand years later than conservative estimates place the occupation of the Andes [52].

The incidence of HAPH is also much lower in Tibetans than in the Han Chinese, a population that recently migrated to the Tibetan plateau [24]. This may reflect a genetic advantage of the Tibetans, who have lower hematocrits [23,71] and reduced pulmonary vascular musculature [27], both of which will minimize pulmonary pressure and are influenced by genetic background (interestingly, reduced pulmonary musculature is a hallmark of altitude adaptation in bovids, such as yaks), in which it is inherited as a simple Mendelian dominant trait.

Polymorphisms are variant sites within genes that originated as a mutation in an individual and have since spread in the population (i.e., is at a frequency greater than what can be accounted for by mutation rates alone). They can be single nucleotide polymorphisms (SNPs) in which one nucleotide base is substituted for another, the insertion or deletion of a single base or a segment of DNA, variations in the length of repeating DNA sequences. Polymorphisms can occur in regulatory regions, where they may affect the activity of the gene (altering either the degree or specificity of expression); in the coding sequences, where they may alter the sequence of the protein (although, as the translational code is redundant, SNPs in the coding sequence are often silent and do not alter the protein sequence); or in introns. For a long time, polymorphisms in introns were assumed to be of no consequence; however, recent observations suggest that introns may play a variety of roles in gene structure, function and regulation [19]. By altering the structure or quantity of a relevant protein, a polymorphism could contribute to the susceptibility to or protection from, altitude-related illnesses. Association studies compare the frequency of alleles at polymorphic loci between groups of people with (i.e., cases) and without (i.e., controls) the condition. An allele that is statistically overrepresented in the affected cohort is said to be associated with the condition. Both to conserve resources and to avoid the statistical problems that arise when performing multiple tests [32], most association studies look at variations in candidate genes, which are genes that encode components of structures, pathways, or processes that are known (or suspected) to be involved in the etiology of the disease. A number of candidate gene polymorphisms have been assessed in the various forms of altitude-related illness.

Vasoactive factors implicated in the pathogenesis of HAPH are endothelin-1, angiotensin converting enzyme (ACE), angiothensin II, serotonin, nitric oxide (NO), bradykinin, prostaglandins and others. For example, we demonstrated an association between the I allele of I/D polymorphism of ACE gene and development of HAPH [6]. Taraseviciene-Stewart et al. (2005) showed that bradykinin B2 agonist demonstrates the capacity to reduce severe pulmonary hypertension, right ventricular hypertrophy and induce apoptosis of hyperproliferative cells in pre-capillary pulmonary arterioles in rats [59]. Eddahibi et al (2000, 2001) showed that serotonin (5-hydroxytryptamine, 5-HT) and its transporter (5-HTT) play a critical role in the pulmonary vascular smooth muscle hyperplasia and vascular remodelling associated with experimental hypoxic pulmonary hypertension (PH) and human primary PH [16,17].

High Altitude Pulmonary Hypertension in the Indigenous Population of Kyrgyzstan

The results of our last 10 years study elucidating the candidate gene polymorphisms involved in genesis HAPH are also presented in this paper.

Ethnic Kyrgyz subjects (all 689 of them) aged 17 to 86 years (mean age 37.8 ± 0.9) who were residents at an altitude 2500–4200 m above sea level in the Naryn and Pamir regions were studied. All subjects underwent health screening by history, physical examination, spirometry, blood pressure measurement and ECG. Right heart catheterization studies were performed in 147 highlanders aged 18–72 years (mean age 34.0 ± 13.1) with symptoms of dyspnea or exercise limitation at altitude, ECG and Echo-signs of HAPH [7,36].

The ethics committee of the National Center of Cardiology and Internal Medicine (Bishkek, Kyrgyz Republic) approved the study and all subjects gave informed consent.

Right heart catheterization was performed when brought to Bishkek (760 m above sea level) with a Swan-Ganz thermodilution catheter introduced via the jugular vein. After 30 minutes of stabilization, baseline measurements were made of systolic, diastolic and mean pulmonary arterial pressure and pulmonary capillary wedge pressure. To assess the magnitude of the pressor response to acute hypoxia, subjects were required to breathe a hypoxic gas mixture (11% oxygen, 89% nitrogen) for 30 minutes, at the end of which hemodynamic measurements were repeated. Arterial oxygen saturation and ECG were monitored throughout. There were no significant complications from right heart catheterization in any of the subjects studied.

High altitude pulmonary hypertension was diagnosed if resting mean PAP was ≥ 25 mmHg [6].

Data are presented as means ± standard error of the mean (SEM). Demographic parameters were compared between groups by unpaired two-sample Student t test. Allele and genotype distributions in the pulmonary hypertensive and control groups were compared using contingency tables, with the Fisher exact test where appropriate. Single factor analysis of variance and the nonparametric Kruskal–Wallis test were employed to compare mean pulmonary artery pressure in patients with different ACE genotypes.

The majority (52.5%) of studied highlanders had normal values for resting mean pulmonary arterial pressure. However, 66 subjects (47.5%) had pulmonary hypertension defined as a mean pulmonary arterial pressure equal to or greater than 25 mm Hg. Inhalation of a hypoxic gas mixture increased pulmonary arterial pressure in most subjects. In 34 subjects (24.5%) with normal resting pressures, there was a greater than twofold increase in pulmonary arterial pressure at acute hypoxia. We referred to this

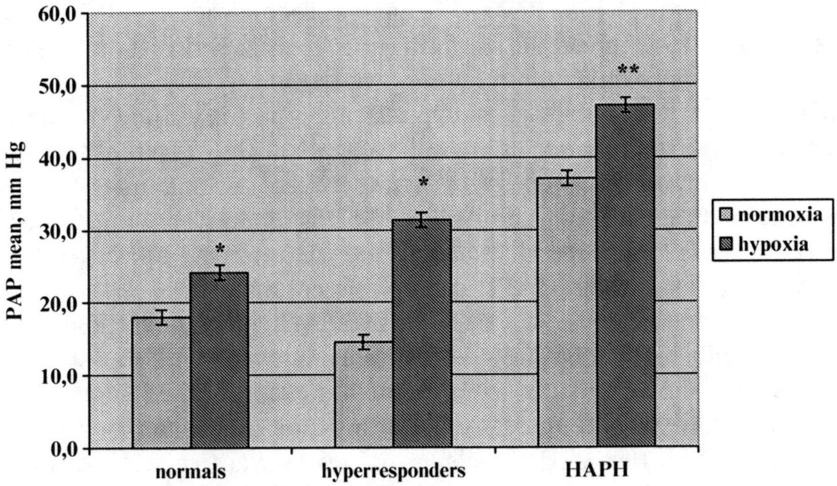

Figure 1. Highlanders could be divided into three groups on the basis of resting pulmonary arterial pressure and response to breathing 11% Oxygen for 30 minutes. $^*p<0.05$, $^{**}p<0.01$ – compared with corresponding normoxic pressure.

group as hyperresponders [6]. Thus, the highlanders could be divided into three groups on the basis of the hemodynamic response to acute hypoxia:

Group 1 - normoresponders, normal resting mean pulmonary artery pressure with a less than twofold increase in MPAP during acute hypoxia;

Group 2 - hyperresponders, normal resting mean pulmonary arterial pressure with a twofold or greater increase in MPAP during acute hypoxia;

Group 3 - HAPH cases, MPAP greater than 25 mm Hg.

The mean pulmonary arterial pressures and response to acute hypoxia for each group are shown in Figure 1.

I/D, G2215A, G2350A polymorphisms of ACE gene, Arg16Gly and Glu27Gln polymorphisms of β_2-adrenoreceptor gene, 4a/b and G894T polymorphisms of eNOS gene, S/L polymorphism of serotonin transporter (5-HTT) gene, C838A polymorphism of p27kip1 gene and C677T polymorphism of methylenetetrahydrofolate reductase (MTHFR) gene were studied in these highlanders with or without HAPH.

Polymorphisms of Ace Gene

Angiotensin-converting enzyme (ACE) could be the candidate gene in the development of HAPH. ACE is a metalloproteinase catalyzing cleavage of dipeptide from angiotensin-1, which produces a very potent vasoconstrictor angiotensin-2 (AT-2). ACE is also known to be involved in degradation of the vasodilator bradykinin. Beyond being a vasoconstrictor, AT-2 stimulates proliferation of endothelial and smooth muscle cells and is therefore one of the key players in vascular remodelling processes [53].

ACE levels fall in response to hypoxia and the magnitude of the fall is greater in individuals that acclimate well to hypoxia [42]. The most commonly studied ACE polymorphism is an insertion (ACE-I) or deletion (ACE-D) of an intronic Alu repeat unit. The ACE-I allele is associated with lower circulating ACE levels [56]. Several studies found the alternate allele (ACE-D) to be more common in their HAPE-susceptible cohort [31,48], although other studies failed to replicate the correlation [14,37,31]. Surprisingly, Tsianos et al. (2005) reported a higher climbing success rate associated with the ACE-I allele and it has been shown to be overrepresented in accomplished climbers [44].

Finally, in our several studies of high altitude pulmonary hypertension, we have found that the ACE-I allele and II homozygote genotype was more common in people with established HAPH [47,6]. It seems very contradictory with the data on the association of ACE-I with better acclimatization to hypoxia and climbing success, but it is rational. In better acclimatization and adaptation to high-altitude, the main aim is to select out the alleles associated with acute and fatal altitude-associated illnesses like HAPE and HACE. ACE is involved in the production of the vasoconstrictor angiotensin-2, degradation of the vasodilator bradykinin and fluid balance regulation. The ACE-D allele associated with higher ACE levels and activity was more common in HAPE-susceptible subjects [31,48]. In a population of highlanders therefore, the ACE-I allele would be beneficial and more common. But HAPH is a more slowly developing disease, which could be established when a subject is older than 30–40 years. The genotypes related to HAPH could be preserved in high-altitude dwellers population. Interestingly, in early 1988 Rabinovitch and co-workers demonstrated that injection of angiotensin-2 prevented development of hypoxic pulmonary hypertension, vascular remodelling and right ventricular hypertrophy in chronically hypoxic rats (Rabinovitch et al., 1988). In COPD patients the DD genotype (higher ACE activity) was also negatively associated with right ventricular hypertrophy in males [62]. Thus the genotype that is beneficial to better acclimatization to a hypoxic environment could be associated with high-altitude related diseases (HAPH) at older ages.

In addition to I/D polymorphism in the ACE gene, there are at least 12 other known variants in the gene, including two (G2215A и G2350A) that have more effect on plasma ACE variation than the I/D locus [74]. For alleles relatively close together, the process of segregation independently in the population can take millennia and until then they are said to be in linkage disequilibrium and move between generations as a haplotype. The haplotype frequencies can vary between populations [55] and the genotype at one polymorphic locus can serve as a marker for all other genotypes on that haplotype. The reason that non-functional variants (e.g., silent polymorphisms of the gene) are sometimes included in association studies is that any observed association could be evidence for a proximal functional variant. Because the interactions between genetic loci likely plays a key role in the development of complex traits, haplotypes, rather than single alleles, may be the critical inherited factors [52]. For example, the combination of the A allele at 2215 and the G allele at the 2350 positions had a greater effect on plasma ACE levels and blood pressure than the individual alleles [74]. There are several combinations of these polymorphisms in different haplotypes of ACE gene.

ACE haplotype frequencies can vary between populations [55], especially those recently founded or isolated and our study was the first to demonstrate this in the Kyrgyz population. We have demonstrated for the Kyrgyz population a linkage disequilibrium of the D allele with A2215 and G2350, whereas the I allele was linked with G2215 and A2350 alleles giving two haplotypes, DAG and IGA. These two haplotypes (DAG and IGA) are the major ACE gene haplotypes found in Kyrgyzs with the frequencies 0.615 for DAG and 0.314 for IGA (Table 1). The frequency of these two haplotypes is 0.93 whereas 5 other haplotypes presented very rarely, with a frequency of less than 0.1.

In Caucasians, IGA and DAG haplotypes have almost the same frequencies and together give a frequency of 0.6 [53]. The ACE gene haplotypes distribution in Kyrgyzs is very different from what was demonstrated for Caucasians with a much higher frequency of IGA and DAG than the other five combinations. This particularity of ACE gene haplotypes distribution we could explain by the relatively high genetic homogeneity of the Kyrgyz population with a prominent "founder effect".

When we studied the distribution of these haplotypes in HAPH patients vs control Kyrgyz highlanders, we found the same pattern as for I and D alleles.

TABLE 1. Distribution of ACE gene haplotypes in Kyrgyz population

Haplotype	I/D	G2215A	G2350A	Frequency
1	I	G	A	0,615
2	D	A	G	0,314
3	D	G	A	0,040
4	D	G	G	0,013
5	D	A	A	0,006
6	I	G	G	0,006
7	I	A	A	0,006

In patients with HAPH the IGA haplotype was more frequent compared to controls (0.73 vs 0.51, respectively). The DAG haplotype was found significantly less in HAPH group (p=0.01, see Table 2). Again, the DAG haplotype had a greater effect on plasma ACE activity and systemic blood pressure than the individual alleles [74] and DD genotype (higher ACE activity) was negatively associated with right ventricular hypertrophy in males with COPD [62]. Thus, our data strongly suggest that the DAG haplotype in Kyrgyz highlanders is negatively associated with the development of HAPH.

Arg16Gly and Gln27Glu Polymorphisms of β_2-Adrenoreceptors Gene

The next candidate gene is the b2-adrenergic receptor (β_2-AR) gene, which is located on chromosome 5. The well-known polymorphisms of this gene are Arg16Gly and Gln27Glu, with allele Gly16 related to desensitization of β_2-AR and the Gln27Gln genotype is associated with decreased vascular response to β-agonists stimulation [13]. Earlier we have demonstrated that severe right ventricular hypertrophy (II and III grade) correlated with b2-adrenergic receptors desensitization [1,2,3]. It was also shown that β_2-AR were desensitized in COPD patients with secondary PH [68]. Therefore, we were very keen to study the association of Arg16Gly and Gln27Glu polymorphisms of the β_2-AR gene with the development of HAPH in Kyrgyz highlanders.

We have found by genotyping study that the highlanders with HAPH have a significantly higher frequency of homozygous genotype Gln27Gln compared to controls (0.61 vs 0.45, respectively, χ^2=6.353, p=0.0415; see table 3). The genotype Glu27Glu was more frequent in healthy highlanders compared to patients with HAPH (0.12 и 0.05, respectively). There was also a trend for the higher frequency of Gln27 allele in the HAPH group compared to controls (0.78 vs 0.66).

As seen in Table 4 the frequencies of Arg16 and Gly16 alleles in HAPH group vs controls were not significantly different. It was also a nonsignificant

TABLE 2. IGA haplotype associated with development HAPH in Kyrgyz highlanders

Groups	Haplotype IGA	Haplotype DAG	Haplotype Other
HAPH	0,73*	0,23	0,04
Healthy	0,51	0,39	0,1

*χ^2=9.028; p=0.01

TABLE 3. Glu27Gln allele and genotype frequencies of β2-adrenoreceptor gene

Group	Genotypes frequency			Alleles frequency	
	Gln27Gln	Gln27Glu	Glu27Glu	Gln	Glu
Healthy	0.45 (28)	0.43 (31)	0.12 (7)	0.66 (87)	0.34 (45)
HAPH	0.61 (50)*	0.34 (23)	0.05 (6)	0.78 (123)	0.22 (47)

* $\chi^2 = 6.353$, $p = 0.0415$

TABLE 4. Arg16Gly allele and genotype frequencies of β2-adrenoreceptor gene

Group	Genotypes frequency			Alleles frequency	
	Arg16Arg	Arg16Gly	Gly16Gly	Arg	Gly
Healthy	0.26 (3)	0.50 (50)	0.24 (2)	0.51 (87)	0.49 (45)
HAPH	0.23 (6)	0.50 (43)	0.27 (8)	0.48 (123)	0.52 (47)

trend of a higher frequency of the Gly16 allele in HAPH patients. But the main genotype in both groups is heterozygous genotype Arg16Gly.

The higher presence of Gln27Gln and Gln27Glu genotypes of β_2-AR gene in HAPH group and findings of our early studies that HAPH patients develop a prominent desensitization of β_2-AR, have proved our suggestion that this desensitization is genetically determined. Desensitization of β_2-AR caused the decreased vasodilatation response of pulmonary arteries to catecholamines and excessive pulmonary vasoconstriction in chronic hypoxia in Gln27 carriers.

We did not find a significant association for Arg16Gly polymorphism with HAPH. Maybe this polymorphism of the β_2-AR gene does not play any functional role in the pathogenesis of HAPH in Kyrgyz highlanders.

C677T Polymorphism of Methylenetetrahydrofolate Reductase Gene

The MTHFR gene has been mapped to the chromosomal region 1p36.3 and is composed of 11 exons [26]. A common mutation of the MTHFR gene is the C to T transition, located at nucleotide 677 (C677T). This results in the amino acid change: alanine to valine. This mutation is associated with increased thermolability and reduced specific activity of the enzyme (mean activity is 65% in the Ala/Val heterozygote and 30% in the Val/Val homozygous state, respectively compared to the mean activity in the Ala/Ala homozygote) [22]. Patients with a deficiency in MTHFR have elevated blood and urinary levels of homocysteine. The MTHFR C677T, causing hyperhomocysteinemia, is an important genetic risk factor for cardiovascular disorders [65]. This is the most common mutation and has prevalence in the general population, 5–10% as TT and up to 40% as CT genotype [35,46]. Nevertheless, due to the high incidence in the general population and its physiological role, the 677C-T mutation may represent an important risk factor of homocystein associated vascular disease [35]. A generally accepted hypothesis is that TT-genotype leads to hyperhomocysteinemia, with a consecutive premature vascular disease and heterozygous carriers have mild hyperhomocysteinemia with a predisposition for accelerated atherosclerosis [18,46].

HAPH is also characterized by remodelling of the pulmonary artery wall compromising intimal thickening and hypertrophy of the tunica media, therefore we have studied the association of C677T polymorphism with HAPH in Kyrgyz highlanders. We have demonstrated that the mutant T allele was significantly more frequent in highlanders with HAPH than in the control group (0.42 vs 0.25, respectively, $\chi^2 = 7.604$, $p = 0.005$). The frequency of homozygous TT-genotype was threefold greater in the HAPH subjects group than in healthy highlanders (0.18 vs 0.06 respectively, $\chi^2 = 8.319$, $p = 0.01$, see table 5).

What could be the rationale for this association? Earlier it was demonstrated that endothelium-dependant vasodilatation driven by NO release has decreased in patients with hyperhomocysteinuria [11]. Six-weeks folate consumption in 5 mg per day doses simultaneously decreased homocysteine levels in blood and increased endothelium-dependant vasodilatation in arteries of healthy volunteers [9]. This effect could be related to the decrease of homocysteine-induced oxidative stress [33]. Antioxidants like ascorbate prevented endothelial dysfunction related to a three-fold increase of homocystein in the blood.

Stuhlinger et al. (2001) have demonstrated that homocysteine inhibited activity of DDAH (the enzyme which degrades asymmetric dimethylarginine, the endogenous inhibitor of NOS). This finding could explain the mechanism of the negative effect of homocysteine on endothelium-dependant

TABLE 5. The C677T polymorphism of MTHFR gene and HAPH

	Genotypes (number of patients)			Alleles (number of alleles)	
Group	677 C/C	677 C/T	677 T/T	C	T
Healthy	0.56 (36)	0.38 (28)	0.06 (3)	0.75 (100)	0.25 (34)
HAPH	0.34 (17)	0.49 (31)	0.18 (8)*	0.58 (65)	0.42 (47)**

*$\chi^2 = 8.319$, $p = 0.01$; ** $\chi^2 = 7.604$, $p = 0.005$

vasodilatation. Thus, we suggest that the association of TT-genotype and T allele with HAPH is related to complication of hypoxia-induced endothelial dysfunction caused by increased homocystein levels in the blood.

C838A Polymorphism of P27kip1 Gene

The balance between cell proliferation and cell quiescence is regulated by a variety of cellular mediators, in which cyclin-dependent kinases and their inhibitors play a very important role. The CDK inhibitor p27 is very important in inhibition of pulmonary artery smooth cell growth, both in vitro and in vivo. In chronically hypoxic mice lungs, hypoxia significantly inhibited p27 expression, showing a 98% decrease in p27 [72]. The inhibition of hypoxic pulmonary vascular remodelling by heparin required the p27 expression [73]. In p27 null mice exposed to hypoxia, heparin did not inhibit cell proliferation in pulmonary vessels. These data strengthen the previous findings that p27 is the only CDK inhibitor involved in hypoxia-induced pulmonary hypertension [73].

Gene encoding p27 is localized on chromosome 12p13. The known C838A polymorphism of p27 gene is associated with decreased activity of promoter region (32). The A838 allele is associated with decreased expression of p27 and cardiovascular diseases. We have demonstrated that genotype A838A was apparently twice as prevalent in highlanders with HAPH than the controls ($\chi^2 = 6.407$, $p = 0.04$). The frequency of the A838 allele was significantly higher in the HAPH group ($\chi^2 = 5.520$, $p = 0.01$, see table 6). These genetic data from human studies strongly support the previous observations made in mice that p27 is the only CDK inhibitor involved in hypoxic pulmonary hypertension.

S/L Polymorphism of 5HTT Gene

In several studies it was shown that serotonin (5-hydroxytryptamine, 5-HT) and its transporter (5-HTT) play a critical role in the pulmonary vascular smooth muscle hyperplasia and vascular remodelling associated with

TABLE 6. C838A polymorphism of p27kip1 gene and HAPH

	Genotypes (number of patients)			Alleles (number of alleles)	
Group	838 C/C	838C/A	838A/A	C	A
Healthy	0.37 (12)	0.48(21)	0.15(4)	0.61(45)	0.39(29)
HAPH	0.20(24)	0.50(52)	0.30(35)*	0.45 (100)	0.55 (122)**

$\chi^2 = 6.407$, $p = 0.04$; ** $\chi^2 = 5.520$, $p = 0.01$.

TABLE 7. 4a/4b polymorphism of eNOS gene and HAPH

	Genotypes (number of patients)			Alleles (number of alleles)	
Group	bb	ab	aa	b	a
Health	0.86 (60)	0.14 (10)	0	0.93 (130)	0.07 (10)
HAPH	0.86 (47)	0.13 (5)	0.005 (1)	0.93 (99)	0.07 (7)

$\chi^2 = 1.93$, $p = 0.38$

experimental hypoxic pulmonary hypertension (PH) and human primary PH [16,17]. High expression of 5-HTT in pulmonary vessels of patients with primary PH was associated with insertion/deletion polymorphisms of promoter region of 5-HTT gene [17]. Insertion is long (L) and deletion is short (S) alleles: the L allele is known to increase the transcription rate of the 5-HTT gene and the S allele is associated with a decreased rate [38]. The LL-genotype is associated with high levels of 5-HTT expression and increased proliferation of PASMC [16,17]. A large cohort study, including 166 cases of familial PAH and 83 idiopathic PAH subjects, has demonstrated that 5HTT gene polymorphism does not correlate with age at diagnosis or survival interval of patients with IPAH and only in FPAH patients does the LL genotype correlate with age at diagnosis [69]. The other large cohort study did not find any significant evidence of association between alleles of the 5HTT gene and familial or idiopathic PAH, nor a relationship with age of onset of a disease [40].

We have found that in the Kyrgyz population the LL –genotype was very rare. We did not find any association of L allele with HAPH (table 7). Moreover, the expression of 5HTT protein in platelets of HAPH patients and healthy Kyrgyz highlanders did not differ.

Glu298Asp Polymorphism of eNOS Gene

Nitric oxide synthase 3 (eNOS). Nitric oxide is a small bioactive molecule that is involved in a variety of physiological functions, including maintaining pulmonary vascular tone, and may play a role in altitude adaptation [70]. Higher levels of NO are naturally exhaled by high-altitude indigenous populations, e.g., Tibetans [8], whereas HAPE-susceptible individuals have lower levels of exhaled NO [10]. NO is synthesized from the amino acid L-arginine by a family of enzymes called nitric oxide synthases (NOS), including NOS3 (or endothelial NOS, eNOS) in the walls of blood vessels. There are known polymorphisms in the NOS3 gene which are associated with a modulation of NO levels and with cardiovascular pathology: 4ab tandem repeats which have been associated with lower exhaled NO [60] and the G894T (mutation

TABLE 8. G894T polymorphism of eNOS gene and HAPH

	Genotypes (number of patients)			Alleles (number of alleles)	
Group	GG	GT	TT	G	T
Health	0.66 (54)	0.30 (33)	0.04 (0)	0.81 (141)	0.19 (33)
HAPH	0.64 (53)	0.32 (28)	0.04 (3)	0.80 (134)	0.2 (34)

χ^2 = 3,36 , p= 0,185

which alters the amino acid sequence Glu298Asp and has been associated with hypertension and preeclampsia; Hingorani, 2003). Association studies of NOS3 alleles distribution in HAPE patients [5,15] reported that the 4a and T894 were more common in Asian subjects with HAPE. Conversely, Weiss et al. (2003) found no association in Caucasians. The reason for this disagreement is unclear because the 4a/b polymorphism was also associated with NO levels in Caucasians [30]. Our study on the Kyrgyz population, which is also from Asian ancestry, has not found any association of 4a and T894 alleles with high-altitude pulmonary hypertension (χ^2= 1.93, p=0.38 and χ^2= 3.36, p= 0.185, respectively; see table 8). Interestingly, that the frequency of mutant eNOS alleles is very low in Kyrgyz highlanders may be due to selection pressure against genotypes associated with HAPE or HACE.

Using the multiple regression analysis, we have studied the association of all these polymorphisms (I/D polymorphism of ACE gene, C677T MTHFR gene polymorphism, C838A polymorphism of p27kip1 gene and G894T polymorphism of eNOS gene) with the development of HAPH. We have found that in all combinations only I allele of I/D polymorphism of ACE gene correlated with the development of high altitude pulmonary hypertension (β=0.26; p=0.03).

Conclusion

High-altitude pulmonary hypertension (HAPH) is a public health problem in the mountainous areas of the world, and because about 10% of the world population is living in the mountains, it could affect millions of people. As recreational travel or industrial development to places such as the Himalayan Plateau, Pamir and Tien-Shan mountains or the Andean Altiplano becomes more common, the number of people experiencing altitude-related illness will increase.

While epidemiological data support the hypothesis that some humans are particularly susceptible to hypoxia, there is only little genetic evidence to support the hypothesis that this is due to innate, inherited factors. Few strong and reliable data exist on familial patterns of susceptibility and, although a number of gene variants have been associated with the conditions, the results are inconsistent among studies. The problem with HAPH is that it is a chronic but not acute illness, with a very slowly developing onset and challenging clinical diagnostics. When the clinical features are established, the parents of the subject usually have been passed and children are too young to be diagnosed. Unfortunately the life expectancy among mountain dwellers is very short and infant mortality is too high, which makes it very difficult to tag the familial patterns of the trait. Generally, it must be remembered that family data for environmentally-related illness can be difficult to obtain and that genetic analysis of HAPH is in its infancy. Many of the studies cited in this paper only relate to a few candidate genes out of the tens of thousands in the human genome and only a few tens of polymorphisms out of millions have been assessed for roles in hypoxia-related diseases.

Coupled with recent genomic developments such as SNP databases and genome-wide haplotype mappings, efficient, new, non-invasive methods of pulmonary arterial pressure study and the increased understanding of the molecular mechanisms of oxygen sensing and hypoxic pulmonary vasoconstriction, the cross-talking of vascular wall cells and mechanisms of hypoxia driven vascular remodelling, this will provide us with opportunities to further our understanding of the pathogenesis of HAPH, its early diagnostics, the biochemistry and physiology of altitude adaptation.

Acknowledgments

The author would like to thank the researchers of my team who conducted the genotyping research on Kyrgyz highlanders: Drs Oleg A. Pak, Jainagul T. Isakova, Eleonora U. Usupova, Mahabat Kochkorova and Dr Baktybek K. Kojonazarov, for helping with the preparation of the manuscript.

References

1. Aldashev, A.A., Borbugulov U., Davletov B., Mirrakhimov M.M. (1989). Human adrenoceptor system response to the development of high altitude pulmonary arterial hypertension. J Mol Cell Cardiol 21(suppl.1): 175–179.
2. Aldashev AA. (1993) High altitude pulmonary hypertension and signal transduction in the cardiovascular system. In: J.S. Brody, D.M. Center, V.A. Tkachuk, eds. Signal Transduction in Lung Cells, Vol. 65. New-York: Lung biology in health and disease, pp 459–482.
3. Aldashev A.A. (2000) High altitude pulmonary hypertension and signal transduction in the cardiovascular system. Recept Signal Transduct Res 20: 255–278.
4. Aguirre J.I., Morrell N.W., Long L., Clift P., Upton P.D., Polak J.M., Wilkins M.R. (2000). Vascular remodeling and ET-1 expression in rat strains with different responses to chronic hypoxia. Am J Physiol 278: 981– 987.

5. Ahsan A., Charu R., Pasha M.A., Norboo T., Charu R., Afrin F., Ahsan A., and Baig M.A. (2004). eNOS allelic variants at the same locus associate with HAPE and adaptation. Thorax 59: 1000–1002.
6. Aldashev A.A., Sarybaev A.Sh., Sydykov A.S., Kalmyrzaev B.B., Kim E.V., Mamanova L.B., Maripov R., Kojonazarov B.K., Mirrakhimov M.M., Wilkins M.R, and Morrell N.W. (2002). Characterization of High-Altitude Pulmonary Hypertension in the Kyrgyz: Association with Angiotensin-Converting Enzyme Genotype. Am J Respir Crit Care Med 166: 1396–1402.
7. Aldashev A.A., Kojonazarov B.K., Amatov T.A., Sooronbaev T.M., Mirrakhimov M.M., Morrell N.W., Wharton J., Wilkins M.R. (2005). Phosphodiesterase type 5 and high altitude pulmonary hypertension. Thorax 60 : 683–687.
8. Beall C.M. (2000). Tibetan and Andean patterns of adaptation to high-altitude hypoxia. Hum Biol 72 : 201–228.
9. Bellamy MF, McDowell IF, Ramsey MW, Brownlee M, Newcombe RG, Lewis MJ. (1999) Oral folate enhances endothelial function in hyperhomocysteinaemic subjects. Eur J Clin Invest 29: 659–662.
10. Busch T., Bartsch P., Pappert D., Grunig E., Hildebrandt W., Elser H., Falke K.J., and Swenson E.R. (2001). Hypoxia decreases exhaled nitric oxide in mountaineers susceptible to high-altitude pulmonary edema. Am J Respir Crit Care Med 163: 368–373.
11. Celermajer DS, Sorensen K, Ryalls M, et al. (1993) Impaired endothelial function occurs in the systemic arteries of children with homozygous homocystinuria but not in their heterozygous parents. J Am Coll Cardiol 22: 854–8.
12. Chou T-C., Knilans T.K. (1996) Right ventricular hypertrophy. In: Electrocardiography in clinical practice, 4th ed. Philadelphia: W.B. Saunders; p. 54–69.
13. Cockcroft JR, Gazis AG, Cross DJ, Wheatley A, Dewar J, Hall IP, Noon JP. (2000). Beta(2)-adrenoceptor polymorphism determines vascular reactivity in humans. Hypertension 36: 371–375.
14. Dehnert C., Weymann J., Montgomery H.E., Woods D., Maggiorini M., Scherrer U., Gibbs J.S., and Bartsch P. (2002). No association between high-altitude tolerance and the ACE I/D gene polymorphism. Med Sci Sports Exerc 34: 1928–1933.
15. Droma Y., Hanaoka M., Hotta J., Katsuyama Y., Ota M., Kobayashi T., and Kubo K. (2003). The r506 Q mutation of coagulation factor V gene in high altitude pulmonary-edema-susceptible subjects. High Alt Med Biol 4: 497–8.
16. Eddahibi S, Hanoun N, Lanfumey L, et al. (2000) Attenuated hypoxic pulmonary hypertension in mice lacking the 5-hydroxytryptamine transporter gene. J Clin Invest 105: 1555–1562.
17. Eddahibi S, Humbert M, Fadel E, et al. (2001) Serotonin transporter overexpression is responsible for pulmonary artery smooth muscle hyperplasia in primary pulmonary hypertension. J Clin Invest 108: 1141–1150.
18. Engbersen AM, Franken DG, Boers GH, Stevens EM, Trijbels FJ, Blom HJ. (1995) Thermolabile 5,10-methylenetetrahydrofolate reductase as a cause of mild hyperhomocysteinemia. Am J Hum Genet 56 :142–50.
19. Fedorova L., and Fedorov A. (2003). Introns in gene evolution. Genetica 118:123–131.
20. Forster P. (1984). Reproducibility of individual response to exposure to high altitude. Br Med J 289:1269.
21. Frid M.G., Aldashev A.A., Nemnoff R.A., Higashito R., Westcott J.Y., Stenmark K.R. (1999) Subendothelial cells from normal bovine arteries exhibit autonomous growth and constitutively activated intracellular signaling. Arterioscler Thromb Vasc Biol 19: 2884 – 2893.
22. Frosst P, Blom HJ, Milos R, et al. (1995) A candidate genetic risk factor for vascular disease: a common mutation in methylenetetrahydrofolate reductase. Nat Genet 10: 111– 113.
23. Garruto R.M., Chin C.T., Weitz C.A., Liu J.C., Liu R.L., and He, X. (2003). Hematological differences during growth among Tibetans and Han Chinese born and raised at high altitude in Qinghai, China. Am J Phys Anthropol 122:171–183.

24. Ge R.-L., and Helun H. (2001). Current concept of chronic mountain sickness: pulmonary hypertension-related high-altitude heart disease. Wilderness Environ Med 12: 190–194.
25. Gonzalez P., Diez-Juan A., Coto E., Alvarez V., Reguero J.R., Batalla A. and Andres V. (2004). A single-nucleotide polymorphism in the human p27kip1 gene (−838C>A) affects basal promoter activity and the risk of myocardial infarction. BMC Biology, 2:5.
26. Goyette P, Summer J.S, Milos R., et al: (1994) Human methylenetetrahydrofolate reductase isolation of cDNA, mapping and mutation identification. Nat Genet 7: 195–200.
27. Gupta M., Rao K., Anand I., Banerjee A., and Boparai M. (1992). Lack of smooth muscle in the small pulmonary arteries of the native Ladakhi. Is the Himalayan highlander adapted? Am Rev Respir Dis 145: 1201–1214.
28. Hackett P. H., and Roach R. C. (2001). High-altitude-related illness. N Engl J Med 345: 107–114.
29. Hingorani A.D. (2003). Endothelial nitric oxide synthase polymorphisms and hypertension. Curr Hypertens Rep 5:19–25.
30. Hoffmann I.S., Tavares-Mordwinkin R., Castejon A.M., Alfieri A.B., and Cubeddu L.X. (2005). Endothelial nitric oxide synthase polymorphism, nitric oxide production, salt sensitivity and cardiovascular risk factors in Hispanics. J Hum Hypertens 19:233–240.
31. Hotta J., Hanaoka M., Droma Y., Katsuyama Y., Ota M., and Kobayashi T. (2004). Polymorphisms of renin–angiotensin system genes with high-altitude pulmonary edema in Japanese subjects. Chest 126: 825–830.
32. Jones R., Pembrey M., Golding J., and Herrick D. (2005). The search for genenotype/phenotype associations and the phenome scan. Paediatr. Perinat. Epidemiol 19: 264–275.
33. Kanani P.M., Sinkey C.A., Browning R.L., Allaman M., Knapp H.R., Haynes W.G. (1999). Role of oxidant stress in endothelial dysfunction produced by experimental hyperhomocyst(e)inemia in humans. Circulation 100: 1161–8.
34. Keavney B., McKenzie C., Connell J., Julier C., Ratcliffe P., Sobel E., Lathrop M., Farral M. Maesured. (1998). Haplotype analyses of the angiotensin I-converting enzyme gene. Human Molecular Genetics 7: 1745–1751.
35. Kluijtmans LA, Blom HJ, Boers GH, van Oost BA, Trijbels FJ, van den Heuvel LP. (1995).Two novel missense mutations in the cystathionine beta-synthase gene in homocystinuric patients. Hum Genet 96: 249–50.
36. Kojonazarov B.K., Imanov B.Zh., Amatov T.A., Mirrakhimov M.M., Naeije R., Wilkins M.R., Aldashev A.A. (2006) Noninvasive and invasive evaluation of the pulmonary arterial pressure in Kyrgyz highlanders. Eur Resp J 1 Nov. Vol 29 : 352–6.
37. Kumar R., Pasha Q., Khan A.P., and Gupta V. (2004). Renin angiotensin aldosterone system and ACE I/D gene polymorphism in high-altitude pulmonary edema. Aviat Space Environ Med 75: 981–983.
38. Lesch K, Bengel D., Heils A., et al. (1996). Association of anxiety-related traits with a polymorphism in the serotonin transporter gene regulatory region. Science 274: 1527–1531.
39. Lin Z.P., Yiao Q.Y., Miao C.Y., and Chen D.S. (1984). Family susceptibility to high altitude heart disease. In: High Altitude Disease, W.Y. Zhang YB, Liu X.L., eds. Qinghai Press, Xining, China; pp. 268–287.
40. Machado RD, Koehler R, Glissmeyer E, Veal C, Suntharalingam J, Kim M, Carlquist J, Town M, Elliott CG, Hoeper M, Fijalkowska A, Kurzyna M, Thomson JR, Gibbs SR, Wilkins MR, Seeger W, Morrell NW, Gruenig E, Trembath RC, Janssen B. (2006). Genetic association of the serotonin transporter in pulmonary arterial hypertension.Am J Respir Crit Care Med 173: 793–7.
41. McKenzie C., Abecasis G., Keavney B., Forrester T., Ratcliffe P., Julier C., ConnelJ., Bennett F., McFarlanca-Anderson N., Lathrop G., Cardon L. (2001). Trans-ethnic fine mapping of quantitative trait locus for circulating angiotensin I-converting enzyme (ACE). Human Molecular Genetics 110: 1077–1084.
42. Milledge J.S., and Catley D.M. (1984). Angiotensin converting enzyme response to hypoxia in man: its role in altitude acclimatization. Clin Sci 67: 453–456.

43. Mirrakhimov M., Winslow R.(1996) The cardiovascular system at high altitude. Environmental physiology / Edited by Fregley M, Blatteal C. Oxford: Oxford University Press;.pp. 1241–58.
44. Montgomery H.E., Marshall R., Hemingway H., Myerson S., Clarkson P., Dollery C.,Hayward M., Holliman D.E., Jubb M., World M., et al. (1997). Human gene for physical performance. Nature 393: 221–222.
45. Moore L.G. (2001). Human genetic adaptation to high altitude. High Alt Med Biol 2: 257–279.
46. Morita H, Taguchi J, Kurihara H, Kitaoka M, Kaneda H, Kurihara Y, Maemura K, Shindo T, Minamino T, Ohno M, Yamaoki K, Ogasawara K, Aizawa T, Suzuki S, Yazaki Y.(1997).Genetic polymorphism of 5,10-methylenetetrahydrofolate reductase (MTHFR) as a risk factor for coronary artery disease. Circulation 95 :2032–6.
47. Morrell N.W., Sarybaev A.S., Alikhan A., Mirrakhimov M.M., and Aldashev A.A. (1999). ACE genotype and risk of high altitude pulmonary hypertension in Kyrghyz highlanders. Lancet 353: 814.
48. Pasha M.A., Charu R., Ahsan A., and Norboo T. (2005). This meeting "High Altitude Medicine and Biology Advanced Research Workshop" Issyk-Kul, june 5–8, 2006. HAPE susceptibility associates with variants of genes of vascular homeostasis. Human Genome Mapping; Genomic Basis of Common Diseases Poster abstract 310.
49. Pei S.X., Chen X.J., Si Ren B.Z., Liu Y.H., Cheng X.S., Harris E.M., Anand I.S., and Harris P.C. (1989). Chronic mountain sickness in Tibet. Q J Med 71: 555–574.
50. Penaloza D, Arias-Stella J, Sime F, Reeavarren S, Marticorena E. (1964). The heart and pulmonary circulation in children at high altitudes: physiology, anatomical and clinical observations. Pediatrics 34: 368–382.
51. Rabinovitch M, Mullen M, Rosenberg HC, Maruyama K, O'Brodovich H, Olley PM. (1988). Angiotensin II prevents hypoxic pulmonary hypertension and vascular changes in rat. Am J Physiol 254: H500–8.
52. Rupert J.L., Koehle M.S. (2006). Evidence for genetic basis for altitude-related illness. High Alt Med Biol 7(2):150–67.
53. Sagnella G.A., Rotwell M..J., Opinipla A.K., Wick P.D., Gook D.G., Capuccio F.P. (1999). A population study of ethnic variations in the angiotensin- converting enzyme I/D polymorphism: relationships with gender, hypertension and impaired qlucose metabolism. J. Hypertens 17: 657–664.
54. Salameh G., Karamsetty R., Warburton R.R., Klinger J.R., Ou L.C., Hill N.S. (1999). Differences in acute hypoxic pulmonary vasoresponsiveness between rat strains: role of endothelium. Am J Physiol 87: 356 – 362.
55. Salisbury B.A., Pungliya M., Choi J.Y., Jiang R., Sun X.J., and Stephens J.C. (2003). SNP and haplotype variation in the human genome. Mutat Res 15 : 53–61.
56. Sayed-Tabatabaei F.A., Schut A.F., Hofman A., Bertoli-Avella A.M., Vergeer J., Witteman J.C., and van Duijn C.M. (2004). A study of gene–environment interaction on the gene for angiotensin converting enzyme: a combined functional and population based approach. J Med Genetics 41: 99–103.
57. Stuhlinger M.C., Tsao P.S., Her J-H., Kimoto M., Balint R.F., and Cooke J.P. (2001). Homocysteine Impairs the Nitric Oxide Synthase Pathway: Role of Asymmetric Dimethylarginine. Circulation 104: 2569–2575.
58. Su B., Xiao C., Deka R., Seielstad M.T., Kangwanpong D., Xiao J., Lu D., Underhill P., Cavalli-Sforza L., Chakraborty R., and Jin L. (2000). Y chromosome haplotypes reveal prehistorical migrations to the Himalayas. Hum Genetics 107: 582–590.
59. Tarasevicíene-Stewart L, Scerbavicius R, Stewart JM, Gera L, Demura Y, Cool C, Kasper M, Voelkel NF. (2005) Treatment of severe pulmonary hypertension: a bradykinin receptor 2 agonist B9972 causes reduction of pulmonary artery pressure and right ventricular hypertrophy. Peptides 1292–300.
60. Thomas S., Bruce C., Birkhead A., and Wang L. (2002). Effect of e NOS polymorphisms and coronary artery disease upon exhaled nitric oxide. J Mol Med 80: 181–186.

61. Tsianos G., Eleftheriou K.I., Hawe E., Woolrich L., Watt M., Watt I., Peacock A., Montgomery H., and Grant S. (2005). Performance at altitude and angiotensin I-converting enzyme genotype. Eur J Appl Physiol 93: 630–633.
62. van Suylen RJ, Wouters EF, Pennings HJ, Cheriex EC, van Pol PE, Ambergen AW, Vermelis AM, Daemen MJ. (1999) .The DD genotype of the angiotensin converting enzyme gene is negatively associated with right ventricular hypertrophy in male patients with chronic obstructive pulmonary disease. Am J Respir Crit Care Med 159: 1791–5.
63. Villard E., Tiret L., Visvikis S., Rakotovao R., Cambien F., Soubrier F. (1996) Identification of new polymorphism of the angiotensin-converting enzyme (ACE) gene, and study of their relationship to plasma ACE levels by two-QTL segregation-linkage analyses. Am J Hum Gent 58: 1268–1278.
64. von Euler US, Liljestrand G. (1946) Observations on the pulmonary aterial blood pressure in the cat. Acta Physiol Scand 12: 301–320.
65. Wald DS, Law M, Morris JK :(2002). Homocysteine and cardiovascular disease: evidence on causality from a meta-analysis. Br Med J 325: 1202.
66. Weir E.K, Tucker A., Reeves J.T., Will D.H., Grover R.F. (1974).The genetic factor influencing pulmonary hypertension in cattle at high altitude. Cardiovasc Res 8: 745 – 749.
67. Weiss J., Haefeli W.E., Gasse C., Hoffmann M.M., Weyman J., Gibbs S., Mansmann U., and Bartsch P. (2003). Lack of evidence for association of high altitude pulmonary edema and polymorphisms of the NO pathway. High Alt Med Biol 4: 355–366.
68. Weitzenblum E, Mammosser M, Ehrhart M.(1986). Evolution and prognosis of pulmonary hypertension in chronic obstructive pulmonary disease. Herz 11:147–154.
69. Willers ED, Newman JH, Loyd JE, Robbins IM, Wheeler LA, Prince MA, Stanton KC, Cogan JA, Runo JR, Byrne D, Humbert M, Simonneau G, Sztrymf B, Morse JA, Knowles JA, Roberts KE, McElroy JJ, Barst RJ, Phillips JA 3. (2005). Serotonin transporter polymorphisms in familial and idiopathic pulmonary arterial hypertension.Am J Respir Crit Care Med 173: 798–802.
70. Wilkins M.R., Aldashev A.A., Morrell N.W. (2002). Nitric oxide, phosphodiesterase inhibition, and adaptation to hypoxic conditions. Lancet 359: 1539–40.
71. Wu T., Wang X., Wei C., Cheng H., Wang X., Li Y., Ge D., Zhao H., Young P., Li G., and Wang Z. (2005). Hemoglobin levels in Qinghai–Tibet: different effects of gender for Tibetans vs. Han. J Appl Physiol 98: 5898–604.
72. Yu L, Quinn DA, Garg HG, Hales CA. (2005). Cyclin-dependent kinase inhibitor p27Kip1, but not p21WAF1/Cip1, is required for inhibition of hypoxia-induced pulmonary hypertension and remodeling by heparin in mice. Circ Res 97:937–45.
73. Yu L, Quinn DA, Garg HG, Hales CA. (2006). Gene expression of cyclin-dependent kinase inhibitors and effect of heparin on their expression in mice with hypoxia-induced pulmonary hypertension. Biochem Biophys Res Commun 345: 1565–72.
74. Zhu X., Bouzekri N., Southam L., Cooper R., Adeyemo A., McKenzie C., Luke A., Chen G., Elston R., Ward R. (2001). Linkage and association analyses of angiotensin I-converting enzyme (ACE) gene polymorphism with ACE concentration and blood pressure. Am J Hum Genet 68: 1139–1148.

CHAPTER 12

GENETIC FACTORS IN THE ACUTE RESPONSE TO HYPOXIA IN ANIMALS MODELS

KINGMAN P. STROHL

Division of Pulmonary and Critical Care Medicine, Department of Medicine, Louis Stokes Department of Veterans Affairs Medical Center, Case Western Reserve University, Cleveland OH

Abstract: The question of whether an inherited effect can be detected has been answered in the affirmative a number of times in human studies showing variations between twin pairs, between families and between populations in Tibet and the Andes. There is now evidence from studies in mice that the adult ventilatory response can be altered by engineered knockout of genes involved in nitric oxide synthase isoforms, as well as knockout models for other proteins. Quantitative and qualitative differences between strains in ventilatory behavior (frequency and tidal volume) before, during and after hypoxia are consistently found by different laboratories. Interbreeding studies have identified chromosomal regions that track with ventilatory behavior during hypoxia, thus suggesting that natural variation acts on hypoxic responsiveness. Further studies will offer opportunity to create a functional map of the connections between genes and ventilatory responses in regard to oxygen homeostasis.

Keywords: ventilation; hypoxia; nitric oxide; chemoreflex; genetics.

Introduction

Ventilatory behavior is one measurable feature in the respiratory system, which in general operates to provide sufficient oxygen to meet cellular metabolic requirements and to remove enough carbon dioxide so that pH is maintained for optimal cell function. Ventilatory behavior also serves in other functions, for instance speech and heat exchange. In mammals, the respiratory control system, consisting of the controller (brain), controlled system (lungs and chest wall), and sensors (e.g., carotid body), acts to maintain arterial Po_2 and Pco_2 within a fairly narrow range despite changes

A. Aldashev and R. Naeije (eds.), Problems of High Altitude Medicine and Biology, 169–184.

in metabolism and environmental conditions with growth, development and extremes of daily activity. For its role in oxygen homeostasis, ventilation, part of the controlled system, is achieved through combinations of tidal volume and frequency [1] and in a given species there is no unique combination that is mechanically most energetically efficient [17,9]. Thus, natural selection has an opportunity to modify ventilatory behavior in a homeostatic manner, without extracting much cost with regard to gas exchange from the lung compartment.

The expected response of ventilation to acute hypoxia is to increase the opportunity for oxygen uptake by an increase in tidal volume and frequency; this increases alveolar oxygen levels by decreasing alveolar carbon dioxide. This effect is important when healthy humans ascend to altitude for recreation or military purposes. In chest diseases where there is a mismatch between respiratory control and ventilatory effects, hypoxia is less avoidable and, indirectly through the increased drive to breathe, is associated with greater feelings of breathlessness or dyspnea [13,82]. In the instance of sleep-disordered breathing, hypoxemia is state-related and intermittent; these disturbances in ventilation fragment sleep and produce hypoxic stress, resulting in daytime symptoms of sleepiness and cardiovascular sequelae [79].

In high altitude native populations exposed to lower inspired oxygen and intermittent hypoxia (due to sleep, exercise, or breath holding), ventilatory control as well as other physiologic elements in oxygen delivery may be engaged to satisfy cellular energy needs for survival [7].

While individual values are modified over time by factors such as chronic exposure to altitude, respiratory loading, physical fitness, age, hormones, sex hormones and sleep [14,81], the focus of this review will be the inheritance of ventilatory traits in response to hypoxia.

Hypoxic Response as a Series of Complex Traits

The ventilation response to hypoxia has several time-domains and points of notable change (Figure 1) [68]. On exposure to hypoxia there is an early peak response followed by a decline in ventilation ("roll-off"). The peak response is thought to originate from the sensor projections from the carotid body [27] while the "roll-off" during hypoxia engages central inhibitory systems by central accumulation and/or release of inhibitory neurotransmitters on respiratory neurons [73]. However, some protein factors, like PDGF and its receptors, affect this response [3,29,97]. The magnitude of both the acute response and "roll-off" differs among species.

Upon reoxygenation there are two broad responses – one called short-term potentiation, where ventilation remains elevated above baseline (pre-hypoxic) values and another called post-hypoxic (frequency or ventilatory)

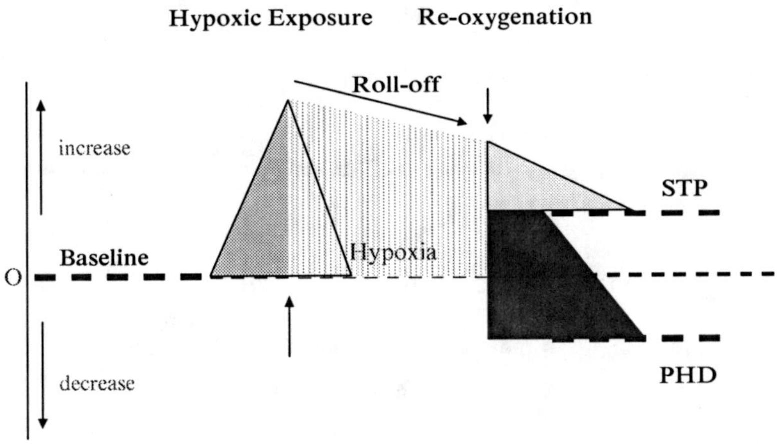

Figure 1. Responses to hypoxia and reoxygenation in the time domain. STP refers to short term potentiation, where the response (frequency or minute ventilation) remains higher than baseline. PHD refers to post hypoxic decline in frequency or minute ventilation, where there occurs an undershoot upon reoxygenation compared to baseline.

decline, where ventilation and/or frequency fall below baseline. Short-term potentiation of ventilation would promote persistence of ventilation [57] and protect against further reductions in drive, potentially leading to apnea [98]. Patients with obstructive sleep apnea, hypopnea syndrome [28] and those with Cheyne-Stokes respiration [2] who regularly experience hypoxia during sleep, often lack short-term potentiation during wakefulness.

Prolonged as well as episodic hypoxemia in animal models will enhance a tendency towards system instability [18,57]. In the awake goat [21,22] and sleeping human [5] unstable breathing develops if a fall in CO_2 (hypocapnia) occurs, thus implying an interplay among chemoreceptors and integration of the response at a brainstem level. Intermittent hypoxia may evoke changes in the operation of respiratory rhythm generation and suggests a system that changes over time in response to hypoxia-reoxygenation cycles [68]. Responses could engage higher brain centers and not just the pons or medulla [56], though a primary role in unstable breathing is not established.

Ventilatory responses to hypoxia (and re-oxygenation) involve interconnected neuronal pools in the medulla and pons [58,61,32]. Central neurotransmitters implicated in re-oxygenation responses include serotonin and adenosine [10,84] and nitric oxide [69]. The pontine A5 region is involved in coordinating this response [94].

The genetic architecture of the hypoxic response is not known but a schematic for the concept is shown in Figure 2. Genes and gene products (mRNA) work at a proteomic and cellular level to form organs that comprise

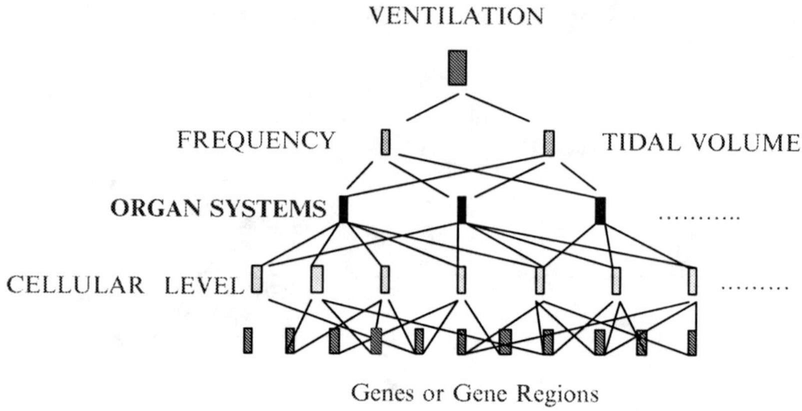

Figure 2. The pathways between genes and the ventilatory traits of respiratory frequency (f) and depth (tidal volume or TV) are complex and involve several levels of cellular and system integration.

the various systems in respiratory control (controllers, controlled systems and sensors). These in turn create the features of respiratory frequency and tidal volume, and comprise minute ventilation of which the important component is alveolar ventilation. In this model the pathways from genes to ventilatory behavior are indirect. No one factor may be necessary or sufficient to explain the hypoxic response and no one gene is necessary or sufficient to produce a variation [54]. As a result, genetic research in humans will require large populations with phenotype collection coordinated among centers in order to identify target regions that might give insight into genes or proteins that affect acute (as well as chronic adaptations) to hypoxia. Complementary to the study of humans is the use of animal models to identify the genomic regions that underlie intermediate traits and are syntenic to humans [75,93]. A reasonable expectation is that natural selection in animals will work on similar pathways if not genes to increase or decrease a trait value, like hypoxic responsiveness, that may operate in human physiology or disease.

Evidence for Inheritance of Ventilatory Traits in Humans

There is "individuality" in respiratory patterning of tidal volume and frequency in humans during both wakefulness and sleep [78]. The shape and timing of tidal breaths are more similar in monozygotic twins than in unrelated individuals not only during breathing at rest but also during behavioral tasks [76]. Respiratory patterning differs in healthy humans and tracks with regions of the genome, especially the trait of breathing frequency during sleep (19]. Differences between humans are presumed to reside in the central patterning of the respiratory rate and regulating the size and pattern of inspiratory and expiratory flow rates [77].

Additional evidence indicates that humans exhibit heritable variations in the response to standard hypoxic challenge. Greater similarities in hypoxic ventilatory responsiveness occur between monozygotic twins than between dyzygotic twins [15,42,45,41,44]. Reports indicate abnormal ventilatory responsiveness to hypercapnia or hypoxia is present in first-degree relatives of patients with excessive hypercapnia, hypoxia,or unexplained respiratory failure [38,59,39,43,40] or those with sleep apnea [71]. In contrast, some but not all studies report concordance of patterns of ventilatory responsiveness to hypercapnia between monozygotic twins [43,52]. This literature forms one basis for concluding that there occurs a rather wide range of variation in hypoxic chemoresponsiveness in the healthy human population, and that such variation to a significant degree is likely to result from heritable factors.

A second line of evidence comes from studies in high altitude natives. The fact that humans live and prosper in moderately low oxygen environments offers natural experiments to examine if or how hypoxic responses are affected by chronic hypoxia. Newcomers acclimatizing to high altitude generally increase hypoxic responses over time [60] but there is a range of response and no instances where inheritance is an explicit part of the experimental protocol. Adult male Tibetan high altitude natives have increased ventilation relative to sea level natives, while reports on Andean and Rocky Mountain high altitude natives show a normal or low normal ventilation [61]. One paper compared resting ventilation and hypoxic ventilatory response of native residents residing at 3,800–4,065 m from the Andes and Tibet, using the same equipment and approach [8]. Within each population, a lower percentage of oxygen saturation of arterial hemoglobin was associated with slightly higher resting ventilation among Tibetans but lower resting ventilation and hypoxic ventilatory responses among Andean women, although the associations accounted for <10% of the variation. Between populations, the Tibetan sample had a 1.5 times higher mean resting ventilation and 2-fold higher hypoxic ventilatory responses. Age being perhaps a surrogate marker for the duration of hypoxia was not a significant factor. AS data had been collected in families, the inherited component was that approximately 35% of the Tibetan, but none of the Andean, variance in resting ventilation could be attributed to genetic factors. With regard to hypoxic ventilatory responses, 31% of the Tibetan, but just 21% of the Andean, variance could be attributed to genetic factors. There are at least two different heritable ventilation phenotypes in human populations living at altitude. The other implication is that lifelong sustained exposure to hypoxia does not favor a unique ventilatory response for survival advantage in humans.

An effort to quantify and identify in humans the chromosomal mechanisms of the hypoxic response is justified. Studies of this issue are likely to provide insight into the influence of natural variation on the physiology of normal breathing, both at sea level and at altitude.

Phenotyping Ventilatory Traits in Small Animals

Studies in nominal models on genetic factors complement studies of cellular and organ system models and precedent exists for identifying phenotype-genotype homologues among rat, mouse and human genomes [55,63], providing an extraordinary opportunity for understanding the evolution of ventilation.

Ideally, one should have collection of phenotype traits or set of traits that are sensitive to single features of the respiratory system-controller, controlled system, or sensor. However, at present this is not the case and our current ability to phenotype living animals cannot isolate each part involved in ventilatory control. The need to study large numbers of small animals and at times permit these test "subjects" to breed has necessitated the use of non-invasive measures of ventilation, namely tidal volume and frequency, using the barometric method (Figure 3) [6]. Compared to the precision

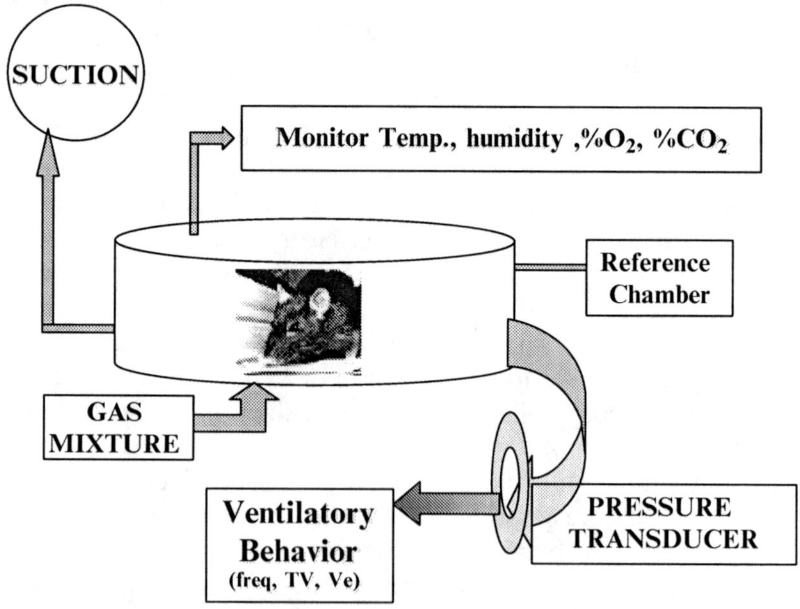

Figure 3. This diagram illustrates the elements of a barometric method for measuring ventilatory behavior in rodents. Not shown in detail is the use of a sealed reference chamber, identical in size to the animal chamber.

available for human monitoring (by facemask and with cooperation with non-invasive monitoring), there are general problems with the barometric approach needed for rodent monitoring [24,36,37,12,20]. While frequency is a very precise value, tidal volume is semi-quantitative [23] and the measurement is affected by body temperature and the temperature and humidity of the chamber [6,31]. The technical errors are manageable (<10%) and enter into non-genetic effects but the strength of this approach is the ability to measure an animal which is relatively unrestrained, and anaesthetized [62]. Variability is induced by environmental factors such as light, smell, noise, etc., but these environmental factors can be reduced by careful attention to the testing chamber protocol [20] and time of day [25,90]. A variation in experimental protocols and testing conditions enters into estimates of the variance attributed to environmental rather than genetic factors. If the environmental effect is too large or uncontrolled, it will obscure detection of even a moderate genetic effect. Other features important to remember in phenotyping for ventilatory behavior are shown in Table 1.

The use of reduced preparations and/or more technologically advanced approaches are effective as second-order phenotyping strategies. The ideal would be to use a reduced preparation in tandem with studies of natural variation to disclose mechanisms for evolutionary fitness. Simultaneous use of proteomics and expression arrays in such models may efficiently screen many biochemical processes that could contribute to trait variance, and can be useful in locating candidate genes within the regions-of-interest identified through the study of inbred lines. This approach is used to identify genomic elements operating in strain differences in sleep in the mouse [96]. Complementary and parallel studies in animals and humans can be more efficient in understanding the biology of the response.

In summary, the key is the knowledge of the trait value and its origins and maintaining the environmental conditions as consistently as possible. Initial results are likely to be confounded by known and unknown sources of variance, not only within a laboratory but also in comparing results from

TABLE 1. Some features to optimize phenotype collection for ventilatory behavior

- Consistent testing facilities with regard to quiet surroundings, odor suppression, and consistency in technical assistance over time
- Standardized protocols for calibration of equipment, testing steps and time of testing
- Appropriate size and shape of barometric chambers to minimize dispersal of pressure and convection effects
- Standardized cleaning of chambers between testing of different animals
- Control and/or knowledge of food vendor and source and other environmental factors used in the housing of animals outside the testing chamber
- Quality control over time using animals from in-bred strains

other laboratories. Bias can be introduced at every level of collection of the phenotype data and will enter into the analysis as an environmental factor, obscuring true linkage. The physiologist will need to prove suspected biological linkage in any number of ways [79].

Evidence for Unequivocal Genetic Effects

The best direct evidence is found in the literature on genetically engineered animals. These studies indicate that genetic background directly influences respiratory frequency, tidal volume, and/or minute ventilation either at rest or with hypoxic challenge.

The studies of nitric oxide synthase (NOS) are one example. There are three isoforms of NOS (N)S-1, NOS-2, and NOS-3) arising from three different regions of the genome and these enzymes are involved in the generation of nitric oxide (NO), a major player in oxygen homeostasis. The concept of genetic transmission of post-hypoxia ventilatory behavior is directly supported by reports of nearly absent respiratory depression in response to brief hyperoxia in nitric oxide synthase (NOS)-3 mutant mice [51]. In addition, an altered breathing pattern occurs in NOS-1 mice where function is eliminated by knock-out [50,46].

There are studies of interesting ‘candidate" genes, believed to influence ventilation as disclosed by reduced preparations or by analogy to other systems. Sometimes insight comes from the availability of a unique strain. These knock-out mouse models report loss of or reduction in hypoxic response attributed to endothelin converting enzyme-1(ECE-1) [72], to endothelin-1 [53], to dopamine [35], to the neutral endopepidase (NEP) [30], and to HIF [47]. However, animals with knocked-out genes for other putative proteins involved in hypoxic responses show no effect on ventilation; this is the case for Endothelin-3 [64].

These studies of knock-out mice underscore the complexity of the genetic architecture for the respiratory network (see Figure 1). Genes may act or more likely interact differently in different stages of development, even altering gain or function in a knock-out model. The reports on the tachykinin NK-1 system show that NK1 receptors are important in the response to acute hypoxia in the adult mouse; however, NK1 receptors are not obligatory for the prenatal development of the respiratory network, for the production of the rhythm, or for the regulation of breathing by short-lasting hypoxia in neonates [70]. When comparisons are made between monoamine oxidase A-deficient transgenic (Tg8) mice with control (C3H) strains, the implication is that an elevated serotonin during the perinatal period alters respiratory network maturation and produces a permanent respiratory dysfunction, whereas a high serotonin level present in adults depresses chemosensation

[11]. Therefore, variation in genetic background can operate to produce effects at a number of developmental time points, suggesting that our cross-sectional studies of humans will be limited in the amount of detail of the longitudinal functions of genes.

The NADPH system is of interest for its presumed role in oxygen sensing at a mitochondrial level. There is a role for the subunit of NADPH, gp91, in cellular sensing of oxygen in airway neuroepithelial cells [26], but not in adrenal cells [95]. Yet in KO models there is little effect on pulmonary vascular [4] or carotid body [33] cellular responses to hypoxia, nor in ventilatory behavior [74].

These knock-out models, while of significant interest, are often not based on proven risk factors for health or disease in the natural world. Evolutionary fitness will require actions of both the real and latent variance in several genes and gene products, respiratory system capacity and learning. Understanding the role of genes in normal and pathologic control of ventilation will require approaches that will accommodate the probable collective effects of multiple loci.

Another way to illuminate genetic influences is to examine drug effects in different strains of rodents. The first study to show an effect of strain on respiratory physiology reported on the effect of brainstem injection of MK-801 to induce apnea. The reproducible effects in Sprague Dawley animals was not found in Wistar rats, animals studied by mistake [16]. The authors were perplexed but noted to their credit that there must be some effect of a genetic background.

We have used this general drug-by-strain approach in unanesthetized animals. As studies in NOS knock-out mice have shown that the nitric oxide system can influence post-hypoxic ventilatory behavior [48,51,49], the question arises whether nitric oxide synthase (NOS) blockade would similarly effect ventilatory behavior in two rat strains. After vehicle, post-hypoxic decline in frequency and minute ventilation is not evident in the Sprague Dawley strain [85]. NOS blockade resulted in a greater increase in resting ventilation in the Sprague Dawley than in the Brown Norway strain, but produced post-hypoxic frequency and ventilatory decline in the Sprague Dawley strain [84]. We have observed a similar effect using a selective neuronal NOS (NOS-1) blocking agent (7-nitroindazole or 7-NI, 60 mg/kg) (K. Strohl, unpublished findings). The results indicate that the various strains do not utilize the NO pathway in the same way with regard to the regulation of ventilatory behavior.

The strength of the knockout approach or drug-by-strain approach is the comfortable connection between a known gene, peptide, or protein and the ability to make a rational connection to ventilatory behavior. However, false-negative as well as false-positive findings may occur due to selection bias and/or over-interpretation of the significance of results from knock-out models, as ventilatory behavior is likely the result of many gene pathways.

Evidence for the Inheritance of Ventilatory Traits in Rodents

In 1984, Ou et al. [66] reported differences in the ventilatory behavior between two colonies of Sprague-Dawley rats in response to chronic exposure to hypoxia. Despite these being out-bred strains (no conscious in-breeding by brother-sister pairing for >20 generations), consistent differences in the ventilatory response to hypoxia before the exposure remained between colonies over the course of several years, and correlated to differences in the erythropoietic and pulmonary vascular pressor responses to chronic hypobaric hypoxia [67]. By the different vendors maintaining closed populations, genetic drift occurred. The problem with the study of these Sprague Dawley strains is that the similarities between the genomes are so great that finding the responsible gene is difficult.

In 1995, Tankersley et al. [89] reported results from the more traditional approach of surveying ventilatory behavior in several in-bred strains of mice. There were significant inter-strain differences in respiratory frequency, hypoxic responsiveness and hypercapnic responsiveness between several strains [88]. Quantitative statistics of animals derived from these strains suggest that the genetic control of hypoxic ventilatory responses exhibits a relatively simple Mendelian inheritance in terms of respiratory timing characteristics. Furthermore, differences in inspiratory time at baseline is linked to a putative genomic region on mouse chromosome 3 [87]; however, a likely candidate gene related to neuronal receptors does not explain this association [91] and this region does not correlate with the variations in lung mechanics between these two strains [92]. Therefore, this study suggests that the phenotypic variation in hypoxic ventilatory response between the two parental strains, especially related to frequency during hypoxia, is possibly regulated by only a few major genetic determinants. This literature encourages the use of functional genomics in an effort to link ventilatory behavior to cellular mechanisms [86].

In 1997, Strohl et al. [83] reported measurements of ventilation and metabolism in four strains of rat, chosen for a wide variation in traits for body weight and/or blood pressure regulation. The conclusion is that strain, more than the effect of body mass or sex, had a major influence on metabolism, the pattern and level of ventilation during air breathing and ventilation during loading or unloading of chemoreceptor input in the unanesthetized rat. A more recent study found similar results in four strains of rat, including a confirmation of the low CO_2 response in the Brown Norway [34]. These strain differences indicate that the ventilatory response to chemosensory input appears to be genetically regulated. (Figure 4)

Inheritance operates on non-steady state responses. Figure 4 illustrated the differences in the ventilatory behavior (frequency, tidal volume

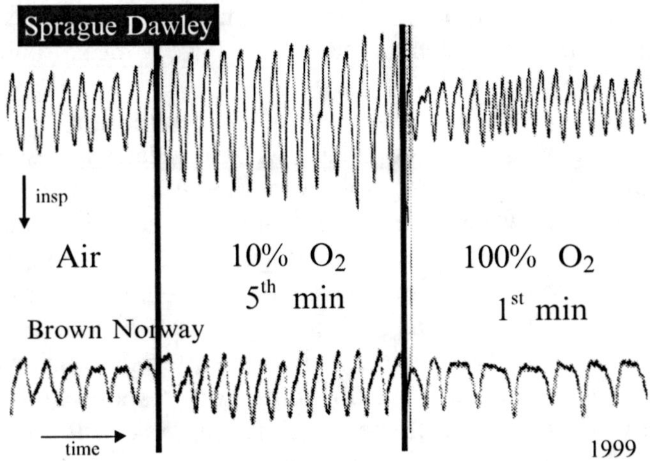

Figure 4. Recordings from two animals (one Sprague Dawley and one Brown Norway) are compared in regard to the pattern of breathing at rest, in the fifth minute of hypoxia and in the first minute or so after re-oxygenation from hypoxia. Adapted from (Subramanian, Han et al. 2001).

and minute ventilation) in Sprague Dawley and Brown Norway animals. Ventilatory decline seen in the Brown Norway in response to 100% oxygen after five minutes of exposure to hypoxic gas (10% oxygen, 90% N_2) was not present in the Sprague Dawley strain but was quite evident in the Brown Norway strain. This study is consistent with the notion that genetic factors not only influence the ventilatory response to hypoxia but also to re-oygenation following hypoxic exposure [85]. Such non-steady state responses could be important intermediate traits relevant to recurrent cycles of hypoxia-reoxygenation present in sleep-disordered breathing.

The above studies in common strains of mice and rats offer the most compelling argument for ventilatory behavior being affected by "natural selection" and offer the foundation for "physiogenomic" studies aimed at elucidating the genetics of these ventilatory control mechanisms [80]. The effects seen in these models can be quite modest and the assignment of cause-and-effect relationships can be complex, given that adjustments in one gene may influence another gene or gene product and one gene can have an influence on more that one trait or part of the system for respiratory control.

Towards a Physiogenetic Map of Ventilatory Behavior

Given the complex nature of ventilatory behavior, it is remarkable that studies of ventilatory behavior have identified any of the genetic effects. Yet a literature on the genetics of ventilatory behavior is emerging with animal models and traits that appear relevant to human pathophysiology. One theme is that a limited number of genes can have a measurable impact on ventilatory behavior in health.

It is likely the genes that not only affect ventilation when breathing is stimulated but also may correlate with regulatory systems for the cardiovascular system, and perhaps even metabolism. This makes sense when one considers how well integrated, from a physiological standpoint, the systems and mechanisms that regulate oxygen homeostasis are. It will, therefore, be important to consider the presence of gene interactions. Such interactions are revealed not only as preliminary data for the mapping of gene loci, but also as a way of gaining insight into the interrelationships and nature of the genetic mechanisms influencing ventilatory responsiveness [80].

Identification of trait-influencing gene regions will be relevant to understanding human diseases characterized by hypo- or hyper-ventilation and/or abnormal respiratory patterns in response to hypoxia. We would have greater opportunity to understand the heterogeneity in responses to environmental influences and, potentially, to develop a set of markers that help to address breathing patterns in human health and disease.

References

1. Agostoni E, Thimm FF, Fenn Wo. (1959). "Comparative features of mechanics of breathing." J Appl Phyisiol 14: 679–683.
2. Ahmed M, Serrette C, Kryger MH, Anthonisen NR. (1994). "Ventilatory instability in patients with congestive heart failure and nocturnal Cheyne-Stokes breathing." Sleep 17: 527–34.
3. Alea, OA, Czapla MA, Lasky JA, Simakajornboon N, Gozal E, Gozal D. (2000). "PDGF-beta receptor expression and ventilatory acclimatization to hypoxia in the rat." Am J Physiol Regul Integr Comp Physiol 279: R1625–33.
4. Archer SL, Reeve HL, Michelakis E, Puttaqunta L, Waite R, Nelson DP, Dinauer MC, Weir EK. (1999). "O2 sensing is preserved in mice lacking the gp91 phox subunit of NADPH oxidase." Proc Natl Acad Sci U S A 96: 7944–9.
5. Badr MS, Skatrud JB, Dempsey JA. (1994). "Effect of chemoreceptor stimulation and inhibition on total pulmonary resistance in humans during NREM sleep." J Appl Physiol 76: 1682–92.
6. Bartlett D Jr, and Tenney SM.(1970). "Control of breathing in experimental anemia." Respir Physiol 10: 384–95.
7. Beall CM. (2000). "Tibetan and Andean contrasts in adaptation to high-altitude hypoxia." Adv Exp Med Biol 475: 63–74.
8. Beall CM, Strohl KP, Blangero J, Williams-Blangero S, Almasy LA, Decker MJ, Worthman CM, Goldstein MC, Vargas E, Villena M, Soria R, Alarcon AM, Gonzales C. (1997). "Ventilation and hypoxic ventilatory response of Tibetan and Aymara high altitude natives." Am J Phys Anthropol 104: 427–47.
9. Bennett FM and Tenney SM (1982). "Comparative mechanics of mammalian respiratory system." Respir Physiol 49: 131–40.

10. Bonham AC (1995). "Neurotransmitters In the CNS Control of Breathing." Resp Physiol 101: 219–230.
11. Burnet H, Bevengut M, Chakri F, Bou-Flores C, Coulon P et al. (2001). "Altered respiratory activity and respiratory regulations in adult monoamine oxidase A-deficient mice." J Neurosci 21: 5212–21.
12. Chaui-Berlinck JG, and Bicudo JE (1998). "The signal in total-body plethysmography: errors due to adiabatic-isothermic difference." Respir Physiol 113: 259–70.
13. Cherniack NS, and Altose MD (1987). "Mechanisms of dyspnea." Clin Chest Med 8: 207–14.
14. CherniackNS, and Longobardo GS (1981). "The chemical control of respiration." Ann Biomed Eng 9: 395–407.
15. Collins DD, Scoggin CH, Zwillich CW, Weil JV. (1978). "Hereditary aspects of decreased hypoxic response." J Clin Invest 70: 105–110.
16. Connelly CA, Otto-Smith MR, Feldman JL. (1992). "Blockade of NMDA receptor-channels by MK-801 alters breathing in adult rats." Brain Res 596: 99–110.
17. Crossfill ML, and Widdicombe J (1961). "Comparative mechanics of the mammalian respiratory system." Resp Physiol 49: 131–140.
18. Dahan A, Berkenbosch A, Degoede J, van den Elsen M, Olievier I, van Kleef J. (1995). "Influence of hypoxic duration and posthypoxic inspired O2 concentration on short term potentiation of breathing in humans." J Physiol (Lond) 488: 803–13.
19. de Geus EJ, Posthuma D, Kupper N, van der Berg M, Willemsen G, Beem AL, Slaqboom PE, Boomsma DI. (2005). "A whole-genome scan for 24-hour respiration rate: a major locus at 10q26 influences respiration during sleep." Am J Hum Genet 76: 100–11.
20. DeLorme MP, and Moss OR (2002). "Pulmonary function assessment by whole-body plethysmography in restrained versus unrestrained mice." J Pharmacol Toxicol Methods 47: 1–10.
21. Engwall MJ, Daristotle L, Niu WZ, Dempsey JA, Bisgard GE. (1991). "Ventilatory afterdischarge in the awake goat." J Appl Physiol 71: 1511–7.
22. Engwall MJ, Smith CA, Dempsey JA, Bisgard GE. (1994). "Ventilatory afterdischarge and central respiratory drive interactions in the awake goat." J Appl Physiol 76: 416–23.
23. Enhorning G, van Schaik S, Lundgren C, Vargas I. (1998). "Whole-body plethysmography, does it measure tidal volume of small animals?" Can J Physiol Pharmacol 76: 945–51.
24. Epstein MA, and Epstein RA. (1978). "A theoretical analysis of the barometric method for measurement of tidal volume." Respir Physiol 32: 105–20.
25. Fenelon K, Seifert EL, Mortola JP. (2000). "Hypoxic depression of circadian oscillations in sino-aortic denervated rats." Respir Physiol 122: 61–9.
26. Fu XW, Wang D, Nurse CA, Dinauer MC, Cutz E. (2000). "NADPH oxidase is an O2 sensor in airway chemoreceptors: evidence from K+ current modulation in wild-type and oxidase-deficient mice." Proc Natl Acad Sci U S A 97: 4374–9.
27. Gauda EB. (2002). "Gene expression in peripheral arterial chemoreceptors." Microsc Res Tech 59: 153–67.
28. Georgopoulus D, Giannouli E, Tsara V, Argiropoulou P, Patakas D, Anthonisen NR. (1992). "Respiratory short-term poststimulus potentiation (after-discharge) in patients with obstructive sleep apnea." Am Rev Respir Dis 146: 1250–5.
29. Gozal D, Simakajornboon N, Czapla MA, Xue YD, Gozal E, Vlasic V, Lasky JA, Liu JY. (2000). "Brainstem activation of platelet-derived growth factor-beta receptor modulates the late phase of the hypoxic ventilatory response." J Neurochem 74: 310–9.
30. Grasemann H, Lu B, Jiao A, Boudreau J, Gerard NP, De Sanctis GT. (1999). "Targeted deletion of the neutral endopeptidase gene alters ventilatory responses to acute hypoxia in mice." J Appl Physiol 87: 1266–71.
31. Hamelmann E, Schwarze J, Takeda K, Oshiba A, Larsen GL, Irvin CG, Gelfand EW. (1997). "Noninvasive measurement of airway responsiveness in allergic mice using barometric plethysmography [see comments]." Am J Respir Crit Care Med 15: 766–75.

32. Haxhiu MA, Mack SO, Wilson CG, Feng P, Strohl KP. (2003). "Sleep networks and the anatomic and physiologic connections with respiratory control." Front Biosci 8: d946–62.
33. He L, Chen J, Dinger B, Sanders K, Sundar K, Hoidal J, Fidone S. (2002). "Characteristics of carotid body chemosensitivity in NADPH oxidase-deficient mice." Am J Physiol Cell Physiol 282: C27–33.
34. Hodges MR, Forster HV, Papanek PE, Dwinell MR, Hogan GE. (2002). "Ventilatory phenotypes among four strains of adult rats." J Appl Physiol 93: 974–83.
35. Huey KA, Low MJ, Kelly MA, Juarez R, Szewczak JM, Powell FL. (2000). "Ventilatory responses to acute and chronic hypoxia in mice: effects of dopamine D(2) receptors." J Appl Physiol 89: 1142–50.
36. Jacky JP. (1978). "A plethysmograph for long-term measurements of ventilation in unrestrained animals." J Appl Physiol 45: 644–7.
37. Jacky JP. (1980). "Barometric measurement of tidal volume: effects of pattern and nasal temperature." J Appl Physiol 49: 319–25.
38. Kafer ER, and Leigh J (1972). "Recurrent respiratory failure associated with the absence of ventilatory response to hypercapnia and hypoxemia." Am Rev Respir Dis 106: 100–8.
39. Kawakami Y, Irie T, Shida A, Yoshikawa T. (1982). "Familial factors affecting arterial blood gas values and respiratory chemosensitivity in chronic obstructive pulmonary disease." Am Rev Respir Dis 125: 420–5.
40. Kawakami Y, Shida A, Yamamoto H, Yoshikawa T. (1985). "Pattern of genetic influence on pulmonary function." Chest 87: 507–11.
41. Kawakami, Y., A. Shida, et al. (1984). "Genetic and environmental influence on inspiratory resistive load detection." Respiration 45: 100–10.
42. Kawakami Y, Yamamoto H, Yoshikawa T, Yamamoto H. (1982). "Respiratory chemosensitivity in smokers. Studies on monozygotic twins." Am Rev Respir Dis 126: 986–90.
43. Kawakami Y, Yamamoto H, Yoshikawa, Shida A. (1984). "Chemical and behavioral control of breathing in twins." Am Rev Respir Dis 129: 703–707.
44. Kawakami Y, Yamamoto H, Yoshikawa T, Shida A. (1985). "Age-related variation of respiratory chemosensitivity in monozygotic twins." Am Rev Respir Dis 132: 89–92.
45. Kawakami Y, Yoshikawa T, Shida A, Asanuma Y, Murao M. (1982). "Control of breathing in young twins." J Appl Physiol 52: 537–42.
46. Kline DD, Overholt JL, Prabhakar NR. (2002). "Mutant mice deficient in NOS-1 exhibit attenuated long-term facilitation and short-term potentiation in breathing." J Physiol 539: 309–15.
47. Kline DD, Peng YJ, Manalo DJ, Semenza GL, Prabhakar NR. (2002). "Defective carotid body function and impaired ventilatory responses to chronic hypoxia in mice partially deficient for hypoxia-inducible factor 1alpha." Proc Natl Acad Sci U S A 15: 15.
48. Kline DD, and Prabhakar NR (2000). "Peripheral chemosensitivity in mutant mice deficient in nitric oxide synthase." Adv Exp Med Biol 475: 571–9.
49. Kline DD, and Prabhakar NR (2001). "Role of nitric oxide in short-term potentiation and long-term facilitation: involvement of NO in breathing stability." Adv Exp Med Biol 499: 215–9.
50. Kline DD, Yang T, Huanq PL, Prabhakar NR. (1998). "Altered respiratory responses to hypoxia in mutant mice deficient in neuronal nitric oxide synthase." J Physiol (Lond) 511: 273–87.
51. Kline DD, Yang T, Premkumar DR, Thomas AJ, Prabhakar. (2000). "Blunted respiratory responses to hypoxia in mutant mice deficient in nitric oxide synthase-3." J Appl Physiol 88: 1496–508.
52. Kobayashi S, Nishimura, Yamamoto M, Akiyama Y, Kishi F, Kawakami Y. (1993). "Dyspnea sensation and chemical control of breathing in adult twins." Am Rev Respir Dis 147: 1192–8.

53. Kuwaki T, Cao WH, Kurihara Y, Kurihara H, Ling GY, Onodera M, Ju KH, Yazaki Y, Kumada M. (1996). "Impaired ventilatory responses to hypoxia and hypercapnia in mutant mice deficient in endothelin-1." Am J Physiol 270: R1279–86.
54. Lander E, and Schork N. (1994). "The genetic dissection of complex traits." Science 265: 2037–2048.
55. Lander ES, and Botstein D. (1989). "Mapping mendelian factors underlying quantitative traits using RFLP linkage maps." Genetics 121: 185–99.
56. Lipton AJ., Johnson MA, Macdonald T, Lieberman MW, Gozal D, Gaston B. (2001). "S-nitrosothiols signal the ventilatory response to hypoxia." Nature 413: 171–4.
57. Menendez AA, Nuckton TJ, Torres JE, Gozal D. (1999). "Short-term potentiation of ventilation after different levels of hypoxia." J Appl Physiol 86: 1478–82.
58. Mironov SL, and Richter DW. (1998). "L-type Ca2+ channels in inspiratory neurones of mice and their modulation by hypoxia." J Physiol 512: 75–87.
59. Moore GC, Zwillich CW, Battaqlia JD, Cotton EK, Weil JV. (1976). "Respiratory failure associated with familial depression of ventilatory response to hypoxia and hypercapnia." N Engl J Med 295(16): 861–5.
60. Moore LG. (2000). "Comparative human ventilatory adaptation to high altitude." Respir Physiol 121: 257–76.
61. Moore LG, Niermeyer S, Zamudio S. (1998). "Human adaptation to high altitude: regional and life-cycle perspectives." Am J Phys Anthropol Suppl 27: 25–64.
62. Mortola JP, and Frappell PB. (1998). "On the barometric method for measurements of ventilation, and its use in small animals." Can J Physiol Pharmacol 76: 937–44.
63. Nadeau JH, Singer JB, Matin A, Lander ES. (2000). "Analysing complex genetic traits with chromosome substitution strains." Nat Genet 24: 221–5.
64. Nakamura A, Kuwaki T, Kuriyama T, Yanaqisawa M, Fukuda Y. (2001). "Normal ventilation and ventilatory responses to chemical stimuli in juvenile mutant mice deficient in endothelin-3." Respir Physiol 124: 1–9.
65. Nattie EE. (2001). "Central chemosensitivity, sleep, and wakefulness." Respir Physiol 129: 257–68.
66. Ou LC, Hill NS, Tenney SM. (1984). "Ventilatory responses and blood gases in susceptible and resistant rats to high altitude." Resp Physiol 58: 161–170.
67. Ou LC and Smith RP. (1983). "Probable strain differences of rats in susceptibilities and cardio- pulmonary responses to chronic hypoxia." Respir Physiol 53: 367–377.
68. Powell FL, Milsom WK, Mitchell GS. (1998). "Time domains of the hypoxic ventilatory response." Respir Physiol 112: 123–34.
69. Price ER, Han F, Dick TE, Strohl KP. (2003). "7-nitroindazole and posthypoxic ventilatory behavior in the A/J and C57BL/6J mouse strains." J Appl Physiol 95: 1097–104.
70. Ptak K, Burnet H, Blanchi B, Sieweke M, De Felipe C, Hunt SP, Monteau R, Hilaire G. (2002). "The murine neurokinin NK1 receptor gene contributes to the adult hypoxic facilitation of ventilation." Eur J Neurosci 16: 2245–52.
71. Redline S, Leitner J, Arnold J, Tishler PV, Altose MD. (1997). "Ventilatory control abnormalities in familial sleep apnea." Am J Respir Crit Care Med 156: 155–160.
72. Renolleau S, Dauger S, Vardon G, Levacher B, Simonneau M, Yanaqisawa M, Gaultier C, Gallego J. (2001). "Impaired ventilatory responses to hypoxia in mice deficient in endothelin-converting-enzyme-1." Pediatr Res 49: 705–12.
73. Richter DW, Ballanyi K, Schwarzacher S. (1992). "Mechanisms of Respiratory Rhythm Generation." Current Opinion in Neurobiology 2: 788–793.
74. Roy A, Rozanov C, Mokashi A, Daudu P, Al-Mehdi AB, Shams H, Lahiri S. (2000). "Mice lacking in gp91 phox subunit of NAD(P)H oxidase showed glomus cell [Ca(2+)](i) and respiratory responses to hypoxia." Brain Res 872: 188–93.
75. Schork NJ, Krieger JE, Trolliet MR, Franchini KG, Koike G, Krieger EM, Lander ES, Dzau VJ, Jacob HJ. (1995). "A biometrical genome search in rats reveals the multigenic basis of blood pressure variation." Genome Res 5: 164–72.

76. Shea SA, Dinh TP, Hamilton RD, Guz A, Benchetrit G. (1993). "Breathing patterns of monozygous twins during behavioural tasks." Acta Genet Med Gemellol (Roma) 42: 171–84.
77. Shea SA and Guz A. (1992). "Personnalite ventilatoire–an overview." Respir Physiol 87: 275–91.
78. Shea SA, Horner RL, Benchetrit G, Guz A. (1990). "The persistence of a respiratory 'personality' into stage IV sleep in man." Respir Physiol 80: 33–44.
79. Society AT. (1999). Finding Genetic Mechanisms in Syndromes of Sleep Disordered Breathing, www.thoracic.org.
80. Stoll M, Cowley AW Jr, Tonellato PJ, Greene AS, Kaldunski ML, Roman RJ, Dumas P, Schork NJ, Wang Z, Jacob HJ. (2001). "A genomic-systems biology map for cardiovascular function." Science 294: 1723–1726.
81. Strohl KP, Cherniack NS, Gothe B. (1986). "Physiologic basis of therapy for sleep apnea." Am Rev Respir Dis 134: 791–802.
82. Strohl KP, and Thomas AJ. (1998). "Breathlessness, anxiety, and respiratory physiology." Psychosom Med 60: 680–1.
83. Strohl KP, Thomas AJ, St Jean P, Schlenker EH, Koletsky RJ, Schork NJ. (1997). "Ventilation and metabolish among rat strains." J Appl Physiol 82: 317–323.
84. Subramanian S, Erokwu B, Han F, Dick TE, Strohl KP. (2002). "L-NAME differentially alters ventilatory behavior in Sprague-Dawley and Brown Norway rats." J Appl Physiol 93: 984–9.
85. Subramanian S, Han F, Erokwu BO, Dick TE, Strohl KP. (2001). "Do genetic factors influence the Dejours phenomenon?" Adv Exp Med Biol 499: 209–14.
86. Tankersley CG. (1999). "Genetic control of ventilation: what are we learning from murine models?" Curr Opin Pulm Med 5: 344–8.
87. Tankersley CG, DiSilvestre DA, Jedlicka AE, Wilkins HM, Zhang L. (1998). "Differential inspiratory timing is genetically linked to mouse chromosome 3." J Appl Physiol 85: 360–5.
88. Tankersley CG, Fitzgerald RS, Kleeberger SR. (1994). "Differential control of ventilation among inbred strains of mice." Am J Physiol 267: R1371–7.
89. Tankersley CG, Fitzgerald RS, Mitzner WA, Kleeberger SR. (1993). "Hypercapnic ventilatory responses in mice differentially susceptible to acute ozone exposure." J Appl Physiol 75: 2613–2619.
90. Tankersley CG, Irizarry R, Flanders S, Rabold R. (2002). "Circadian rhythm variation in activity, body temperature, and heart rate between C3H/HeJ and C57BL/6J inbred strains." J Appl Physiol 92: 870–7.
91. Tankersley CG, Kulaga H, Wang MM. (2001). "Inspiratory timing differences and regulation of Gria2 gene variation: a candidate gene hypothesis." Adv Exp Med Biol 499: 477–82.
92. Tankersley CG, Rabold R, Mitzner W. (1999). "Differential lung mechanics are genetically determined in inbred murine strains." J Appl Physiol 86: 1764–9.
93. Thibonnier M, and Schork NJ (1995). "The genetics of hypertension." Curr Opin Genet Dev 5: 362–70.
94. Thoby-Brisson M, and Ramirez JM. (2000). "Role of inspiratory pacemaker neurons in mediating the hypoxic response of the respiratory network in vitro." J Neurosci 20: 5858–66.
95. Thompson RJ, Farragher SM, Cutz E, Nurse CA. (2002). "Developmental regulation of O(2) sensing in neonatal adrenal chromaffin cells from wild-type and NADPH-oxidase-deficient mice." Pflugers Arch 444: 539–48.
96. Tononi G, and Cirelli C. (2001). "Modulation of brain gene expression during sleep and wakefulness: a review of recent findings." Neuropsychopharmacology 25: S28–35.
97. Vlasic V, Simakajornboon N, Gozal E, Gozal D. (2001). "PDGF-beta receptor expression in the dorsocaudal brainstem parallels hypoxic ventilatory depression in the developing rat." Pediatr Res 50: 236–41.
98. Younes M. (1989). "The physiologic basis of central apnea and periodic breathing." Current Pulmonology 10: 265–326.

CHAPTER 13

WHO GETS HIGH ALTITUDE PULMONARY EDEMA AND WHY?

PETER BÄRTSCH[1], CHRISTOPH DEHNERT[2], HEIMO MAIRBÄURL[1], MARC MORITZ BERGER[2]

[1]*Medical University Clinic, Dept. of Internal Medicine VII, Div. of Sports Medicine, Heidelberg, Germany*
[2]*Medical University Clinic, Department of Anesthesiology, Heidelberg, Germany*

Abstract: This paper focuses on high altitude pulmonary edema (HAPE) that occurs in individuals who are free of any pre-existing disease. An exaggerated hypoxic pulmonary vasoconstriction (HPV) is a hallmark of susceptibility to HAPE. In addition, a low hypoxic ventilatory response and defective sodium-dependent absorption of water from the alveoli may contribute to HAPE-susceptibility. However, excessive pulmonary artery hypertension appears to be crucial for the development of HAPE, since lowering pulmonary artery pressure by drugs, such as nifedipine or tadalafil (phospho-diesterase-5-inhibitor), will in most cases prevent HAPE. There is increasing evidence that the excessive pulmonary artery pressure response in HAPE-susceptible individuals is due to a reduced NO bioavailability. HAPE-susceptible individuals show an endothelial dysfunction in the systemic circulation in hypoxia. Lower levels of exhaled NO in hypoxia before and during HAPE in susceptible individuals suggest that this abnormality also occurs in the lungs and polymorphisms of the eNOS gene are associated with susceptibility to HAPE in the Indian and Japanese population.

Keywords: high altitude pulmonary edema; hypoxia; pulmonary circulation; endothelial dysfunction; NO; pathophysiology

High altitude pulmonary edema is a non-cardiogenic pulmonary edema that occurs in non-acclimatized previously healthy, often young individuals within 2 – 4 days after rapid ascent above altitudes of 3500 – 4000 m [1,2]. A typical radiographic appearance is shown in figure 1. This presentation focuses on the role of exaggerated hypoxic pulmonary vasoconstriction (HPV) as the cause of HAPE and discusses potential mechanisms accounting for the pulmonary leak and for the abnormal pulmonary pressure

A. Aldashev and R. Naeije (eds.), Problems of High Altitude Medicine and Biology, 185–195.

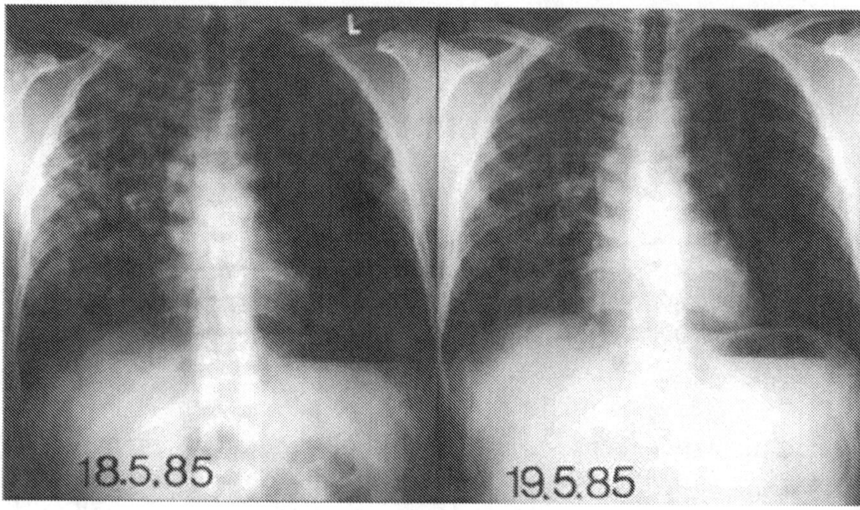

Figure 1. Radiograph of a 25-year-old mountaineer who developed HAPE after an ascent to 4559 m within 2 days (left side). The edema regresses significantly within 1 day without treatment at low altitude (right side).

response. More extensive reviews on this subject have been published recently [3,4].

Who Gets HAPE?

Individuals who develop HAPE have an increased HPV. Pulmonary artery pressure is about 30 – 50% higher in individuals who are prone to HAPE compared with non-susceptible controls at an altitude of 4559 m, and this higher pressure precedes edema formation [5] (figure 2). The increased HPV can also be demonstrated at low altitude by a brief hypoxic challenge [6,7]. Furthermore, HAPE-susceptible individuals show also an abnormally high rise of pulmonary artery pressure during exercise in normoxia, suggesting that the pulmonary vessels also have an increased vasoconstrictor response to increased flow [8,9]. Differences in pulmonary artery pressure between HAPE-susceptible individuals and non-susceptible controls in normobaric hypoxia ($FIO2 = 0.12$) or during normoxic exercise can be detected non-invasively by Doppler echocardiography (10), which shows little overlap of pulmonary artery pressure between groups (figure 3). Invasive studies [8,9] have demonstrated that this abnormal pressure response is attributable to an increased resistance and not to differences in pulmonary blood flow.

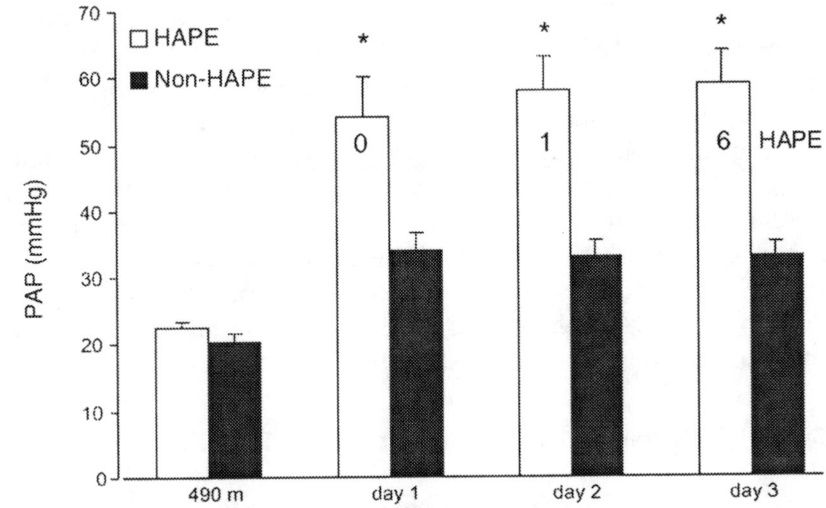

Figure 2. Systolic pulmonary artery pressure (mean values ± SEM) measured by Doppler echocardiography in 7 subjects developing HAPE (empty bars) and in 7 mountaineers not susceptible to HAPE (black bars) at low altitude and on the first, second and third day at an altitude of 4559 m. The numbers in the white bars indicate that HAPE was diagnosed in 1 subject on day 2 and in 6 subjects on day 3. Data from reference (5).

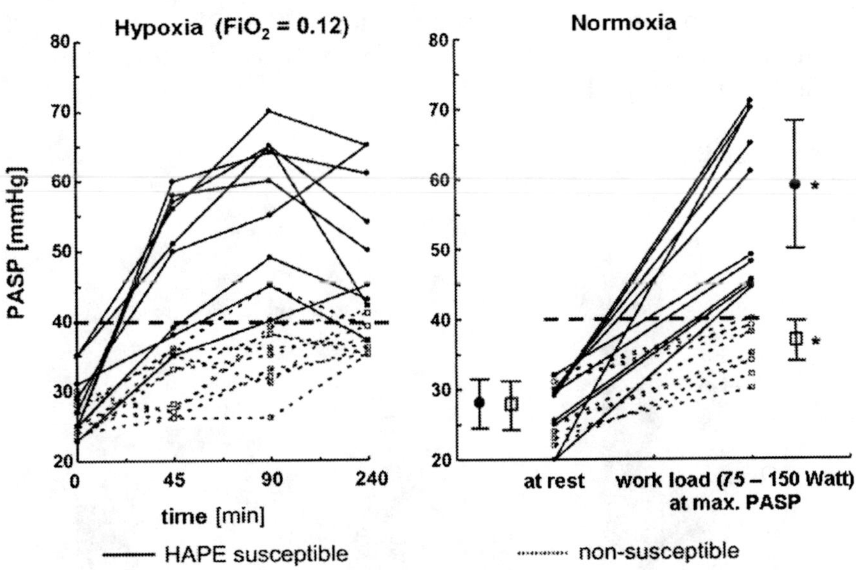

Figure 3. Pulmonary systolic artery pressure (PASP) in HAPE-susceptible individuals (solid lines and filled symbols) and in non-susceptible controls (dashed lines and open symbols) during exposure to normobaric hypoxia (left panel) and before and during exercise on a bicycle ergometer (right panel). The highest PASP recordings during exercise (75 – 150 Watt) are shown. FIO2: fraction of inspired O2.*: $p < 0.005$ compared with pre-exercise values within groups and with post-exercise values between groups. Data from reference (10).

The importance of an excessive rise of pulmonary artery pressure for the development of HAPE is underlined by the fact that lowering pulmonary artery pressure during ascent to high altitude can prevent HAPE. In placebo-controlled double-blind studies, a non-specific pulmonary vasodilator (3×20 mg nifedipine) [5] or the phosphodiesterase-5-inhibitor tadalafil (2×10 mg) [11], a selective pulmonary vasodilator reduces the prevalence of pulmonary edema in HAPE-susceptible individuals after rapid ascent to 4559 m from 60 to 70% to about 10%. Furthermore, the significant preventive effect of 2×8 mg dexamethasone per day could also predominantly be attributed to pulmonary vasodilation [11], since this drug unexpectedly lowered pulmonary artery pressure at high altitude as much as tadalafil.

Why does High Pulmonary Artery Pressure Cause HAPE?

Recent studies performed in the Capanna Regina Margherita (4559 m) have shown that the leak of HAPE is caused by increased capillary pressure and not by an inflammatory process. The study of Maggiorini et al. using right-heart catheterization confirmed the abnormal increase of pulmonary artery pressure and a normal wedge pressure in individuals developing HAPE (figure 4) and in addition demonstrated by the single occlusion method that capillary pressure is also elevated to 20 – 25 mmHg [12], exceeding threshold values of 17 – 24 mmHg for edema formation established in dog models [13].

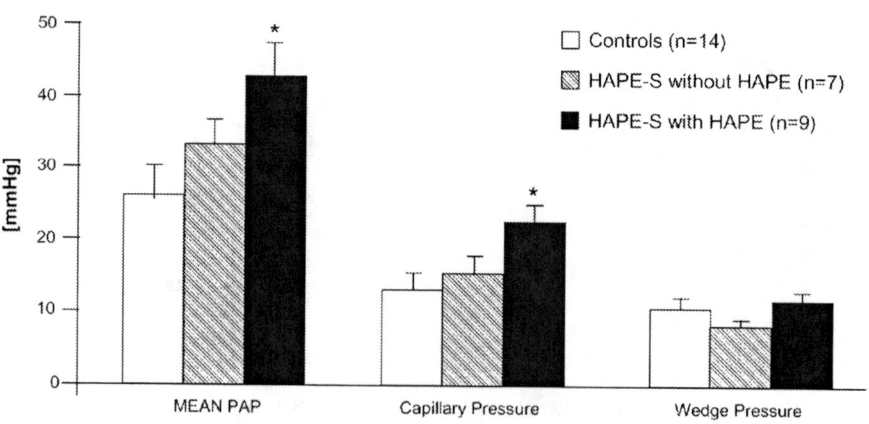

Figure 4. Pulmonary vascular pressures (mean ± SD) measured by right-heart catheterization in 14 controls and 16 HAPE-susceptible (HAPE-S) individuals on the second day at 4559 m. HAPE-S are further divided in those who did and did not develop HAPE during the study. *: $p < 0.005$ vs. control and HAPE-S without HAPE. Data from reference (12).

Broncho-alveolar lavage (BAL), performed within a day after ascent to 4559 m, revealed elevated red blood cell counts and serum-derived protein concentration in BAL fluid (table 1) in subjects developing HAPE [14]. There was no increase of inflammatory cells or pro-inflammatory mediators in HAPE-susceptible individuals compared to controls and baseline (table 1). BAL in more advanced or longer lasting HAPE showed in some but not all cases elevated pro-inflammatory cytokines, leukotriene B4 and increased granulocytes [15,16]. Furthermore, urinary leukotriene E4 excretion was increased in patients with HAPE reporting to clinics in the Rocky Mountains [17]. These observations suggest that inflammation is absent in early HAPE and may occur as a consequence of alveolar edema or the process that leads to edema formation.

The increased capillary pressure and the absence of inflammation in early HAPE suggest that there is a partial disruption of the alveolar-capillary barrier. Whether ruptures of basement membranes as suggested by West et al. [18] or non-traumatic, dynamic, pressure-sensitive stretching of pores or opening of fenestrae [1] account for the leak, is a question of debate which has been discussed in detail in a recent, more extensive review on HAPE [4].

TABLE 1. Broncho-alveolar lavage at low and high altitude

	490 m		4559 m		
	CONT	HAPE-S		HAPE-S	HAPE-S
	(n=8)	(n=9)	CONT	(well) (n=6)	(ill) (n=3)
Cell count ($\times 10^4$/ml)	8.1	6.3	9.5	8.1	9.8
Macrophages (%)	94	95	93	92	88
Neutrophils (%)	1	0	0	0	1
Red cells (% BAL cells)	1	4	6	51*	74*
Total protein (mg/dl)	1	2	14	13	163*
Albumin (ug/ml)	34	29	42	127*	402*
PAP systolic	22	26	37	61*	81*
IL-1 (pg/ml)	ND	ND	ND	ND	ND
IL-6 (pg/ml)	ND	ND	ND	ND	176*
IL-8 (pg/ml)	0.1	0.1	0.2	0.2	0.2
TNF-α (pg/ml)	ND	ND	ND	ND	ND
LTB_4 (pg/ml)	547	521	499	537	512
PGE-2 (pg/ml)	13	14	13	19	18
Thromboxane (pg/ml)	24	14	43	28	51

* $p < 0.05$ compared to control (CONT) and values at low altitude indicate that subjects developed HAPE in the 24 hours following the BAL, ill indicates that HAPE was present at the time of the lavage. Data from reference (14).

Several mechanisms have been suggested to explain how high PAP can account for high capillary pressure in HAPE. The most widely favored hypothesis of inhomogeneous HPV [20] has received experimental support from animal studies using fluorescent microbeads [21] and from human lung perfusion analysis by MRI [22,23], as discussed earlier. High flow in areas of low vasoconstriction can raise capillary pressure due to venous resistance and cause extravascular fluid accumulation as shown in animal experiments [24]. In addition, transarteriolar leakage [25] and hypoxic venoconstriction [26] have been suggested. These two mechanisms, alone or in combination, cannot explain the often patchy radiographic appearance of early HAPE on chest radiographs or CT scans, unless there is additional regional heterogeneity of HPV. Branching of capillaries directly from larger arterioles, suggested as an alternative or additional mechanism [27] or transarteriolar leakage, might give an explanation for the less frequent cases of HAPE with early perihilar manifestations. The similarity of the radiographic appearance between 2 different episodes of HAPE in the same individual is random, suggesting that structural abnormalities do not account for edema location [28].

What is the Cause of the Abnormal Vasoreactivity of the Pulmonary Circulation in HAPE-Susceptible Individuals?

Mechanisms that could contribute to the exaggerated pressure response of the pulmonary circulation of individuals susceptible to HAPE are listed in table 2. Several observations suggest that decreased NO bioavailability may account for the abnormal pulmonary vascular response in susceptible individuals. Figure 5 shows that NO concentrations are decreased in exhaled air in HAPE-susceptible individuals during a 4-hour hypoxic exposure at low altitude [29] and during the development of HAPE at high altitude [30]. Furthermore, concentrations of nitrate and nitrite in broncho-alveolar lavage fluid were lower in mountaineers who developed HAPE compared to controls [14] and HAPE-S have an impaired endothelium-dependent vasodilator response to acetylcholine in the systemic circulation (figure 6) [31]. The abnormal rise of PAP to exercise in normoxia (8–10) might be explained by

TABLE 2. Potential mechanisms contributing to susceptibility for HAPE

1. Increased vasoconstriction to hypoxia
• Decreased bioavailability of NO
• Increased activity of sympathetic nervous system
2. Low hypoxic ventilatory response
3. Low to normal lung volume and reduced compliance
4. Reduced alveolar sodium clearance

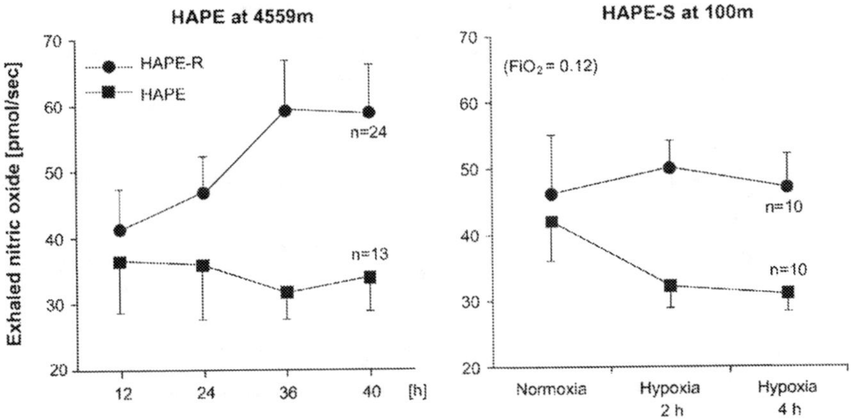

Figure 5. Left: exhaled nitric oxide (NO) after 40 h at 4559 m in individuals developing HAPE and in individuals not developing HAPE (HAPE-R) despite identical exposure to high altitude (30). Right: exhaled NO in HAPE-susceptible subjects (HAPE-S) and HAPE-R individuals after 4 h of exposure to hypoxia (FIO2 = 0.12) at low altitude (elevation 100 m). n: number of subjects. Data from reference (29).

an impaired endothelial NO release in response to increased blood flow in the pulmonary circulation. In accordance with this hypothesis, inhalation of 15 – 40 ppm NO lowered PAP and improved gas exchange in subjects with HAPE to control levels [32,33] and the phosphodiesterase-5 inhibitor tadalafil, which increase the cyclic GMP in lung tissue by inhibition of its degradation, lowered PAP and prevented HAPE [11].

It is likely that additional factors, such as increased sympathetic activity [34] or other vasoconstrictors such as angiotensin II [35], endothelin [36] or arachadonic or acid metabolites contribute to the increased PAP in HAPE-susceptible subjects. Increased skeletal muscle sympathetic activity [15] and increased plasma and/or urinary levels of norepinephrine compared to controls were found during hypoxia at low altitude or before and during [35,37] HAPE.

Additional Factors Contributing to HAPE-Susceptibility

LOW HYPOXIC VENTILATORY RESPONSE AND LUNG VOLUME

Both a low hypoxic ventilatory drive leading to increased pulmonary vasoconstriction and smaller lungs in relation to body size (decreased pulmonary vascular cross-sectional area) are factors known to increase pulmonary arterial pressure and hence, susceptibility to HAPE [4]. The considerable overlap for both factors between HAPE-susceptible and resistant individuals [38]

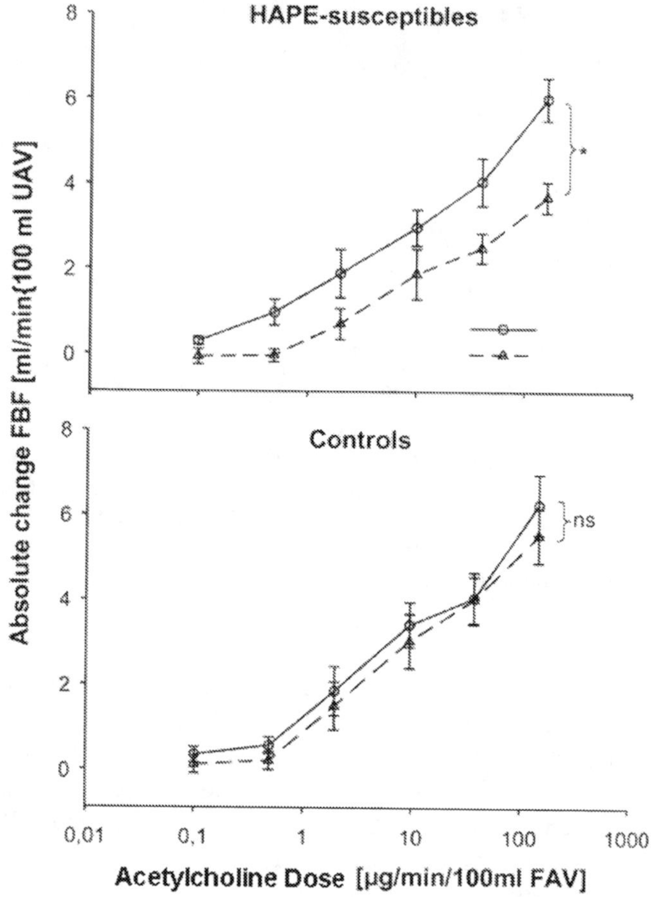

Figure 6. Forearm blood flow (FBF) response to acetylcholine after exposure to normoxia and hypoxia in 9 mountaineers susceptible to high altitude pulmonary edema (HAPE-S) and 9 mountaineers not susceptible to HAPE (controls). Data are expressed as mean absolute change from baseline FBF (± SEM). *: $p = 0.01$ between normoxia and hypoxia (ANOVA). Data from reference (31).

suggests that they are at best contributory but not essential for susceptibility to HAPE.

REDUCED FLUID CLEARANCE FROM THE ALVEOLAR SPACE

Hypoxia impairs fluid clearance from the alveoli by inhibiting activity and expression of various Na-transporters [39] [40]. It was suggested that a decreased capacity of epithelial Na-reabsorption might predispose to HAPE. This hypothesis is compatible with the finding that inhalation of high dose salmeterol, a beta-2 agonist which enhances transepithelial sodium transport [41], can prevent HAPE in some susceptible individuals [42]. Because of multiple actions of this drug, like lowering pulmonary artery pressure, increasing ventilatory response to hypoxia and tightening cell-to-cell contacts, we need, however, more specific drugs for a precise evaluation of the role of alveolar fluid clearance from the alveoli for the pathophysiology of HAPE.

References

1. Bärtsch P (1999) High altitude pulmonary edema. Med Sci Sports Exer. 31(1):S23–S27.
2. Hackett PH, Roach RC (2001) High-altitude illness. N Engl J Med. 345:107–14.
3. Schoene, R. B.; Swenson, E. R.; Hultgren, H. N (2001) High-altitude pulmonary edema (Chapter). In: Hornbein, T. F.; Schoene, R., eds. High altitude - an exploration of human adaptation. New York: Marcel Dekker Inc. pp. 777–814. (LENFANT, C., exec. ed. Lung biology in health and disease; v. 161).
4. Bärtsch P, Mairbäurl H, Maggiorini M, Swenson E (2005) Physiological aspects of high-altitude pulmonary edema (Invited Review). J Appl Physiol. 98:1101–10.
5. Bärtsch P, Maggiorini M, Ritter M, Noti C, Vock P, Oelz O (1991) Prevention of high-altitude pulmonary edema by nifedipine. N Engl J Med. 325:1284–9.
6. Viswanathan R, Jain SK, Subramanian S, Subramanian TAV, Dua GL, Giri J. (1969) Pulmonary edema of high altitude II. Clinical, aerohemodynamic, and biochemical studies in a group with history of pulmonary edema of high altitude. Am Rev Respir Dis. 100:334–41.
7. Hultgren HN, Grover RF, Hartley LH.(1971) Abnormal circulatory responses to high altitude in subjects with a previous history of high-altitude pulmonary edema. Circulation 44:759–70.
8. Kawashima A, Kubo K, Kobayashi T, Sekiguchi M.(1989) Hemodynamic responses to acute hypoxia, hypobaria, and exercise in subjects susceptible to high-altitude pulmonary edema. J Appl Physiol 67(5):1982–9.
9. Eldridge MW, Podolsky A, Richardson R.S., Johnson DH, Knight DR, Johnson EC, Hopkins SR, Michimata H, Grassi B, Feiner J, et al.(1996) Pulmonary hemodynamic response to exercise in subjects with prior high-altitude pumonary edema. J ApplPhysiol 81(2):911–21.
10. Grünig E, Mereles D, Hildebrandt W, Swenson ER, Kübler W, Kuecherer H, Bärtsch P.(2000) Stress doppler echocardiography for identification of susceptibility to high altitude pulmonary edema. J Am Coll Cardiol. 35:980–7.
11. Maggiorini M , Brunner-La Rocca H-P, Peth S, Fischler M, Böhm T, Bernheim A, Kiencke S, Bloch KE, Dehnert C, Naeije R, et al.(2006) Both tadalafil and dexamethasone may reduce the incidence of high-altitude pulmonary edema. Ann Intern Med. 145:497–506.
12. Maggiorini M , Mélot C, Pierre S, Pfeiffer F, Greve I, Sartori C, Lepori M, Hauser M, Scherrer U, Naeije R.(2001) High-altitude pulmonary edema is initially caused by an increase in capillary pressure. Circulation 103:2078–83.
13. Homik LA, Bshouty RB, Light RB, Younes M.(1988) Effect of alveolar hypoxia on pulmonary fluid filtration in in situ dog lungs. J Appl Physiol 65:46–52.
14. Swenson ER, Maggiorini M, Mongovin S, Gibbs JSR, Greve I, Mairbäurl H, Bärtsch P. (2002) Pathogenesis of high-altitude pulmonary edema: Inflammation is not an etiologic factor. JAMA 287:2228–35.

15. Schoene RB, Swenson ER, Pizzo CJ, Hackett PH, Roach RC, Mills WJ, Henderson WR, Martin TR.(1988) The lung at high altitude: bronchoalveolar lavage in acute mountain sickness and pulmonary edema. J App Physiol 64:2605–13.
16. Kubo K, Hanaoka M, Hayano T, Miyahara T, Hachiya T, Hayasaka M, Koizumi T, Fujimoto K, Kobayashi T, Honda T.(1997) Inflammatory cytokines in BAL fluid and pulmonary hemodynamics in high-altitude pulmonary edema. Respir Physiol 111:301–10.
17. Kaminsky DA, Jones K, Schoene RB, Voelkel NF. (1996)Urinary leuktriene E (4) levels inhigh-altitude pulmonary edema: A possible role for inflammation. Chest 110(4):939–45.
18. West JB, Tsukimoto K, Mathieu-Costello O, Prediletto R. (1991)Stress failure in pulmonary capillaries. J Appl Physiol 70:1731–42.
19. Neal CR, Michel CC. (1996) Openings in frog microvascular endothelium induced by high intravascular pressures. J Physiol 492(1):39–52.
20. Hultgren, H. N.(1978) High altitude pulmonary edema. In: Staub, N. C., ed. Lung Water and Solute Exchange. New York: Marcel Dekker; pp. 437–64.
21. Hlastala MP, Lamm WJE, Karp A, Polissar NL, Starr IR, Glenny RW. (2004) Spatial distribution of hypoxic pulmonary vasoconstriction in the supine pig. J Appl Physiol 96(5):1589–99.
22. Hopkins SR, Garg J, Bolar DS, Balouch J, Levin DL.(2005) Pulmonary blood flow heterogeneity during hypoxia and high altitude pulmonary edema. Am J Respir Crit Care Med. 171:83–7.
23. Dehnert C, Risse F, Ley S, Kuder TA, Buhmann R, Puderbach M, Menold E, Mereles D, Kauczor H-U, Bärtsch P, et al.(2006) Magnetic resonance imaging of uneven pulmonary perfusion in hypoxia in humans. Am J Respir Crit Care Med. 174:1132–8.
24. Younes M, Bshouty Z, Ali J.(1987) Longitudinal distribution of pulmonary vascular resistance with very high pulmonary flow. J Appl Physiol 62:344–58.
25. Whayne Jr. TF, Severinghaus JW.(1968)Experimental hypoxic pulmonary edema in the rat. J Appl Physiol 25:729–32.
26. Zhao Y, Packer CS, Rhoades RA. (1993) Pulmonary vein contracts in response to hypoxia. Am J Physiol 1993;265:L87–L92.
27. Goetz AE, Kuebler WM, Peter K. (1996) High-altitude pulmonary edema. N Engl J Med. 335:206–7.
28. Vock P, Brutsche MH, Nanzer A, Bartsch P.(1991) Variable Radiomorphologic Data of High Altitude Pulmonary Edema - Features from 60 Patients. Chest 100(5):1306–11.
29. Busch T, Bärtsch P, Pappert D, Grünig E, Elser H, Falke KJ, Swenson ER.(2001) Hypoxia decreases exhaled nitric oxide in mountaineers susceptible to high altitude pulmonary edema. Am J Respir Crit Care Med. 163:368–73.
30. Duplain H, Sartori C, Lepori M, Egli M, Allemann Y, Nicod P , Scherrer U. (2000) Exhaled nitric oxide in high-altitude pulmonary edema: role in the regulation of pulmonary vascular tone and evidence for a role against inflammation. Am J Respir Criti Care Med. 162:221–4.
31. Berger M, Hesse C, Dehnert C, Siedler H, Kleinbongard P, Bardenheuer HJ, Kelm M, Bärtsch P, Haefeli WE. (2005) Hypoxia impairs systemic endothelial function in individuals prone to high-altitude pulmonary edema. Am J Respir Criti Care Med. 172:763–7.
32. Scherrer U, Vollenweider L, Delabays A, Savcic M, Eichenberger U, Kleger G-R, Firkrle A, Ballmer P, Nicod P, Bärtsch P. (1996) Inhaled nitric oxide for high-altitude pulmonary edema. N Engl J Med. 334:624–9.
33. Anand IS, Prasad BAK, Chugh SS, Rao KRM, Cornfield DN, Milla CE, Singh N, Singh S, Selvamurthy W.(1998) Effects of inhaled nitric oxide and oxygen in high-altitude pulmonary edema. Circulation 98:2441–5.
34. Duplain H, Vollenweider L, Delabays A, Nicod P, Bärtsch P, Scherrer U. (1999) Augmented sympathetic activation during short-term hypoxia and high-altitude exposure in subjects susceptible to high-altitude pulmonary edema. Circulation 99:1713–8.

35. Bärtsch P , Shaw S, Franciolli M, Gnädinger MP, Weidmann P.(1988) Atrial natriuretic peptide in acute mountain sickness. J Appl Physiol 65:1929–37.
36. Sartori C, Vollenweider L, Löffler B-M, Delabays A, Nicod P, Bärtsch P, Scherrer U.(1999) Exaggerated endothelin release in high-altitude pulmonary edema. Circulation 99:2665–8.
37. Cunningham WL, Becker EJ, Kreuzer F. (1965) Catecholamines in plasma and urine at high altitude. J Appl Physiol 20:607–10.
38. Hohenhaus E, Paul A, McCullough RE, Kücherer H, Bärtsch P. (1995) Ventilatory and pulmonary vascular response to hypoxia and susceptibility to high altitude pulmonary oedema. Eur Respir J. 8:1825–33.
39. Planes C, Escoubet B, Blot-Chabaud M, Friedlander G, Farman N, Clerici C. (1997) Hypoxia downregulates expression and activity of epithelial sodium channels in rat alveolar epithelial cells. Am J Respir Cell Mol Biol. 17:508–18.
40. Mairbäurl H, Weymann J, Möhrlein A, Swenson ER, Maggiorini M, Gibbs JSR, Bärtsch P. (2003) Nasal epithelium potential difference at high altitude (4,559 m). Am J Respir Criti Care Med. 167:862–7.
41. Matthay MA, Clerici C, Saumon C. (2002) Active fluid clearance from distal airspaces. J Appl Physiol 93:1533–41.
42. Sartori C, Allemann Y, Duplain H, Lepori M, Egli M, Lipp E, Hutter D, Turini P, Hugli O, Cook S, et al. (2002) Salmeterol for the prevention of high-altitude pulmonary edema. N Engl J Med. 346:1631–6.

CHAPTER 14

EFFECTS OF INHALED NITRIC OXIDE AND OXYGEN IN HIGH ALTITUDE PULMONARY EDEMA

INDER S. ANAND

Department of Cardiology, VA Medical Center and University of Minnesota, Minneapolis, USA

Abstract: The use of inhaled nitric oxide in acutely ill patients with high altitude pulmonary edema was first reported in 1998. We demonstrated that both nitric oxide and oxygen cause an acute decrease in pulmonary artery pressure, intrapulmonary shunting and improvement in oxygenation. There appears to be an additive effect on pulmonary hemodynamics and an even greater effect on gas exchange when both oxygen and nitric oxide are delivered simultaneously. While further studies are necessary to determine the potential long-term benefits or adverse sequelae associated with nitric oxide use, this report suggests that there may be significant benefits for patients who are acutely ill with high altitude pulmonary edema. This report may also provide some insight into the mechanism whereby nitric oxide and oxygen improve gas exchange in a hypoxic hypobaric atmosphere.

Keywords: Nitric oxide; hypoxic; high altitude pulmonary edema.

High altitude pulmonary edema (HAPE) is a life threatening condition [13] characterized by pulmonary hypertension, increased pulmonary capillary permeability, and hypoxemia [9, 12, 19]. Although the mechanisms responsible for the development of HAPE are not entirely clear, measurements of pulmonary hemodynamics in patients with HAPE or incipient HAPE suggest that edema is caused by uneven severe hypoxic pulmonary vasoconstriction and an increase in pulmonary artery pressure in the lungs without elevation of left atrial pressure. This results in leakage of large-molecular-weight proteins and erythrocytes across the alveolar capillaries in areas of the lung that are not vasoconstricted [2, 6, 11, 15]. Earlier studies of broncho alveolar lavage (BAL) fluid had suggested that inflammation may play a role in the genesis of HAPE [19]. More recent studies have, however, disproved any role of inflammation in its pathogenesis [19,20,21]. Taken together, these studies strongly suggests that high capillary hydrostatic pressure induces a high-permeability type lung edema in the absence of inflammation, a

A. Aldashev and R. Naeije (eds.), Problems of High Altitude Medicine and Biology, 197–209.

concept first introduced by John West under the term "stress failure" [22]. Moreover, observations that lowering pulmonary arterial pressure with a vasodilator like nifedipine improves symptoms, further strengthens the role of pulmonary hypertension [9, 14]. Therefore, the logical treatment of HAPE is to increase alveolar PO_2 either by administration of oxygen or by descent to lower altitude. Unfortunately, the option of immediate descent is often not available because of severe weather and rugged mountain conditions. Alternative solutions are therefore required.

Scherrer et al [18] were the first to report that inhaled nitric oxide (NO) decreased pulmonary arterial pressure and improved ventilation-perfusion mismatch in HAPE-prone subjects exposed to high altitude in a controlled experimental setting. Whether use of inhaled NO might be a viable solution for patients with HAPE in the field remained to be determined. Experimental studies have also shown that oxygen and NO cause pulmonary vasodilatation through the activation of different K^+ channels in the pulmonary artery smooth muscle [3,4]. Hence, there are theoretical grounds for believing that the vasodilatory effects of oxygen and NO could be additive. In this paper we summarize the results of a study that was designed to test the effects of NO and to explore the hypothesis that combined use of NO and oxygen has an additive effect in reducing pulmonary artery pressures in patients with HAPE [1]. To determine the separate and interactive effects of oxygen and inhaled NO, we treated HAPE patients with NO alone, oxygen alone and NO plus oxygen. Since the investigations were carried out in the field, it was hoped that the results would also prove of practical help in the treatment of HAPE.

Methods

The studies were carried out on 14 male soldiers (age 29 ± 2 years, mean $\pm$ SEM), who developed symptoms of HAPE in the Ladakh region of Kashmir in the Western Himalayas, at altitudes of 3,500 to 6,000 meters (Table 1). Most patients were airlifted by helicopters, from various locations in the Western Himalayas, down to the High Altitude Medical Research Center, attached to a hospital in Leh, Ladakh (3,600 m; barometric pressure, 500 mmHg), where they were investigated. All subjects were residents of low altitude and were posted to high altitude on combat duty.

The clinical severity of HAPE was assessed using the Lake Louise acute mountain sickness (AMS) scoring system [17]. Briefly, patients were assessed for the presence of 5 symptoms: headache; gastrointestinal upset; fatigue, weakness or both; dizziness, lightheadedness or both; and difficulty in sleeping. Change in mental status, ataxia and peripheral edema were also assessed. Each of these symptoms and signs were rated between 0 and 3. A score of 0 indicated no symptoms, 1 mild symptoms, 2 moderate symptoms, and 3 severe

TABLE 1. Baseline data on 14 patients with HAPE breathing room air

NAME	AGE	AMS Score	RR (/min)	HR (b/min)	PAP (mmHg)	PaO_2 (mm Hg)	SaO_2 (%)	$A\text{-}aDO_2$ (mmHg)	Hb (g/dl)
KD	36	4	28	127	37	28	58	29	12.8
GP	24	7	32	114	46	37	63	20	15.1
AGN	28	7	20	107	33	-	60	-	16.6
BKS	38	3	20	110	40	-	81	-	14.0
CS	21	5	30	133	34	26	59	28	13.8
KKP	32	7	21	104	20	43	80	20	14.6
AMP	29	5	32	101	20	36	76	25	14.2
KS	24	7	34	119	17	31	76	34	14.6
RGS	30	3	32	109	35	46	76	18	15.0
UK	22	9	56	138	39	49	71	16	14.6
BBD	34	6	29	99	36	33	70	29	15.0
DC	36	9	27	110	34	53	83	10	15.4
MR	28	6	35	111	46	20	46	39	14.6
SC	20	12	36	113	35	21	40	46	15.0
Mean	28.7	6.4	30.9	113.9	33.7	35.3	67.1	26.2	14.7
SD	5.7	2.4	8.7	11.2	8.6	10.3	12.7	9.8	0.8

AMS, acute mountain sickness score.

symptoms. AMS score is the sum of scores of all the eight symptoms and signs. A chest X-ray was taken and arterial blood gas measured. Only patients with an AMS score >3, alveolar to arterial oxygen tension difference ($A\text{-}aDO_2$) > 10 mmHg and evidence of pulmonary edema on chest x-ray were studied.

Pulmonary hemodynamics (Right atrial, pulmonary arterial and pulmonary arterial wedge pressures) were measured by Swan-Ganz thermodilution catheters and systemic hemodynamics by an intra-arterial cannula. Pulmonary artery and systemic pressures and pulse oximetry were monitored continuously. Cardiac output was measured by thermodilution. Arterial and mixed-venous blood gas tension hemoglobin concentration, hemoglobin oxygen saturation and methemoglobin levels were measured at regular intervals. The partial pressure of alveolar oxygen (P_AO_2) was calculated from the alveolar gas equation: $P_AO_2 = PIO_2 - PaCO_2/R$. The calculated alveolar to arterial oxygen tension difference ($A\text{-}aDO_2$) and PaO_2 were used to assess changes in oxygenation.

Administration of Inspired Gases

The effect of four different gas mixtures was tested in these patients. Ambient air (FiO_2, 0.21, $PIO_2 \sim 90$ mmHg), nitric oxide at a concentration of 15 parts per million (ppm) in air (FiO_2 0.21), oxygen (FiO_2, 0.50) and a mixture of nitric oxide (15 ppm) and oxygen (FiO_2, 0.50). A system was

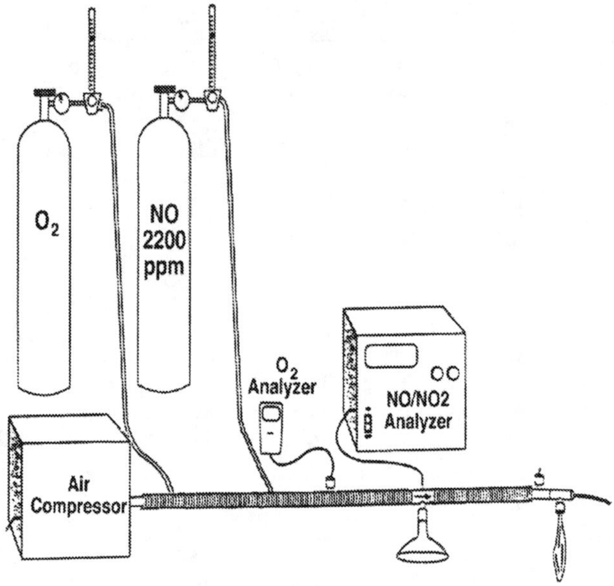

Figure 1.. Diagram of the set-up used to deliver different gas mixtures.

designed to alter NO or oxygen concentrations of the gas mixture independently, without affecting minute ventilation or airway pressure (Figure 1). Briefly, patients were asked to breath spontaneously through a snugly fitted facemask coupled to a one-way inspiratory valve. Humidified room air from a compressor was delivered, at flow rates two to three times the patient's minute ventilation, to the inspiratory valve via a T tube connector. The other end of the T tube was connected to a 6-foot long, 1.5 inch wide, corrugated tube to vent expiratory gases to the outside. An in-line oxygen analyzer (MiniOX I, Catalyst Research, Owings Mills, MD) was used to control the FiO_2 delivered. Nitric oxide (Puritan Bennett, Lenexa, KS) was supplied in a concentration of 2200 ppm and was delivered using a sensitive direct reading flow meter (0–300 ml/min, Cole-Parmer Instrument Co. Vernon Hills, IL). The concentration of inhaled nitric oxide was monitored just proximal to the facemask with a commercially available nitric oxide monitor, using electrochemical detectors (NOxBOX, Bedfont Scientific USA, Medford, NJ) and maintained at 15 ppm. High flow rates of gas mixtures helped to avoid formation of nitrogen dioxide and prevent rebreathing.

Study Design

After recording baseline measurements on room air, the effects of NO (15 ppm in room air, FiO_2 0.21), oxygen (FiO_2 0.50) and a mixture of NO and oxygen (15 ppm NO and 0.50 FiO_2) were tested. To exclude the cumulative effects of these gases, the inhalation of each gas mixture was followed by a period breathing room air. Moreover, the sequence of administration of gases was randomized. The effects of 4 different treatment conditions were tested in each patient: room air and the 3 different gas mixtures. Each treatment lasted approximately 30 minutes and measurements were performed in the last 10 minutes, when the hemodynamic and gas exchange variables were stable. In between treatments, a 30-minute period of exposure to room air was introduced as a "washout period", at the end of which hemodynamic and gas exchange measurements were repeated. Thus, a total of 7 measurements were made on each patient. Four on room air and 3 on the gas mixtures. In two patients, blood gas measurements could not be recorded because of equipment failure. In these patients, only hemodynamic data were available. At the end of the study, which lasted approximately 4 hours, patients were treated in the routine manner with supplemental oxygen (35% O_2 by face mask) until symptoms and signs of HAPE had completely resolved. Patients were then transported to low altitude. No complications occurred during the study.

Results

All patients in this study had moderate to severe HAPE with a mean ± SEM AMS score of 6.4 ± 0.7, radiographic evidence of pulmonary edema and significant arterial hypoxemia (Table 1). Hemodynamic measurements confirmed the presence of pulmonary arterial hypertension, with normal pulmonary capillary wedge pressures and normal systemic hemodynamics (Table 2, measurements on room air). Blood gas analysis revealed severe hypoxemia and increased A-aDO_2. Pulmonary artery pressure correlated inversely with arterial oxygen saturation ($r=-0.64$, $p<0.01$, Figure 2) and arterial oxygen tension ($r=-0.34$, $p=0.017$) and directly with A-aDO_2 ($r=0.30$, $p=0.04$). The effects of the 7 gas mixtures on hemodynamics and gas exchange are shown in Figure 3. Notice that after exposure to NO, oxygen and NO + oxygen, all variables returned to baseline values when subjects were placed back on room air. The measurements obtained during the room air periods were therefore averaged for each subject and compared to the data obtained during treatment with each of the gases.

Effect of Inhaled Nitric Oxide

Inhalation of NO at 15 ppm caused a prompt reduction in pulmonary artery pressure by a mean of 11.1 ± 1.5 mmHg ($p<0.001$) and in pulmonary vascular resistance by 36% ($p<0.001$). The mean PaO_2, $PaCO_2$, and SaO_2 increased slightly (all $p<0.01$, Table 2 and Figure 4). A decrease in A-aDO_2 was also

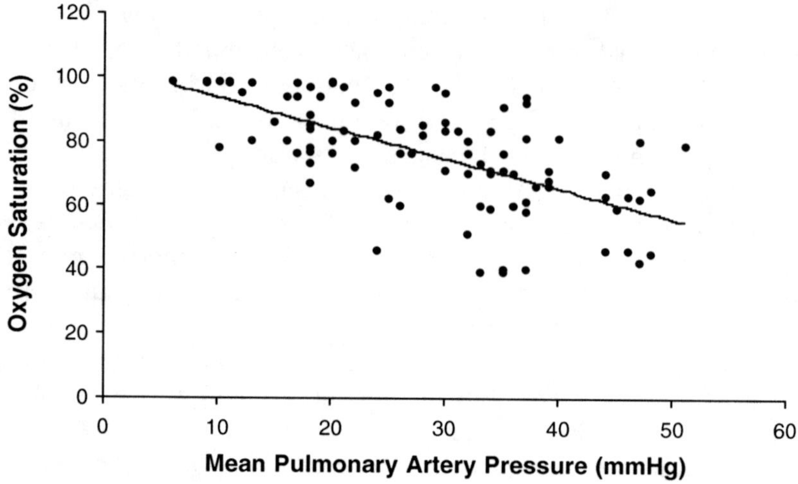

Figure 2. Scatter plot showing the relationship between mean pulmonary pressure and hemoglobin oxygen saturation. The scattergram includes values of pulmonary artery pressure and oxygen saturation at baseline and during treatment with different gas mixtures.

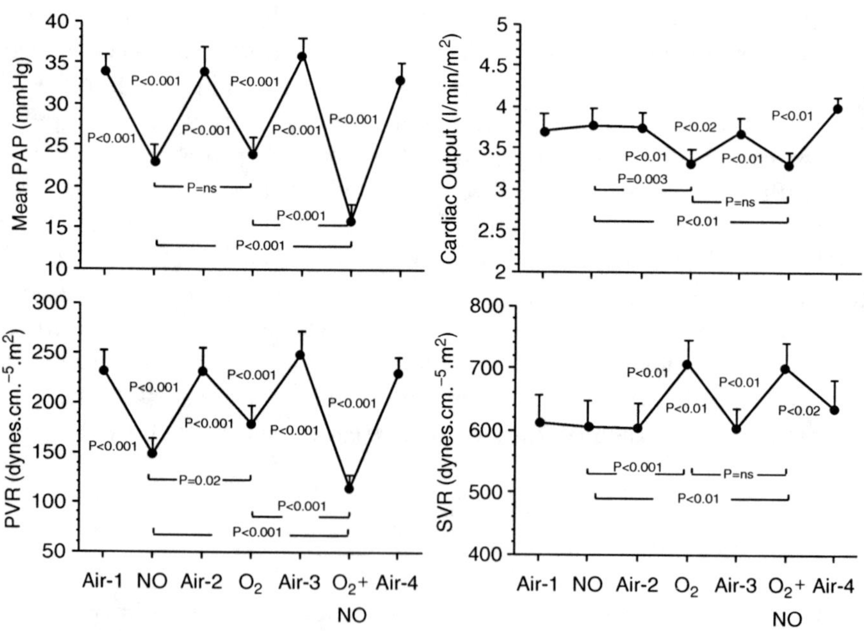

Figure 3. Effect of different gas mixtures on hemodynamic and gas exchange. Note how all the variable return to baseline when subjects are placed back on room air.

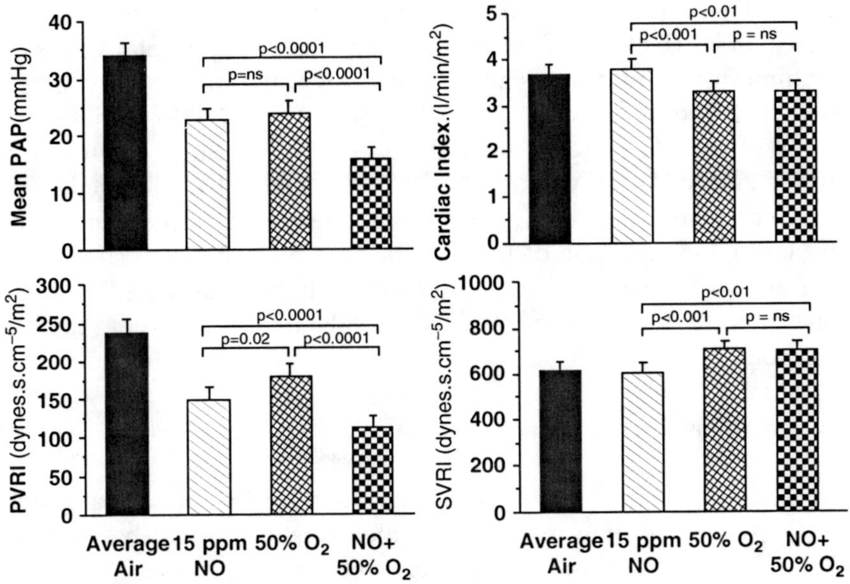

Figure 4. Effect of the 3 different gas mixture on pulmonary and systemic hemodynamic parameters as compared with the average of 4 episodes to room air.

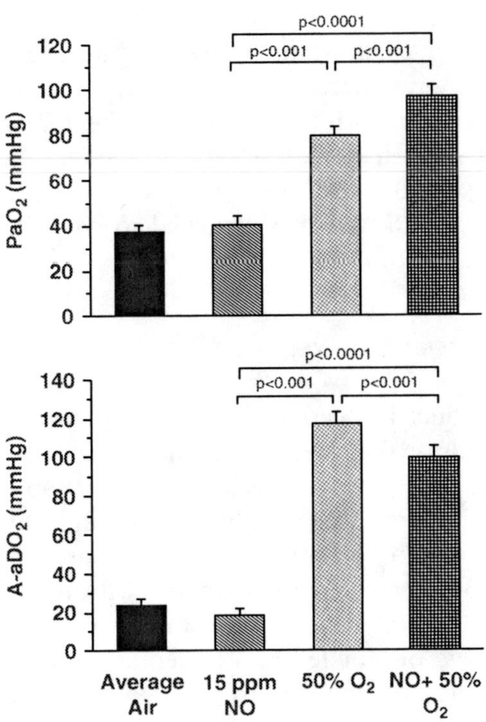

Figure 5. Effect of the 3 different gas mixture on gas exchange parameters as compared with the average of 4 exposures to room air.

noted ($p<0.01$, Table 2 and Figure 5). Since PAO_2 was virtually unchanged, the decrease in A-aDO_2 may be interpreted as indicating a relative decrease in intrapulmonary shunting. The decrease in pulmonary artery pressure correlated with the decrease in A-aDO_2 ($r=0.59$, $P=0.028$). Inhalation of NO had no effects on systemic hemodynamics (Table 2 and Figure 4); cardiac output and systemic vascular resistance remained unchanged ($p>0.5$ for both). The heart rate did not change but respiratory rate decreased by 6.5% ($p<0.05$). On cessation of nitric oxide inhalation and return to breathing room air, all the hemodynamic and gas exchange variables returned to baseline values. Throughout the study, the methemoglobin level in the blood never exceeded 2%.

Effect of Breathing Oxygen

Oxygen inhalation caused a significant decrease in pulmonary artery pressure (10.6 ± 1.2 mmHg, $p<0.001$), which was similar to that seen after inhalation of NO ($p=0.49$ for the difference between treatments, Table 2 and Figure 4). In contrast to NO, however, oxygen produced a decrease in cardiac output (11.4%, $p=0.003$). Therefore, the calculated pulmonary vascular resistance fell by a smaller amount after inhalation of oxygen than after inhalation of NO (23% vs. 36%, $p=0.02$ for the difference between treatments, Table 2 and Figure 4). In addition, treatment with oxygen increased systemic vascular resistance by 14.7% ($p<0.001$) and decreased the heart rate by 11.8% ($p<0.001$). The respiratory rate decreased by 9.4% ($p=0.002$) but this decrease was comparable to that seen with NO ($p=0.6$ for the difference between treatments). As expected, oxygen increased PaO_2 and SaO_2 to a greater extent than inhalation of NO ($p<0.001$ for both differences between treatments, Table 2 and Figure 5). Again, all variables returned to baseline values after resumption of breathing room air.

Effect of Breathing Nitric Oxide Combined with Oxygen

The combination of NO and oxygen produced a decrease in pulmonary artery pressure and pulmonary vascular resistance that was greater than that seen with NO or oxygen alone ($p<0.0001$ for differences between treatments, Table 2 and Figure 4). The effect of the combination was simply additive and not interactive, i.e., the effect due to the joint action of both gases was not greater than the sum of the effect of each gas considered separately ($p=0.11$ for interaction). The responses seen in systemic hemodynamics were similar to those seen after treatment with oxygen: cardiac output fell and systemic vascular resistance increased, and both effects were not significantly different ($p>0.5$)

TABLE 2. Hemodynamic and Gas Exchange data on 14 patients during short-term inhalation of room air, nitric oxide (15 ppm), 50 % oxygen, and a mixture of nitric oxide (15 ppm) and 50 % oxygen

	AIR-1 Mean ± SEM	NO 15 ppm Mean ± SEM	AIR-2 Mean ± SEM	50 % O2 Mean ± SEM	AIR-3 Mean ± SEM	NO + 50% O2 Mean ± SEM	AIR-4 Mean ± SEM
Heart rate (beats/min)	114 ± 3.1	112 ± 3.5	119 ± 4.0	105 ± 3.4	119 ± 2.3	101 ± 2.8	116 ± 3.0
RAP (mm Hg)	2 ± 0.9	1 ± 1.0	2 ± 1.1	2 ± 1.0	2 ± 1.1	2 ± 0.9	2 ± 0.8
PAP (mm Hg)	34 ± 2.4	23 ± 2.1	34 ± 2.8	24 ± 2.4	36 ± 2.4	16 ± 1.7	33 ± 2.3
PCWP (mm Hg)	4 ± 1.0	3 ± 1.1	3 ± 1.1	3 ± 0.9	3 ± 1.0	3 ± 1.2	3 ± 1.1
SAP (mm Hg)	80 ± 3.1	80 ± 3.0	81 ± 3.3	84 ± 2.7	80 ± 3.0	82 ± 2.5	83 ± 3.2
Cardiac Index (liters/m/m^2)	3.71 ± 0.2	3.78 ± 0.2	3.76 ± 0.2	3.33 ± 0.2	3.69 ± 0.2	3.31 ± 0.2	4 ± 0.2
PVRI (dynes.sec.cm^{-5}.M^2)	233 ± 19.8	149 ± 16.1	233 ± 22.4	179 ± 17.7	250 ± 22.9	114 ± 12.9	230 ± 16.4
SVRI (dynes.sec.cm^{-5}.M^2)	613 ± 44.5	606 ± 41.1	604 ± 40.5	708 ± 37.7	604 ± 33.4	702 ± 41.2	637 ± 45.9
RR (per min)	31 ± 2.4	29 ± 2.2	32 ± 2.3	29 ± 2.1	32 ± 2.3	27 ± 2.1	32 ± 2.5
PaO_2 (mm Hg)	35 ± 3.1	40 ± 3.6	37 ± 3.4	81 ± 5.5	38 ± 3.1	98 ± 6.1	39 ± 3.2
$PaCO_2$ (mm Hg)	26 ± 0.8	28 ± 0.8	27 ± 0.7	27 ± 0.7	26 ± 0.7	27 ± 0.7	26 ± 0.5
SaO_2 (mmHg)	67 ± 3.5	72 ± 3.6	67 ± 3.8	94 ± 1.1	68 ± 3.6	96 ± 1.3	70 ± 3.7
PIO_2 (mm Hg)	94 ± 0.4	93 ± 0.4	94 ± 0.5	231 ± 1.5	94 ± 0.5	227 ± 3.3	94 ± 0.4
PAO_2 (mmHg)	61 ± 1.1	59 ± 0.9	60 ± 0.8	197 ± 2.1	61 ± 0.6	193 ± 3.5	61 ± 0.7
A-aDO_2	26 ± 3.0	18 ± 3.1	23 ± 3.4	116 ± 6.2	23 ± 2.9	95 ± 5.5	22 ± 3.3

RAP, mean right atrial pressure; PAP, mean pulmonary arterial pressure; PCWP, mean pulmonary capillary wedge pressure; SAP, mean systemic arterial pressure; PVRI pulmonary vascular resistance index; SVRI, systemic vascular resistance index; RR, respiratory rate.

from those seen with oxygen alone. With respect to gas exchange, while NO caused only a small increase in PaO_2, combined treatment with NO and oxygen increased PaO_2 considerably more than with oxygen alone ($p<0.0001$ vs. oxygen, Table 2 and Figure 4, $p<0.001$ for interactive effect of combination). The combined treatment decreased A-aDO_2 from that seen after treatment with oxygen alone ($p<0.001$ vs. oxygen alone, Table 2 and Figure 5).

Discussion

In this paper we summarize our previous report of the first use of inhaled nitric oxide at high altitude in patients who were severely ill with HAPE, using invasive hemodynamics[1]. We found that inhaled NO improved arterial oxygenation and diminished pulmonary arterial pressure in patients with profound hypoxemia, moderately severe pulmonary hypertension and overtly symptomatic pulmonary edema. While treatment with either inhaled nitric oxide or oxygen acutely improved oxygenation and lowered pulmonary artery pressure, the use of inhaled nitric oxide and oxygen together caused an additive effect on pulmonary hemodynamics and an even greater effect on gas exchange.

In contrast to other vasodilator agents that have been used at altitude, [5,10,14] inhaled NO improved ventilation-perfusion mismatch and decreased venous admixture, as documented by a decrease in A-aDO_2, both on room air and at 50% FIO_2. This may be attributed to the fact that inhaled NO selectively vasodilates only those portions of the pulmonary vasculature that are ventilated, resulting in more optimally matched ventilation and perfusion. This report, therefore, extends observations of previous investigators who also demonstrated decrease in pulmonary artery pressure (by Doppler echocardiography) and improvement in ventilation-perfusion mismatch with inhaled NO (40 ppm), on ventilation-perfusion scans [18]. There are, however, a number of significant differences between the two studies [1,18]. The earlier study was done on HAPE-prone subjects in the controlled environment of a laboratory at high altitude [18]. Only 10 of the 18 subjects developed radiographic evidence of pulmonary edema and even in those, the A-aDO_2 was only modestly increased (15 ± 4 mmHg). We investigated severely ill patients who had developed HAPE during routine activities at high altitude and obtained hemodynamic and gas exchange data using invasive monitoring [1]. This study therefore, underscores the feasibility of using inhaled NO in the setting of a field hospital, provided the equipment can be miniaturized. Moreover, a lower dose of NO was used (15 ppm) and the effects of inhaled NO, oxygen and their combination were compared. The interpretation of this data is that ventilation and perfusion were better matched in the presence of NO and oxygen than with either of these two gases alone.

The observation that NO and oxygen interact to improve oxygenation and decrease pulmonary arterial pressure suggests that these two gases act on separate but complementary mechanisms, to cause pulmonary vasodilation at high altitude. Normally, the pulmonary vasculature is able to sense a decrease in oxygen tension and respond with vasoconstriction, due to inactivation of oxygen sensitive potassium (K^+) channels in pulmonary artery smooth muscle cells [16,23]. Both oxygen and nitric oxide cause pulmonary vasodilation, at least in part, through activation of K^+ channels. The additive effects of NO and oxygen, when given together, may derive from activation of different K^+ channels. Oxygen appears to activate predominantly the voltage-dependent K^+ channels, whereas NO activates a Ca-sensitive K^+ ($K_{Ca}{}^{++}$) channel [3,4,23]. Thus, while both NO and oxygen are capable of independently causing significant pulmonary vasodilatation and subsequent increases in oxygenation, their additive effects may be more profound than their effect alone.

The synergistic effects of NO and oxygen on gas exchange are not surprising. Inhaled NO, when given alone, improves oxygenation presumably by increasing blood flow through the well-ventilated parts of the lungs that are exposed to room air. With combined NO and oxygen, not only is blood flow to the ventilated parts of the lung expected to be greater, it is also exposed to a much higher oxygen tension. Therefore, the improvement in gas exchange parameters with the combined use of NO and oxygen are greater than the additive effects of the individual gases.

Since the publication of the two reports demonstrating a beneficial effect of the use of NO in HAPE, [1,18] a number of studies have suggested that lack of or reduced availability of NO may be an important cause of excessive hypoxic pulmonary hypertension in patients with HAPE. First, HAPE susceptible subjects have low levels of NO in exhaled air [8]. Second, the bronchoalveolar lavage (BAL) fluid, in patients with HAPE have low levels of nitrites and nitrates, as compared to normal [5]. Both these findings suggest inadequate NO production in the lungs of HAPE susceptible subjects. Finally, NO-dependent endothelial vasodilation in the forearm of HAPE-susceptible individuals is markedly decreased [7]. Hence, there may be more than one reason to treat HAPE patients with inhaled NO.

In summary, the original publication of this report in 1998 represents the first report of the use of inhaled NO in acutely ill patients with HAPE at altitude [1]. We demonstrate that both NO and oxygen cause an acute decrease in pulmonary artery pressure, intrapulmonary shunting and improvement in oxygenation. There appears to be an additive effect on pulmonary hemodynamics and an even greater effect on gas exchange when both oxygen and NO are delivered simultaneously. While further studies are necessary to determine the potential long-term benefits or adverse sequelae associated with NO use, this report suggests that there may be significant benefits for patients who are acutely ill with high altitude pulmonary edema. Finally, this report may provide some insight into the mechanism whereby NO and oxygen improve gas exchange in a hypoxic hypobaric atmosphere.

References

1. Anand, I.S., B.A. Prasad, S.S. Chugh, K.R. Rao, D.N. Cornfield, C.E. Milla, N. Singh, S. Singh, and W. Selvamurthy. (1998) Effects of inhaled nitric oxide and oxygen in high-altitude pulmonary edema. Circulation. 98:2441–5.
2. Antezana, G., G. Leguia, A. Morales Guzman, J. Coudert, and H. Spielvogel. (1982) Hemodynamic study of high altitude pulmonary edema (12,200 ft). In High altitude physiology and medicine. Vol. 232. W. Brendel and R. Zink, editors. Springer-Verlag, New York. 41.
3. Archer, S., J. Huang, V. Hampl, D. Nelson, P. Shultz, and E. Weir. (1994) Nitric oxide and cGMP cause vasodilation by activation of a charybdotoxin-sensitive K channel by cGMP-dependent protein kinase. Proc Natl Acad Sci. 91:7583–7587.
4. Archer, S., J. Huang, H. Reeve, V. Hampl, S. Tolarova, E. Michelakis, and E. Weir. (1996) Differential distribution of electrophysiologically distinct myocytes in conduit and resistance arteries determines their response to nitric oxide and hypoxia. Circ Res. 78:431–442.
5. Bartsch, P., M. Maggiorini, M. Ritter, C. Noti, P. Vock, and O. Oelz. (1991) Prevention of high-altitude pulmonary edema by nifedipine. N Engl J Med. 325:1284–1289.
6. Bartsch, P., H. Mairbaurl, M. Maggiorini, and E.R. Swenson. (2005) Physiological aspects of high-altitude pulmonary edema. J Appl Physiol. 98:1101–10.
7. Berger, M.M., C. Hesse, C. Dehnert, H. Siedler, P. Kleinbongard, H.J. Bardenheuer, M. Kelm, P. Bartsch, and W.E. Haefeli. (2005) Hypoxia impairs systemic endothelial function in individuals prone to high-altitude pulmonary edema. Am J Respir Crit Care Med. 172:763–7.
8. Duplain, H., C. Sartori, M. Lepori, M. Egli, Y. Allemann, P. Nicod, and U. Scherrer. (2000) Exhaled nitric oxide in high-altitude pulmonary edema: role in the regulation of pulmonary vascular tone and evidence for a role against inflammation. Am J Respir Crit Care Med. 162:221–4.
9. Hackett, P., and R. Roach. (1990) High altitude pulmonary edema. J Wilderness Med. 1:3–26.
10. Hackett, P., R. Roach, G. Hartig, E. Greene, and B. Levine. (1992) The effect of vasodilators on pulmonary hemodynamics in high altitude pulmonary edema: A Comparison. Int J Sports Medicine. 13:S68–S71.
11. Hultgren, H. (1978) High altitude pulmonary edema. In Lung water and solute exchange. Vol. 7. N. Staub, editor. Mercel Dekker, New York. 437–469.
12. Hultgren, H., C. Lopez, E. Lundberg, and H. Miller. (1964) Physiologic studies of pulmonary edema at high altitude. Circulation. 29:393–408.
13. Lobenhoffer, H., R. Zink, and W. Brendel. (1982) High altitude pulmonary edema: analysis of 166 cases. In High altitude physiology and medicine. W. Brendel and R. Zink, editors. Springer-Verlag, New York. 219–231.
14. Oelz, O., C. Noti, M. Ritter, R. Jenni, and P. Bartsch. (1989) Nifedipine for high altitude pulmonary oedema. Lancet. ii:1241–1244.
15. Penaloza, D., and F. Sime. (1969) Circulatory dynamics during high altitude pulmonary edema. Am J Cardiol. 23:369–378.
16. Post, J., J. Hume, S. Archer, and E. Weir. (1992) Direct role for potassium channel inhibition in hypoxic pulmonary vasoconstriction. Am J Physiol. 262:C882–C890.

17. Roach, R., P. Bartsch, P. Hackett, O. Oelz, and Lake Louise AMS Scoring Committee. (1993) The Lake Louise acute mountain sickness scoring system. In Hypoxia and Mountain Medicine. J. Sutton, C. Houston, and G. Coates, editors. Queen City Printers, Burlington, Vt. 272–274.
18. Scherrer, U., L. Vollenweider, A. Delabays, M. Savcic, U. Eichenberger, G.-R. Kleger, A. Fikrle, P. Ballmer, P. Nicod, and P. Bartsch. (1996) Inhaled nitric oxide for high altitude pulmonary edema. N Eng J Med. 334:624–629.
19. Schoene, R., E. Swenson, C. Pizzo, and et al. (1988) The lung at high altitude: bronchoalveolar lavage in acute mountain sickness and pulmonary edema. J Appl Physiol. 64:2605–2613.
20. Schoene, R.B. (2004) Unraveling the mechanism of high altitude pulmonary edema. High Alt Med Biol. 5:125–35.
21. Swenson, E.R., M. Maggiorini, S. Mongovin, J.S. Gibbs, I. Greve, H. Mairbaurl, and P. Bartsch. (2002) Pathogenesis of high-altitude pulmonary edema: Inflammation is not an etiologic factor. JAMA. 287:2228–35.
22. West, J.B., G.L. Colice, Y.J. Lee, Y. Namba, S.S. Kurdak, Z. Fu, L.C. Ou, and O. Mathieu-Costello. (1995) Pathogenesis of high-altitude pulmonary oedema: direct evidence of stress failure of pulmonary capillaries. Eur Respir J. 8:523–9.
23. Yuan, X.-J., W. Goldman, M. Tod, L. Rubin, and M. Blaustein. (1993) Hypoxia reduces potassium currents in cultured rat pulmonary but not mesenteric arterial myocytes. Am J Physiol. 264:L116–L123.

CHAPTER 15

ALTERED AUTOREGULATION OF CEREBRAL BLOOD FLOW IN HYPOXIA

Relevance to the Pathophysiology of Acute Mountain Sickness

ROBERT NAEIJE, AURELIE VAN OSTA

From the Department of Physiology, Faculty of Medicine of the Free University of Brussels, Belgium

Abstract: Acute mountain sickness (AMS) is a syndrome of headache, anorexia, nausea and fatigue, which commonly occurs with rapid ascent to high altitudes. The pathogenesis of AMS remains incompletely understood. A leading theory has been that AMS could be an early stage manifestation of high altitude cerebral edema, which sometimes complicates AMS and is of poor prognosis. There has indeed been recent reports of magnetic resonance imaging (MRI) evidence of hypoxia-induced reversible brain edema in healthy volunteers. Interestingly, in these studies, brain edema was both vasogenic and cytotoxic but with only the MRI cytotoxicity signals correlated to AMS symptomatology. Studies in volunteers exposed to normobaric or hypobaric hypoxic conditions have disclosed a hypoxia-induced alteration of the autoregulation of cerebral blood flow in proportion to the severity of oxygen deprivation and to AMS symptoms. The alteration of cerebral autoregulation contributes to breathing instability during sleep and may thereby promote periodic breathing and nocturnal oxygen desaturation. The alteration of cerebral autoregulation could also be a cause of overperfusion of cerebral capillaries and vasogenic edema during exercise and/or cold exposure. A common cause for altered cerebral autoregulation and cytotoxic brain edema could be hypoxia-induced release of oxygen free radicals. Thus, AMS is likely the result of a dynamic interaction between hemodynamic and cytotoxic events.

Keywords: Altitude; brain; cerebral blood flow; acute mountain sickness; cerebral edema

Introduction

Acute mountain sickness (AMS) is a syndrome of headache, anorexia, nausea, vomiting, fatigue, insomnia, dyspnea, ataxia, oliguria and edema, which occurs with rapid ascent to high altitudes [30]. The pathogenesis of

A. Aldashev and R. Naeije (eds.), Problems of High Altitude Medicine and Biology, 211–220.

AMS remains incompletely understood. A leading theory has been that hypoxia-induced cerebral vasodilatation and high cerebral blood flow (CBF) could increase cerebral capillary pressure to cause a "vasogenic cerebral edema" due to excessive capillary filtration and capillary injury [6]. However, although it has been shown that CBF increases with acute exposure to high altitudes and tends to follow the same time course as AMS symptoms [30], some studies reported on an increase in CBF in subjects with AMS [3,9,22] but others did not find any relationship [4,17,24]. These discrepancies might be explained by the fact that AMS could be caused by an impairment of cerebral autoregulation rather than by absolute changes in CBF [15,28].

Cerebral autoregulation describes the inherent ability of the cerebral blood vessels to maintain a constant CBF despite changes in blood pressure. The function of cerebral autoregulation is to protect the brain against oxygen deprivation at low perfusion pressures, and against the risk of brain edema at high perfusion pressures [14]. In addition, cerebral autoregulation may help to prevent periodic breathing and sleep apneas by limiting oscillations in central chemoreceptor stimulation [1]. Hypoxia has been shown to impair cerebral autoregulation in experimental animals [8,13] and in man [10,28,29]. If an altered cerebral autoregulation were to be the main determinant of a vasogenic edema caused by an increased capillary filtration pressure, any increase in blood pressure should be an aggravating circumstance. This is indeed the case, as field studies clearly show that physical exercise and/or cold increase the incidence and severity of AMS [26,30]. Alternatively, hypoxia-induced impairment of CBF autoregulation could be coincidental, as static cerebral autoregulation is recently reported to be similarly impaired in newcomers at high altitudes and Sherpas [10].

Another possible mechanism leading to AMS could be a hypoxia-induced decrease in cerebral critical closing pressure (CCP), that is, the effective backpressure of the cerebral circulation. Cerebral closing pressure is the minimum pressure the inflow pressure (blood pressure) must overcome to generate a flow. Since the pressure-flow relationship in the cerebral circulation is adequately described by a linear approximation, CCP can be estimated from the extrapolation to the pressure axis of pressure-flow plots [25]. Hypercapnia decreases CCP and thereby increases cerebral blood volume [23]. Hypoxia has been reported to decrease CCP in rabbits [27] and in normal human subjects [29].

Recent Studies on the Effects of Hypoxia on CBF Autoregulation

Cerebral autoregulation can be studied in static or in dynamic conditions. Static autoregulation refers to changes in steady-state CBF recorded after an increase in blood pressure induced by the infusion of a vasopressor drug [10].

Dynamic autoregulation refers to continuous changes in CBF either in natural conditions, by the calculation of a transfer function from the spectral analysis of blood pressure and flow signals [37], or by the calculation of a rate of correction of flow per unit of change in blood pressure [27]. While static and dynamic cerebral autoregulation measurements have shown to be correlated [27], the agreement of both approaches in hypoxia is not known and it remains uncertain whether pharmacological manipulations of blood pressure might be without intrinsic influence on the autoregulation process. Therefore, it seems preferable to evaluate cerebral autoregulation in dynamic rather than in static conditions.

Van Osta et al. investigated the effects of hypoxic breathing on dynamic cerebral autoregulation and CCP in 15 normal volunteers and correlated the results to an AMS score obtained after 6 hours of hypoxic exposure in a hypobaric chamber [29]. Cerebral blood flow velocity was measured by transcranial Doppler and blood pressure by finger plethysmography in normoxia (fraction of inspired O_2, FIO_2 0.21) and after a short period of hypoxic breathing (FIO_2 0.12). A dynamic CBF autoregulation index (ARI) and a CCP were calculated from continuous recordings of CBF velocity and blood pressure during transient hypotension induced by the sudden release of inflated bilateral thigh cuffs.

In such experiments, blood pressure falls 15 to 25% for 20 to 30 s, while the CBF initially follows in parallel but returns to baseline in 5 to 7 s. The normal response of CBF to a fall in blood pressure is a 20% correction per second, yielding an ARI of around 5 [19]. An ARI of 10 corresponds to a perfect autoregulation and an ARI of 0 to no autoregulation at all [19]. The same measurements allow the plotting of blood pressure as a function of CBF, as both are initially rapidly decreased after cuff release. The first seconds of these pressure and flow changes are passive and are best described by a linear approximation. The extrapolation of linear pressure-flow relationships to the pressure axis defines a critical closing pressure. The experimental setting with pressure and flow recordings for the calculations of both ARI and CCP, in normoxia and in hypoxia, is illustrated in figures 1 to 3.

Van Osta et al. correlated these measurements to an AMS score sampled after 6 hours in a hypobaric chamber at a simulated altitude of 4260 m. Hypoxia decreased CCP from by 18% ($p < 0.05$) and ARI by 17% ($p < 0.05$). There was a negative correlation between baseline normoxic ARI and AMS score ($r = -0.54$, $p < 0.05$) and a positive correlation between ARI and CCP in hypoxia ($r = 0.61$, $p < 0.05$). These results suggested that hypoxia-induced impairment of cerebral hemodynamics might play a role in the pathogenesis of AMS [29].

Van Osta et al. then measured CBF, blood pressure, ARI and CCP at 490 m and 20 hours after arrival at 4559 m, in 35 healthy volunteers [28]. These

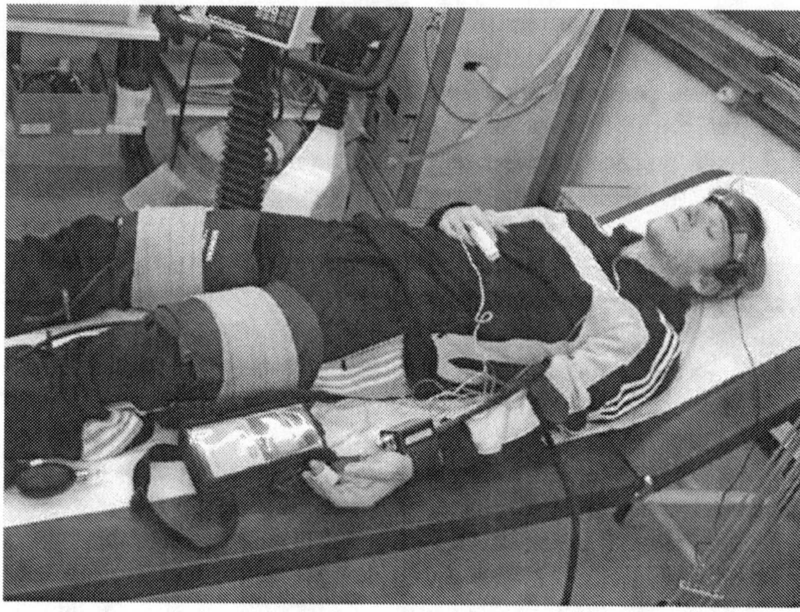

Figure 1. Measurement of cerebral autoregulation in a volunteer, equipped with cuffs placed around the thighs for manipulation of blood pressure, a finger plethysmograph for continuous measurement of blood pressure, and a cerebral Doppler probe positioned next to the middle cerebral artery.

subjects had been randomized to tadalafil, dexamethasone or placebo as part of a study on the pharmacological prevention of high-altitude pulmonary edema [18]. Altitude was associated with an increase in a cerebral sensible AMS (AMS-C) score ($p<0.001$), without change in average CBF, ARI, or CCP. However, the AMS-C score was negatively correlated to ARI ($r = -0.47$, $p<0.01$). The ARI and CCP were positively correlated to arterial oxygenation. The AMS-C score was lower in dexamethasone-treated subjects compared to high-altitude pulmonary edema-sensible controls. A stepwise multiple linear regression analysis on arterial PCO_2, SaO_2, and baseline or altitude ARI, identified altitude ARI as the only significant predictor of the AMS-C score ($p=0.01$). These results supported the notion that impaired dynamic autoregulation of CBF could play a role in AMS symptomatology [28].

Thus cerebral hemodynamic studies so far fit with the notion that AMS and high altitude cerebral edema are at the extremes of a spectrum of progressively severe hypoxia-induced vasogenic cerebral edema. This would explain the striking clinical similarities between of AMS and cerebral edemas of other causes, such as cerebral vein thrombosis. This would certainly account for the efficacy of therapies aimed at the decrease of vasogenic cerebral edemas, such as high doses of corticosteroids [11].

3. Recent imaging studies in hypoxic volunteers

Progress in magnetic resonance imaging (MRI) technology have allowed for accurate determinations of brain volume and of the vasogenic and cytotoxic components of brain edema in hypoxic studies with and without AMS symptomatology. Hackett et al. reported on an intense transverse relaxation rate (T2) signal in white matter, mainly in the splenium of the corpus callosum, and no grey matter abnormalities in 7 of 9 patients with high altitude cerebral edema, investigated after evacuation from high-altitude locations [7].

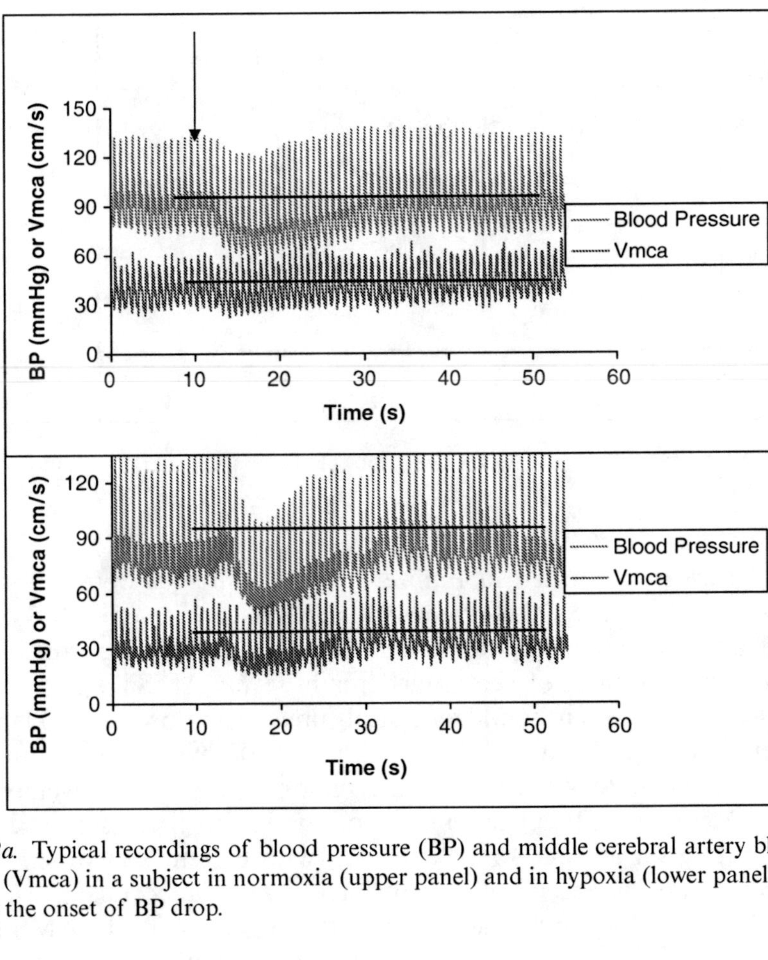

Figure 2a. Typical recordings of blood pressure (BP) and middle cerebral artery blood flow velocity (Vmca) in a subject in normoxia (upper panel) and in hypoxia (lower panel). Arrows indicate the onset of BP drop.

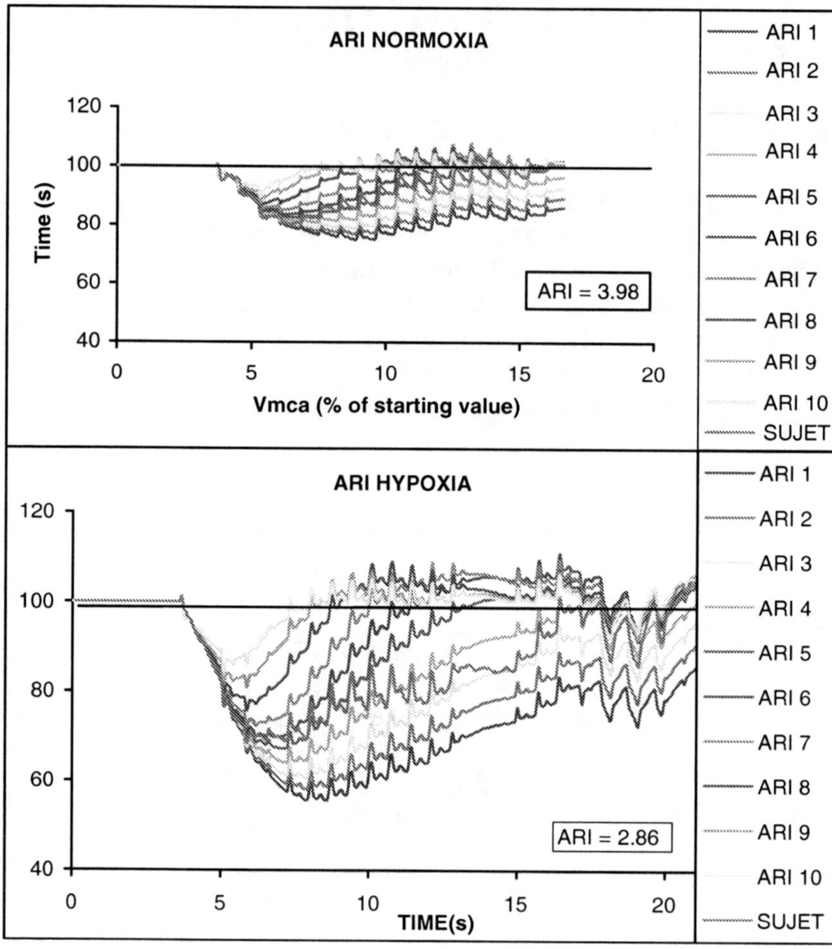

Figure 2b. Autoregulation index (ARI) calculations in normoxia (upper panel) and in hypoxia (lower panel).

A typical case is illustrated in Figure 4. Similar images were reported by Matsuzawa et al. in the sickest four of 7 subjects with severe AMS after 24 hours of altitude exposure [20]. These results are in keeping with previous CT scan demonstrations of cerebral edema in severe AMS [16].

However, more recently, Morocz et al. imaged the brains of 11 healthy volunteers before and after 32 hours of hypobaric hypoxic exposure to an altitude equivalent to 4572m, and the majority of whom developed significant AMS scores [21]. The volumes of the brains increased by 2 to 3% (corresponding on average to 24 to 37ml, with extremes at of 2.5ml and 71ml) due to an increased volume of cortical and subcortical grey matter and no change in the white matter and without correlation to AMS scores. The T2 signals in the white matter, which are normally increased in focal

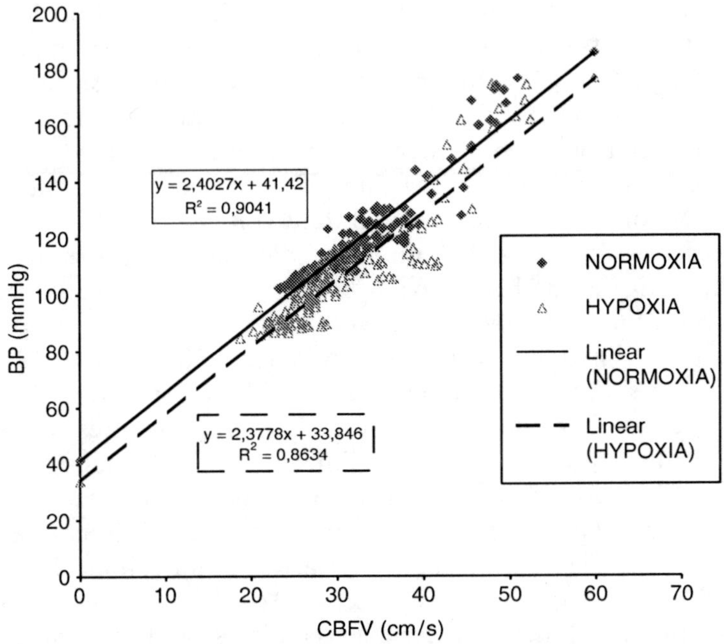

Figure 3. Blood pressure and blood pressure (BP) versus middle cerebral artery velocity (CBFV) in a subject in normoxia and in hypoxia. A cerebral closing pressure (CCP) is estimated by the extrapolation of a linear approximation describing pressure-flow plots. Hypoxia decreased CCP.

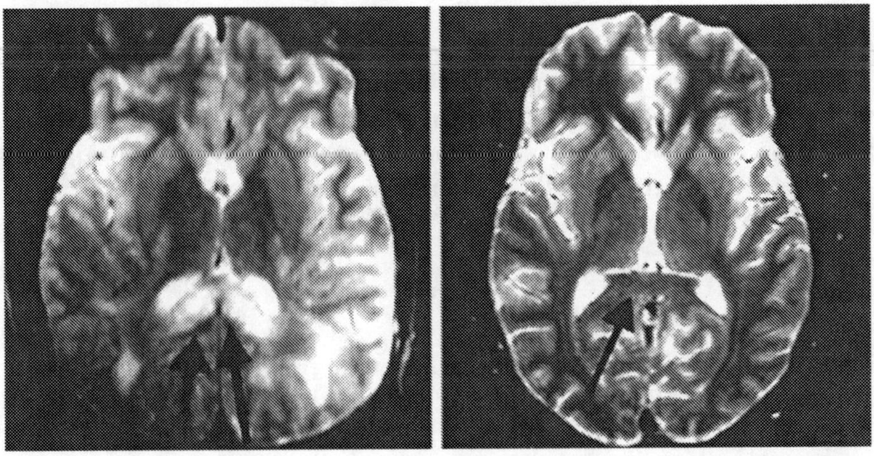

Figure 4. Left, Axial T_2-weighted magnetic resonance image of a patient with high altitude cerebral edema showing markedly increased signal in corpus callosum (arrows), including both the genu and the splenium, as well as increased signal of periventricular and subcortical white matter. Right, Axial T_2-weighted magnetic resonance image of the same patient 5 weeks after original presentation, demonstrating no residual abnormality in splenium (arrow). (From reference 7, with permission).

brain edema, remained unchanged. Fischer et al. reported on MRI of the brains of 10 subjects exposed to a simulated altitude of 4500 m for 10 hours after the administration of either a placebo, theophylline or acetazolamide [5]. Although 8 of the 10 subjects presented with moderate to severe AMS, there was no MRI of cerebral edema, irrespective of the medication taken. However, there was a moderate swelling of the brain, as indicated by a significant reduction of the inner cerebral fluid volume.

Most recently, Bailey et al. combined molecular and neuroimaging techniques to investigate whether hypoxia-induced release of oxygen free radicals might account for vasogenic edema and increased intracranial pressure in AMS [2]. Twenty-two subjects were exposed for 18 hours to 12% oxygen breathing, with sampling of blood and spinal fluid for oxygen free radicals measurements, lumbar puncture to estimate intracranial pressure, and MRI at the end of the hypoxic exposure. A clinical AMS was diagnosed in 50% of the subjects. Electron paramagnetic resonance spectroscopy identified a clear increase in blood and spinal fluid oxygen free radicals. Intracranial pressure remained normal. There was a slight increase in brain volume, by an average of 7 ml (0.6%) with no evidence of edema. There was tendency for greater increase in brain volume in the sickest subjects, without relationship to oxidative stress or intracranial pressure.

The experiment was repeated by Kallenberg et al., who applied T2- and diffusion-weighted MRI to 22 subjects exposed during 12 hours to a 12% oxygen, corresponding to the altitude of 4500 m [12]. A clinical AMS was diagnosed in 50% of the subjects. Hypoxia was associated with an increase in brain volume, increased T2 and a general trend towards an increase in the diffusion coefficient, indicating both vasogenic and cytotoxic edema. While thus there was cerebral edema as a cause of increased volume of the brain, only the diffusion coefficient (cytotoxic edema) was correlated to AMS symptomatology. The authors concluded that a tightly-fitting brain caused by both vasogenic and cytotoxic edema may prove of pathophysiological importance in AMS.

Conclusions

Altogether, these results are compatible with brain edema as a common determinant to AMS and high altitude cerebral edema. Disturbed cerebral autoregulation could be the cause of the vasogenic component of cerebral edema in severe AMS. Since head trauma with cerebral edema is known to be associated with an alteration in cerebral autoregulation, and since oxygen free radicals are a cause of abnormal vasoreactivity, there would be a vicious circle as illustrated in figure 5, where increased blood pressure with exposure to cold and/or exercise would understandably intervene as aggravating factors.

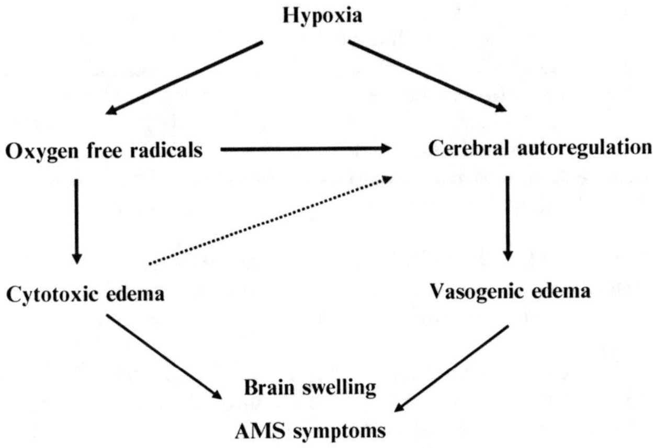

Figure 5. Pathogenesis of acute mountain sickness and high altitude cerebral edema.

The cause of both cytotoxic edema and abnormal CBF regulation could be the hypoxia-induced release of oxygen free radicals.

References

1. Ainslie PN, Burgess K, Subedi P, Burgess KR. Alterations in cerebral dynamics at high altitude following partial acclimatization in humans: wakefulness and sleep. J Appl Physiol epub ahead of print.
2. Bailey DM, Roukens R, Knauth M, Kallenberg K, Christ S, Mohr A, Genius J, Storch-Hagenlocher B, Meisel F, McEneny J, Young IS, Steiner T, Hess K, Bartsch P. (2006) Free radical-mediated damage to barrier function is not associated with altered brain morphology in high-altitude headache. J Cereb Blood Flow Metab. 26 : 99–111. 3. Baumgartner RW, Bärtsch P, Maggiorini M, Waber U, Oelz O. (1994) Enhanced cerebral blood flow in acute mountain sickness. Aviat Space Environ Med 65, 726–729.
4. Baumgartner RW, Spyridopoulos I, Bärtsch P, Maggiorini M, Oelz O. (1999) Acute mountain sickness is not related to cerebral blood flow: a decompression chamber study. J Appl Physiol 86: 1578–1582.
5. Fischer R, Vollmar C, Thiere M, Born C, Leitl M, Pfluger T, Huber RM. (2004) No evidence of cerebral oedema in severe acute mountain sickness. Cephalalgia 24: 66–71.
6. Hackett PH. (1999) High altitude cerebral edema and acute mountain sickness. A pathophysiology update. Adv Exp Med Biol 474: 23–45.
7. Hackett PH, Yarnell PR, Hill R, Reynard K, Heit J, McCormick J. (1998) High-altitude cerebral edema evaluated with magnetic resonance imaging. JAMA 280: 1920–1925.
8. Häggendal E, Johansson B. (1965) Effects of arterial carbon dioxide tension and oxygen saturation on cerebral blood flow autoregulation in dogs. Acta Physiol Scand 66: 27–53.
9. Jansen GF, Krins A, Basnyat B. (1999) Cerebral vasomotor reactivity at high altitude in humans. J Appl Physiol 86: 681–686.
10. Jansen GFA, Krins A, Basnyat B, Bosxh A, Odoom JA. (2000) Cerebral autoregulation in subjects adapted and not adapted to high altitude. Stroke 31: 2314–2318.

11. Johnson TS, Rock PB, Fulco CS, Trad LA, Spark RF, Maher JT. (1984) Prevention of acute mountain sickness by dexamethasone. N Engl J Med 310: 683–686.
12. Kallenberg K, Bailey DM, Christ S, Mohr A, Roukens R, Menold E, Steiner T, Bartsch P, Knauth M. (2006) Magnetic resonance imaging evidence of cytotoxic cerebral edema in acute mountain sickness. J Cereb Blood Flow Metab epub ahead of print.
13. Kogure K, Scheinberg P, Fujishima M, Busto R, Reinmuth OM. (1970) Effects of hypoxia on cerebral autoregulation. Am J Physiol 219: 1393–1396.
14. Lassen NA. (1959) Cerebral blood flow and oxygen consumption in man. Physiol Rev 39: 183–238.
15. Lassen NA, Harper AM. (1975) High-altitude cerebral oedema. Lancet. 2: 1154.
16. Levine BD, Yoshimura K, Kobayashi T, Fukushima M, Shibamoto T, Ueda G. (1989) Dexamethasone in the treatment of acute mountain sickness. N Engl J Med 321: 1707–1713.
17. Lysakowski C, Von Elm E, Dumont L, Junod J-D, Tassonyi E, Kayser B, Tramer MR. (2003) The effects of magnesium, high altitude, and acute mountain sickness on blood flow velocity in the middle cerebral artery. Clin. Sci. (Lond) 106: 279–285.
18. Maggiorini M, Brunner-La occa P, Peth S, Fischler M, Bohm T, Bernheim A, Kiencke S, Bloch KE, Dehnert C, Naeije, Lehmann T, Bartsch P, Mairbaurl H. (2006) Both tadalafil and dexamethasone may reduce the incidence of high-altitude pulmonary edema: a randomized trial. Ann Intern Med. 145: 497–506.
19. Mahoney PJ, Panerai RB, Deverson ST, Hayes PD, Evans DH. (2000) Assessment of the thigh cuff technique for measurement of dynamic cerebral autoregulation. Stroke 31: 476–480.
20. Matsuzawa Y, Kobayashi T, Fujimoto K, Shinozaki S, Yoshikawa S. Cerebral edema in acute mountain sickness. In Reeves JT, Sekigushi M, editors, (1992) High Altitude Medicine, Matsumoto, Japan, Shinshu University, 300–304.
21. Morocz IA, Zientara GP, Gudbjartsson H, Muza S, Lyons T, Rock PB, Kikinis R, Jolesz FA. (2001) Volumetric quantification of brain swelling after hypobaric hypoxia exposure. Exp Neurol 168: 96–104.
22. Otis SM, Rossman ME, Scneider PA, Rush M P, Ringelstein EB. (1989) Relationship of cerebral blood flow regulation to acute mountain sickness. J. Ultrasound Med. 8: 143–148.
23. Panerai RB, Deverson ST, Mahony P, Hayes P, Evans DH. (1999) Effects of CO2 on dynamic cerebral autoregulation measurement. Physiol Meas 20: 265–275.
24. Reeves JT, Moore LG, McCullough RE, McCullough RG, Harrison G, Tranmer BI, Micco AJ, Tucker A, Weil JV. (1985) Headache at high altitude is not related to internal carotid arterial blood velocity. J Appl Physiol 59: 909–915.
25. Richards HK, Czosnyka M, Pickard JD. (1999) Assessment of critical closing pressure in the cerebral circulation as a measure of cerebrovascular tone. Acta Neurochirurgica. 141: 1221–1227.
26. Roach R, Maes D, Sandoval D, Robergs RA, Icenogle M, Hinghofer-Szalkay H, Lium D, Loeppky JA. (2000) Exercice exacerbates acute mountain sickness at simulated high altitude. J Appl Physiol 88: 581–585.
27. Tiecks FP, Lam AM, Aaslid R, Newell DW. (1995) Comparison of Static and dynamic cerebral autoregulation measurements. Stroke 26: 1014–1019.
28. Van Osta A, Moraine JJ, Melot C, Mairbaurl H, Maggiorini M, Naeije R.. (2005) Effects of high altitude exposure on cerebral hemodynamics in normal subjects. Stroke 36: 557–560.
29. Van Osta A, Moraine JJ, Berre J, Melot C, Naeije R. Hypoxia alters dynamic cerebral autoregulation and decreases cerebral closing pressure in normal volunteers. Submitted.
30. Ward MP, Milledge JS, West JB. (2000) High altitude medicine and physiology (2nd ed). Chapman and Hall Medical, London, pp 388–411.
31. Zhang R, Zuckerman JH, Giller CA, Levine BD. (1998) Transfer function analysis of dynamic cerebral circulation in humans. Am J physiol 274: H233–241.

CHAPTER 16

CARDIAC LIMITATION TO EXERCISE CAPACITY AT HIGH ALTITUDES

SANDRINE HUEZ, ROBERT NAEIJE,
VITALIE FAORO

Department of Physiology, Faculty of Medicine of the Free University of Brussels, Belgium

Abstract: Exposure to high altitude is associated with a decrease in aerobic exercise capacity. This is explained by a decrease in oxygen delivery to the tissues or the product of cardiac output by arterial oxygen content. Arterial oxygen content is decreased at altitude because of a reduced inspired partial pressure of oxygen. However, this limited by the hypoxic chemoreflex, which increases ventilation and decreases alveolar partial pressure of carbon dioxide, thereby improving alveolar partial pressure of oxygen. In addition, there is a renal synthesis and release of erythropoietin, which increases the hemoglobin content of the blood. Both adaptations bring arterial oxygen content back to its pre-hypoxic exposure sea-level value in 2 to 3 weeks at altitudes up to 5000 m, without, however, restoring exercise capacity. Altitude is also associated with a decrease in maximum cardiac output. The mechanisms of hypoxia-induced decrease in maximum cardiac output remain incompletely understood. Previously proposed explanations have been a decreased peripheral demand due to altered matching of diffusional and convectional oxygen delivery processes, a decrease in the chronotropic reserve or a decreased central nervous system output to the heart. Pharmacological studies in hypoxic volunteers suggest that at least part of the limitation of cardiac output at high altitude might be related to hypoxic pulmonary hypertension, as a cause of excessive right ventricular afterload. This notion has recently been confirmed by Doppler echocardiographic studies, which suggest that high altitude-induced right heart failure (HARHF) might be more common than previously assumed.

Keywords: altitude, exercise; heart; pulmonary hypertension; hypoxic pulmonary vasoconstriction; right heart failure

A. Aldashev and R. Naeije (eds.), Problems of High Altitude Medicine and Biology, 221–229.

Introduction

Reduced exercise tolerance at high altitudes has long puzzled scientists. Horace-Benedict de Saussure, who was a professor of philosophy at the university of Geneva and led the second ascent to the Mont Blanc (4807 m) in 1787, recorded his pulse, respirations, temperature and symptoms, and wrote: "The sort of weariness which proceeds from the rarity of the air is absolutely insurmountable; when it is at its height, the most imminent peril will not make you move a step faster... Since the air had hardly more than half of its usual density, compensation had to be made for the lack of density by the frequency of respirations. That is the cause of the fatigue that one experiences at great heights. For while the respiration is accelerating, so is the circulation" [6].

De Saussure correctly assigned the decreased exercise capacity at altitude to the respiratory and cardiovascular effects of reduced atmospheric pressure. It took, however, an additional century to realize that the cause of it all was a decreased inspired PO_2 (PIO_2) [25]. Since then, expeditions and hypobaric chamber experiments have gathered the data showing altitude-related exponential decrease in maximum O_2 consumption (VO_2max), along with decreased PIO_2, but whether the main limiting factor is pulmonary, cardiac or muscular remains disputed [9].

The limitation in aerobic exercise capacity at high altitude is illustrated in figure 1, which represents measurements of VO_2, carbon dioxide production

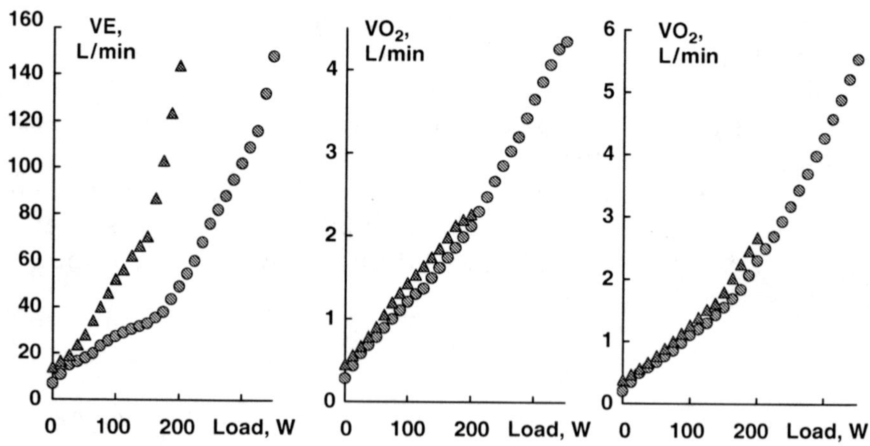

Figure 1. Cardiopulmonary exercise tests in a normal volunteer at sea level (red circles) and after two weeks acclimatization (blue triangles), at the altitude of 5000 m. Altitude was associated with decreases in workload and VO_2max, while maximum ventilation (V_E) was unchanged in the face of increased ventilatory equivalent for CO_2.

(VCO_2) and ventilation as a function of progressively increased workload in a subject at sea level and again after two weeks at an altitude of 5000 m on Mount Chimborazo. The altitude of 5000 m was associated with decreases in maximum workload and VO_2max by approximately 40%, with a maintained VO_2/workload ratio and a preserved maximum ventilation in spite of a markedly increased ventilatory equivalent for CO_2.

Mechanisms of Decreased Exercise Capacity at High Altitude

Altitude is associated with a decrease in inspired partial pressure of O_2 because of a decrease in barometric pressure. Therefore, altitude decreases alveolar PO_2, which limits the oxygenation of mixed venous blood in the pulmonary capillaries. As long as alveolar PO_2 is maintained to values equal or higher than 55 to 60 mmHg, the oxygenation of hemoglobin is maintained at more than 90 % and O_2 delivery to the tissues is preserved. Altitude exposure is associated with a peripheral chemoreflex-mediated increase in alveolar ventilation, which also helps to maintain alveolar PO_2. However, as altitude increases, a decrease in alveolar PO_2 is unavoidable and accordingly, maximum O_2 delivery decreases because of a decrease in arterial O_2 content [9].

At acute exposure to altitudes up to 4000 m or equivalent hypoxia induced by a decreased fraction of inspired O_2 from normal 0.21 to 0.12, maximum cardiac output is similar to that attained during normoxic exercise and decreased VO_2max has indeed been found to be essentially explained by a decrease in arterial O_2 content. However, more severe hypoxia is also associated with a decreased maximum cardiac output and flow to exercising muscles, leading to a decrease in VO_2max that is out of proportion to decreased arterial O_2 content [9,25]. It has been estimated that two thirds of the decrease in VO_2max at 5300 m, the altitude of Mount Everest base camp, can be accounted for by a decreased arterial O_2 content, and one third by a limitation of cardiac output [3].

Half of the decrease in CaO_2 measured during acute hypoxic exercise is attributable to decreased PIO_2 and the other half to increased alveolo-to-arterial PO_2 gradient [3]. Hypoxic exercise is known to decrease arterial oxygenation because of a diffusion limitation for O_2 and altered ventilation/perfusion (VA/Q) matching, with diffusion limitation playing a proportionally more important role as PIO_2 decreases [24]. The diffusion limitation is due to a combination of decreased pulmonary capillary erythrocyte transit time and decreased driving pressure for alveolo-capillary transfer of O_2. Altered VA/Q matching is more difficult to understand but may be related to hypoxia-induced interstitial edema and perhaps, to inhomogenous hypoxic pulmonary vasoconstriction.

More chronic hypoxic exposure restores CaO_2 to sea-level values, due to polycythemia and hyperventilation but is not associated with a recovery of

VO_2max [4]. This is explained by persistent failure of peak cardiac output to normalize and preferential distribution of cardiac output to non-exercising tissues [4].

The mechanisms of decreased maximum cardiac output in hypoxia remain incompletely understood. Maximum heart rate progressively decreases with increasing altitudes, down to around 120 beats/min at the summit of Mount Everest [19]. However, decreased chronotropic response to exercise is unlikely to play a major role, as vagal blockade with glycopyrrolate in subjects exposed during 9 weeks to the altitude of 5260 m was recently shown to restore maximum heart rate to sea-level values, without affecting peak cardiac output, work rate or VO_2max [2]. Profound hypoxia in vitro is associated with a decreased myocardial fibre contractility, but systolic function has been reported to be well preserved and actually even enhanced, up to the altitude of Mount Everest in acclimatized volunteers [19, 22]. There has been suggestion of a role for decreased central command by the effect of decreased PO_2 on medullary neurons projecting to a brainstem "cardiovagal center" [15], but there is little experimental evidence that this might play a role in the limitation of aerobic exercise capacity.

As nothing appears to be intrinsically wrong with the heart at high altitudes, attention has rather focused on the role of peripheral limitation of the diffusion of O_2. At tissue level, transfer of O_2 from the capillaries to the mitochondria is determined by an optimal matching between convectional O_2 transport (Fick principle) and diffusional transport (Fick's law of diffusion), which can be graphically demonstrated to occur at a lower cardiac output in hypoxia [23]. There is experimental evidence that muscle capillary PO_2 can be approximated by venous PO_2, and that mitochondrial PO_2 is between 1 and 2 mmHg. Accordingly, it is reasonable to assume that muscle VO_2 is directly proportional to venous PO_2 times and a diffusion constant. However, any increase in venous oxygenation decreases the arterio-venous O_2 content difference and thereby also decreases O_2 delivery to the tissues. As illustrated in figure 2, there is only one value for venous PO_2 and a corresponding cardiac output at which these two mechanisms of O_2 transport to muscle mitochondria can be coupled. According to the same analysis, any increase in cardiac output increases venous PO_2, but this cannot increase VO_2 because of a necessarily associated decreased muscle diffusion for O_2.

Right Ventricular Limitation to Exercise Capacity at High Altitudes

Exposure to hypoxia induces pulmonary vasoconstriction. Hypoxic pulmonary vasoconstriction serves to maintain a high PVR during the aquatic fetal life, when there is no need for pulmonary gas exchange, and helps to maintain the matching of perfusion to ventilation in case of regional

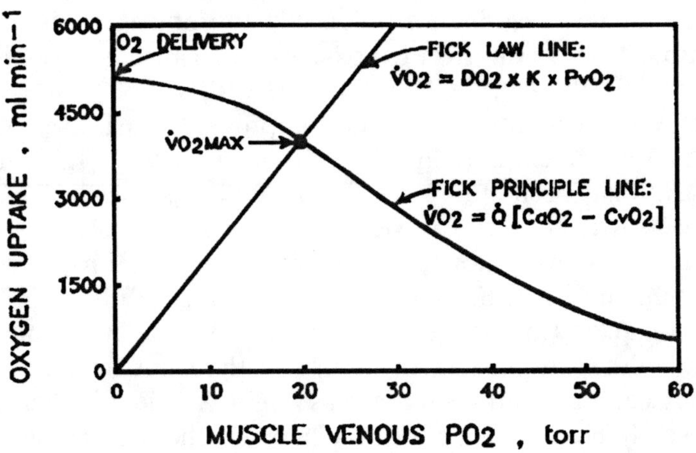

Figure 2. Graphical analysis of the coupling between convectional and diffusional oxygen (O_2) transport mechanisms. Q: cardiac output; a: arterial; v: venous. From reference 23, with permission

decrease in PO_2 in atmospheric postnatal normal life [18]. However, whole lung hypoxic vasoconstriction serves no purpose and can actually be deleterious by causing lung edema, right heart failure or both [25]. The notion of hypoxic pulmonary hypertension as a cause of limitation to exercise capacity due to afterload-induced right heart failure was recently introduced, in relation to the advent of efficacious pharmacological therapies for pulmonary hypertension at high altitudes. Ghofrani et al. reported that the intake of the phosphodiesterase-5 (PDE-5) inhibitor sildenafil increased exercise capacity at the base camp of Mount Everest [11]. This remarkable observation was confirmed on the slopes of the Mont Blanc, by Richalet et al. [20], and in the Kyrgyz mountains, by Aldashev et al. [1]. The authors agreed that the most likely explanation for performance-enhancing effects of sildenafil at high altitudes would be a decrease in PVR, allowing for an increased maximum cardiac output and O_2 uptake [1,11,20]. Sildenafil has been extensively used as an effective treatment for erectile dysfunction [5] but has long been known to be a potent pulmonary vasodilator, and has actually been shown by a randomized controlled trial to be effective in the treatment of pulmonary arterial hypertension [10].

However, this notion will have to be confirmed. In the study by Ghofrani et al. [11], pulmonary artery pressures during exercise in hypoxia were actually not much higher than the upper limit of normal in normoxic healthy people [17]. There are preliminary reports that sildenafil intake may improve hypoxic exercise capacity in relation to both an improvement in arterial oxygenation and a decrease in PVR [7]. Fischler et al. reported in a preliminary study that pulmonary vasodilation induced by the intake of tadalafil, another PDE-5 inhibitor, does not affect hypoxic exercise capacity in subjects prone to high altitude pulmonary edema (HAPE) with severe pulmonary hypertension [8]. It may be that sildenafil also improves hypoxic exercise capacity through an improvement in pulmonary diffusion capacity [12]. On the other hand, sildenafil has been reported to improve the distance walked in 6 minutes in subjects with chronic hypoxic pulmonary hypertension [1], very much as reported in those with more severe pulmonary arterial hypertension [10]. Along the same line, it is likely that right ventricular failure contributes to limit exercise capacity in subacte mountain sickness and in chronic mountain sickness [25], although this has not been directly investigated or tested with pharmacological interventions to decrease right ventricular afterload.

Most recently, Huez et al. reported on Doppler echocardiography with tissue Doppler imaging (TDI) in a normal subject who developed severe pulmonary hypertension after arrival on the Bolivian Altiplano [14]. This subject had a previous history of HAPE but had since repeatedly been at high altitudes with

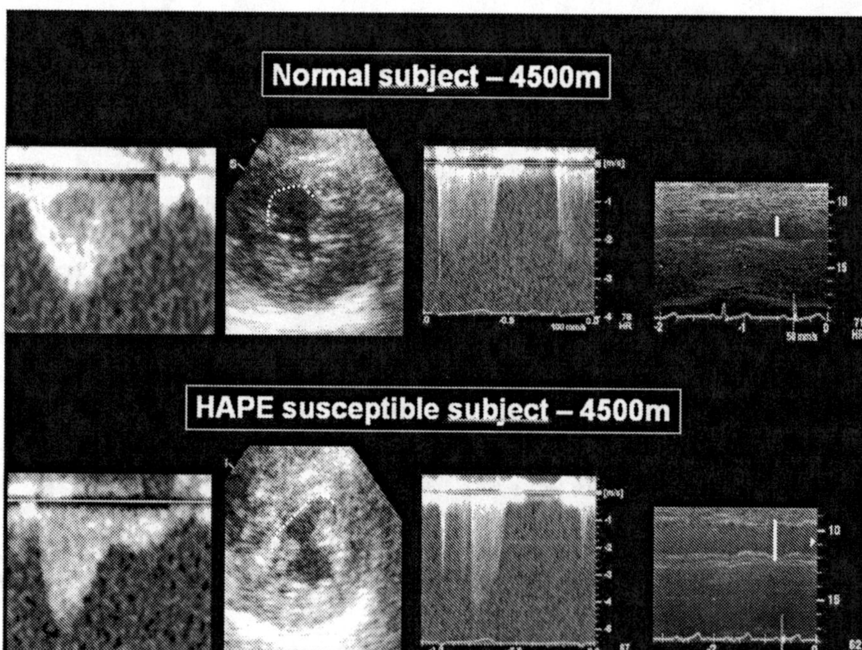

Figure 3. Doppler echocardiography and tissue Doppler imaging in a subject susceptible to high altitude pulmonary edema (HAPE-s) and in a control, at sea level and after acclimatization at 4300 m. The HAPE-s subject developed severe pulmonary hypertension with right heart failure or HARHF (see text), while the control developed a moderate increase in pulmonary artery pressures with no change in right ventricular function. After reference 14, with permission.

no recurrence because of appropriate acclimatization. His clinical examination was unremarkable and he was asymptomatic except for a question of being somewhat more dyspneic than usual at exercise. Sea-level measurements were normal, with normal right heart chamber dimensions and contractility, trans-tricuspid and mitral flow patterns, acceleration time of pulmonary arterial flow and maximum velocity of tricuspid regurgitation, normal inferior vena cava diameter with inspiratory collapse and unremarkable TDI. However, at the altitude of 4500 m, the right ventricle and right atrium showed increased sizes with septal displacement, the maximum velocity of the tricuspid regurgitation was increased and the pulmonary arterial flow pattern was abnormal because of a shortened acceleration time and midsystolic deceleration; the inferior vena cava was dilated with no inspiratory collapse (Figure 3). Most remarkably, TDI disclosed a "postsystolic shortening" wave as previously reported in ischemic left ventricles, quite suggestive of ventricular failure [14].

The acute medical complications of high-altitude exposure are generally believed to be essentially cerebral or pulmonary, with subjects exposed to the risk of acute mountain sickness (AMS), HAPE and/or high-altitude cerebral edema (HACE) [13]. Huez et al. suggest that high altitude-induced right heart failure (HARHF) should be added to the list [14]. They argue that the condition has gone unnoticed until now because of the known paucity of clinical symptoms of right ventricular failure on excessive afterload in patients with severe pulmonary hypertension, and that the advent of performant portable Doppler echocardiography equipment will make the diagnosis of HARHF common clinical practice under field conditions. It remains to be seen how often HARHF really occurs and to what extent moderate levels of right ventricular dysfunction relate to decreased exercise capacity.

Conclusions

Aerobic exercise capacity is decreased at high altitudes, in relation to decreased inspired oxygen, pulmonary diffusion limitation and VA/Q imbalance and altered convectional and diffusional oxygen transport mechanisms. Recent echocardiographic studies have disclosed a component of relative right heart failure, or HARHF, that may be amenable to pharmacological interventions.

References

1. Aldashev AA, Kojonazarov BK, Amatov TA, Sooronbaev TM, Mirrakhimov MM, Morrell NW, Wharton J, Wilkins MR. (2005) Phosphodiesterase type 5 and high altitude pulmonary hypertension. Thorax 60: 683–687.
2. Boushel R, Calbet JA, Radegran G, Sondergaard H, Wagner PD, Saltin B. (2001) Parasympathetic neural activity accounts for the lowering of exercise heart rate at high altitude. Circulation 104: 1785–1791.

3. Calbet JA, Boushel R, Radegran G, Sondergaard H, Wagner PD, Saltin B. (2003) Determinants of maximal oxygen uptake in severe acute hypoxia. Am J Physiol Regul Integr Comp Physiol. 284: R291–303.
4. Calbet JA, Boushel R, Radegran G, Sondergaard H, Wagner PD, Saltin B. (2003) Why is VO2 max after altitude acclimatization still reduced despite normalization of arterial O2 content? Am J Physiol Regul Integr Comp Physiol. 2003; 284: R304–316.
5. Carson CC 3rd. Sildenafil: a 4-year update in the treatment of 20 million erectile dysfunction patients. Curr Urol Rep. 4: 488–496.
6. De Saussure, HB. (1998) Voyages dans les Alpes. Edited by Louis Fauche-Borel, imprimeur du Roi, Neuchatel, Switzerland, 1796. Cited by Houston CS, in: Going Higher. Oxygen, Man and Mountains. 4th edition. Publishes by The Mountaineers, Seattle.
7. Faoro V, Lamotte M, Deboeck G, Pavelescu A, Huez S, Guenard H, Martinot JB, Naeije R. (2007) Effects of sildenafil on exercise capacity in hypoxic normal subjects. High Alt Med Biol in press.
8. Fischler M, Dorschner L, Debrunner J, Brunner-La Rocca HP, Kliencke S, Birheim A, Bloch K, Mairbaurl H, Maggiorini M. (2005) Maximum exercise capacity at high altitude is not influenced by prophylaxis with dexamethasone or tadalafil in HAPE-susceptible subjects. Abstract presented at the 14th International Hypoxia Symposium, Lake Louise, Alberta, Canada, February 22–27.
9. Fulco CS, Rock PB, Cymerman A. (1998) Maximal and submaximal exercise performance at altitude. Aviat Space Environ Med. 69 : 793–801.
10. Galie N, Ghofrani HA, Torbicki A, Barst RJ, Rubin LJ, Badesch D, Fleming T, Parpia T, Burgess G, Branzi A, Grimminger F, Kurzyna M, Simonneau G. (2005) Sildenafil Use in Pulmonary Arterial Hypertension (SUPER) Study Group. Sildenafil citrate therapy for pulmonary arterial hypertension. N Engl J Med 353; 2148–2157.
11. Ghofrani HA, Reichenberger F, Kohstall MG, M:rosek EH, Seeger T, Olschewski H, Seeger W, Grimminger F. (2004) Sildenafil Increased Exercise Capacity during Hypoxia at Low altitudes and at Mount Everest Base Camp, Ann Intern Med 141:169–77.
12. Guazzi M, Tumminello G, Di Marco F, Fiorentini C, Guazzi MD. (2004) The Effects of Phosphodiesterase-5 Inhibition with sildenafil on pulmonary hemodynamics and diffusion capacity, exercise ventilatory efficiency, and oxygen uptake kinetics in chronic heart failure. J Am Coll Cardiol 44:2339–48.
13. Hackett PH, Roach RC. (2001) High-altitude illness. N Engl J Med 345:107–14.
14. Huez S, Faoro V, Vachiery JL, Unger P, Martinot JB, Naeije R. (2007) High altitude induced right heart failure. Circulation 115: 108–109.
15. Kayser B. (2003) Exercise begins and ends in the brain. Eur J Appl Physiol 90: 411–419.
16. Maggiorini M, Mélot C, Pierre S, Pfeiffer F, Greve I, Sartori C, Lepori M, Hauser M, Scherrer U, Naeije R. (2001) High altitude pulmonary edema is initially caused by an increased capillary pressure. Circulation 103: 2078–2083.
17. McQuillan BM, Picard MH, Leavitt M, Weyman AE. (2001) Clinical correlates and reference intervals for pulmonary artery systolic pressure among echocardiographically normal subjects. Circulation. 104:2797–2802.
18. Naeije R. (2004) Pulmonary vascular function. In: Pulmonary Circulation. Siseases and their Treatment. Edited by AJ Peacock and LJ Rubin. Arnold, London, chap 1, pp 3–13.
19. Reeves JT, Groves BM, Sutton JR, Wagner PD, Cymerman A, Malconian MK, Rock PB, Young PM, Houston CS. (1987) Operation Everest II: preservation of cardiac function at extreme altitude. J Appl Physiol. 63: 531–539.
20. Richalet JP, Gratadour P, Robach P, Pham I, Dechaux M, Joncquirt-Latarjet A, Mollard P, Brugniaux J, Cornolo J. (2005) Sildenafil Inhibits Altitude-induced Hypoxemia and pulmonary Hypertension. Am J Respir Crit Care Med 171:275–81.
21. Rubin LJ, Naeije R. (2004) Sildenafil for enhanced performance at high altitude? Ann Intern Med. 141: 233–235.

22. Suarez J, Alexander JK, Houston CS. (1987) Enhanced left ventricular systolic performance at high altitude during operation Everest II. Am J Cardiol 60: 137–142.
23. Wagner PD. (2000) Reduced maximal cardiac output at altitude – mechanisms and significance. Respir Physiol 120: 1–11.
24. Wagner PD. (2001) Gas exchange. In: High Altitude. An Exploration of Human adaptation, edited by Hornbein TF and Schoene RB. Lung Biology in Health and Disease, executive director C Lenfant, volume 161. Marcel Dekker, New York, chap 8, pp 199–234.
25. West JB. (2004) The physiologic basis for high altitude diseases. Ann Intern Med 141: 789–800.

CHAPTER 17

PEDIATRIC HIGH ALTITUDE HEART DISEASE: A HYPOXIC PULMONARY HYPERTENSION SYNDROME

TIANYI WU

National Key Laboratory of High Altitude Medicine of the Ministry of Science and Technology, People's Republic of China. Department of Hypoxic Physiology and Mountain Sickness, High Altitude Medical Research Institute, Xining, Nanchua West Road #344, Qinghai, 810012, P.R.C.

Abbreviations: PHAHD: pediatric high altitude heart disease; ISMS: subacute infantile mountain sickness; SHAPH: symptomatic high altitude pulmonary hypertension; HAHD: high altitude heart disease; MPAP: mean pulmonary artery pressure; PPH: primary pulmonary hypertension; CMS: chronic mountain sickness.

Abstract: Previous studies suggest that Tibetans as the oldest mountainous population are better adapted to high altitude. We hypothesized that Tibetans have an unusually small degree of hypoxic pulmonary vasoconstriction (HPV) compared with Han newcomers from the lowlands acclimatized to high altitude. We have studied the pulmonary hemodynamics in healthy Tibetan highlanders and Han newcomers in Qinghai-Tibet. Data were collected from right cardiac catheterization. Cardiac output (CO), pulmonary artery wedge pressure and pulmonary artery pressure were measured in all volunteers at various altitudes. At a given altitude, Tibetans show a lower mean pulmonary artery pressure (MPAP) than Han subjects at rest. During exercise, MPAP in Tibetans increased slightly with a significantly increased cardiac output (CO), whereas the Han showed an obviously increased MPAP both at 2,261m and 3,950 m with a slightly increased CO. Tibetans have a much higher exhaled nitric oxide (NO) than lowlanders. The pulmonary hypertension was relived by oxygen breathing in Han newcomers who has migrated to altitude not more than one month previously indicated that the pulmonary hypertension was due to HPV. But with hypoxic pulmonary hypertension (HPH) in two-year Han immigrants the response to oxygen was less apparent because of vascular remodeling. The pulmonary arterial vasculature studies showed that in normal Tibetan infants over the age 4 months, their small pulmonary arteries are thin-walled and the pulmonary arterioles have thin walls consisting of single elastic laminae. In contrast, in Han Chinese children who were born and raised at high altitude in Tibet until the age of 4 years, the small pulmonary

A. Aldashev and R. Naeije (eds.), Problems of High Altitude Medicine and Biology, 231–247.

arteries retain a thick smooth muscle. It is usually noted that at high altitude the muscularity in Han infant pulmonary arteries fails to regress, as it does at sea level. The evolutionary pressure for the phenomenon of HPV presumably comes from its value in the perinatal period. We remain emphatic on the point that the pulmonary hypertension at high altitude has no useful function but in fact is deleterious because it is usually associated with several altitude diseases – high altitude pulmonary edema, subacute mountain sickness (infantile and adult) and chronic mountain sickness. Indeed, Tibetans having a normal PAP and a minimal HPV, as well as a marked increase in exercise CO is indicative of remarkable high altitude adaptation. Tibetans are though to have the longest residence at high altitude and more genetically homogenous than Han Chinese, suggesting an evolutionary effect on the genetic control of HPV.

Keywords: pulmonary hemodynamics, Tibetan natives, Han lowlanders, genetic adaptation

Introduction

Children, especially during the first year of life, are faced with a more rigorous test of altitude hypoxia. Historically, there have been two periods of large movement of the human population from low to high altitude. From the fifteenth to sixteenth centuries, the Spaniards who first colonized the Andes became well aware that their infants did not thrive if born and raised at high altitude [24]. Some four hundred year later, by the middle of the 20th century, a large number of lowland Han Chinese began migrating to Qinghai-Tibet. The Han men and their wives believed that they could give birth to children on the plateau as at sea level. However, not long after, many infants and young children died of illness due to a congestive heart failure. Wu and Liu (1955) [37] first reported a Han infant aged 11 months born at Lhasa (3658 m) presenting dyspnea, cyanosis and congestive cardiac failure. She died because evacuation to a lower altitude was delayed. At necropsy, marked right ventricular hypertrophy and muscular thickening of the peripheral pulmonary arteries was found. The pathology ruled out other diagnoses such as congenital heart disease and the authors named this "pediatric high-altitude heart disease"(PHAHD). The term was accepted by the Chinese medical Association for High Altitude Medicine in 1995.

Subsequently other, similar cases were reported in Qinghai-Tibet. Among them, Sui et al (1988) [35] studied the pathology of the disease and termed it "subacute infantile mountain sickness" (ISMS), he and other two collaborators, Heath and Anand both used this term and one after another published in English, which exerted a great influence in the west [2, 10]. Now, more than one thousand cases of PHAHD or ISMS have been reported from the Qinghai-Tibetan plateau, the Karakoram and Tien-Shan mountainous areas, but this new syndrome is found most commonly in China [3, 7].

However, it is not as some authors suggest that ISMS was virtually confined to the Himalayan area or Tibet [7, 11]. There have been some reports from the Andes. Infantile or children with severe pulmonary hypertension was found in Morococha (4540 m) and La Oroya (3730 m) in Peru [12, 13, 37]. A series of similar cases was reported in La Paz (3600–4200 m) Bolivia [4, 14, 29, 30]. The condition is also recognized in Leadville, Colorado (3100 m) in North America [8, 17, 30]. These data are important and indicate that the disease may affect the health of high-altitude pediatric populations all over the world [45].

Definition and Nomenclature

PHAHD, also named ISMS, is a syndrome, which is the occurrence of symptomatic, severe pulmonary hypertension in infants or young children who were born or brought up at high altitude above 3000 m; symptoms result from an excessive increase in pulmonary artery pressure and right heart failure. These infants often died if continuously exposed to high altitude and autopsy revealed extreme medial hypertrophy of the pulmonary arteries and an increased muscularization of the pulmonary arterioles, as well as right ventricular dilatation and hypertrophy, attributed to secondary to pulmonary vascular disease. The cure for this syndrome is oxygen administration and early evacuation.

Various authors use different terms to denote identical altitude illnesses. Since Wu and Liu in 1955 [37] first used the term "pediatric high altitude heart disease, PHAHD", it is now well accepted for this syndrome in China [44]. After that, in the year 1988, Sui GJ, a Chinese pathologist and his colleagues, in collaboration with an English research group in Lhasa, Tibet, noted that it is an often fatal disease affecting infants and manifesting itself over a period of weeks and months rather than days or years, it came to be designated as "subacute infantile mountain sickness" [35]. Otherwise, because it is known that mild pulmonary hypertension without symptoms is one of the common features of altitude residents, to draw a clear distinction between physiologic and pathologic pulmonary hypertension, a term "symptomatic high altitude pulmonary hypertension" (SHAPH) was first proposed by Jones et al. (1982) [16], then by Pollard and Niermeyer (2002) [33]. Furthermore, Niermeyer (2003) [30] suggest the term of SHAPH includes acute exacerbation of pulmonary hypertension and the subacute form. In this regard, Hultgren (1997) [13] suggested this asymptomatic condition is best defined as "high altitude pulmonary hypertension" whereas in those with symptomatic cases, a more appropriate term would be "accelerated pulmonary hypertension of high altitude". The lack of a common term has always confused scientists. In August 2004, the VI World Congress on Mountain Medicine and High Altitude Physiology was held in Xining, Qinghai, China. An International Working Group reached agreement on the "Consensus Statement by and Ad Hoc Committee of the International Society for Mountain Medicine on Chronic High Altitude Diseases". Of these, PHAHD or ISMS was defined as "A subacute clinical syndrome characterized by severe pulmonary hypertension leading in infant (or adult) lowlanders who migrate to high altitude to congestive failure of the right heart within weeks or months". And the term for the syndrome was proposed as "Cardiac subacute mountain sickness" [19].

Incidence and Importance

In Qinghai-Tibet the incidence or prevalence of PHAHD or ISMS is corresponding higher. From 1978 to 1985, an epidemiological study on PHAHD among 6,823 Han infants and children (after birth to 14 years of age) was carried out on the Qinghai-Tibetan plateau. The diagnosis of PHAHD was based on history, symptoms, clinical examination, electrocardiography (ECG), echocardiography, chest radiography, blood count and arterial oxygen saturation (see below). Incidence was 3.66% among Han infants and 1.52% in Han children at 3050 to 5226 m. The incidence increased with increasing altitude and decreased with increasing age [41].

In the 70s to 80s of the 20th century in Tibet, a very high prevalence of PHAHD was also represented by the hospital pediatric population. In the Tibetan People's Hospital in Lhasa (3658 m), a total of 238 patients with PHAHD had been admitted to the hospital, during the period from 1/1962 to 12/1963, making a prevalence of 20.7% for the disease in the total hospital pediatric population [47]. During the period from 1/1974 to 12/1975, a total of 412 patients with PHAHD were admitted to the same hospital, accounting for 16.2% of pediatric cases hospitalized during the same period [15]. All the above patients were of Han origin except two, who were native Tibetans.

Over the next two decades, more effective prevention among the altitude children was performed in Tibet, but the incidence of the disease decreased slowly because changing poor acclimatization of the Han children is difficult and takes time.

We found no clear data on the incidence of PHAHD or ISMS in South and North American children. However, more than ten million children have been born and live permanently above 3000 m in the mountainous areas of the world. In addition, several million individuals visit high altitudes annual for work or for recreation, some of them with their children and thus the risk of acute and subacute mountain sickness in these children will increase. Therefore, questions about the altitude tolerance of children are receiving increasing attention.

Population Differences

Wu et al. (1983) [40] presented a comparative study performed in the Qingnan area and Aljin Mountains at altitudes between 3050 m and 5188 m. Four different ethnic pediatric populations (from birth to 14 years of age) who have been at altitude for varying lengths of time but reside at equal altitudes were studied. It is interesting to note that there is a relationship between population prevalence of PHAHD and duration of altitude residence. The prevalence of PHAHD is markedly lower among native Tibetan children than in Han, Kazakhi or Mongolian children at comparable altitudes in Tibet (Table 1).

Tibetans are the oldest population living permanently on the high Tibetan plateau for between 25,000 and 50,000 years or more, their children yielding the lowest prevalence of 0.27%. By the early thirteenth century, some Mongolian tribes migrated from Mongolia to the Tibetan plateau over about 700 years and their children presented a moderate prevalence of 0.85%. The Kazakhi herdsmen from Balikul (550 m) have migrated to Tibet for about 50 years with a nomadic life. The Han are typical lowland population who have migrated to high altitude in Tibet only within the last 50 years [25, 40, 42]. Both Kazakhi and Han children have a high prevalence of 2.95% and 2.07%, respectively, almost ten times higher than the Tibetan children. Among all populations at high altitude, those living there the longest have the lowest prevalence of PHAHD, whereas those living there the shortest have the highest prevalence. Thus, it appears that prevalence of PHAHD is a function of the length of time of residence at high altitude of one's ethnic ancestry. This may be explained by genetic differences.

Low Birth Weight Increases PHAHD

A recent study among 42 Han and 36 Tibetan infants was performed in the Goluok area at an altitude of 3750 m. All Han mothers studied had resided in Goluok for more than two years at the time of their delivery, Tibetan

TABLE 1. Prevalence of pediatric high altitude heart disease among four pediatric ethnic populations

	Infants and children			
Ethnic Group	Surveyed (n) Subjects (n)	Patients (%)	Prevalence	The length of time of altitude residence (yr)
Han (Chinese)	4773	99	2.06	Not more than 50
Kazakh	508	15	2.95	About 50
Mongolian	828	7	0.85	About 700
Tibetan	2227	6	0.27	25000–50000

Statistical differences: Han vs. Kazakh $P>0.05$; Han vs. Mongolian $P<0.O5$; Han vs. Tibetan $P<0.01$; Kazakh vs. Mongolian $P<0.01$; Kazakh vs. Tibetan $P<0.01$; Mongolian vs. Tibetan $P<0.05$.

mothers were living in their native place. After birth, the mean birth weight (± SD) in Han and Tibetan newborns was 3014±42 g and 3448±48g, respectively (P<0.05). The percentages of low birth weight (LBW, <2500gm) in Han and Tibetan newborns were 19% (n=8) and 3% (n=1), respectively (P<0.05). During the 2-year follow-up periods, the incidence of ISMS was 12% (n=5, three were LBW) in Han infants but none in Tibetan infants. In the Han group, three LBW infants died at two years, two due to congestive cardiac failure and one had a lung infectious cause. No deaths occurred in Tibetan babies (Xue and Wu, unpublished observations).

These observations point out an increased incidence of PHAHD or ISMS contributed to altitude–associated LBW. Oxygenation appears to be a determinant of infant birth weight. As compared to Han pregnant women, Tibetan mothers during pregnancy have a higher ventilation and increased acute hypoxic ventilatory responsiveness, greater distribution of common iliac blood flow to the uterine artery and higher arterial oxygen saturation, perhaps helping to provide a better fetal oxygen supply and protection from interuterine growth restriction (IUGR) and thus obtaining heavier birth weights in infants [26, 27]. Also Han infants compared to Tibetan babies presented a lower arterial oxygen saturation, with a greater vulnerability to incomplete or disrupted cardiopulmonary transition, which resulted in severe pulmonary hypertension [28, 30]. Clearly, these are important factors for the occurrence of PHAHD in Han infants.

Clinical Features

As a consequence of the rich accumulation of epidemiological and clinical data, we have strong evidence that in Tibet, high altitude heart disease (HAHD) has no age limit and cases have been described in infants, children and adolescents as well as adults [21, 38, 40, 41, 44, 45], with the highest incidence occurring in infants (89.5–92.0% of all cases). Most infants and children affected by this illness were of Han origin (over 97 percent were of lowland Han ancestry) [21, 23]. PHAHD or ISMS developed rarely in Tibetan infants. There are three conditions in the occurrence of PHAHD or ISMS among children in Tibet. 1). Infants born at high altitude and remaining there since birth (accounting for 57% in Tibet and 73.7% in Qinghai); 2). Infants born at low altitude and later brought up to high altitude (36% in Tibet and 16.1% in Qinghai); and 3). Children with parents who migrated from an intermediate altitude to a higher altitude (7% in Tibet and 10.2% in Qinghai) [23,39]. PHAHD or ISMS is rarely experienced below 3000 m but becomes increasingly common over 3500 m.

Early symptoms were restlessness, nocturnal crying, irritability, sleeplessness, anorexia, coughing, and hoarseness. Not long afterwards, they presented depression, tachycardia, tachypnoea, marked cyanosis, oliguria, peripheral and facial edema, live enlargement, rales in the lung and fever. The neck veins were distended. On auscultation an accentuated or splitting second pulmonary sound was heard, a soft pulmonic systolic or diastolic murmur; at the apex of the heart, a low-pitched, soft, blowing systolic murmur was heard.

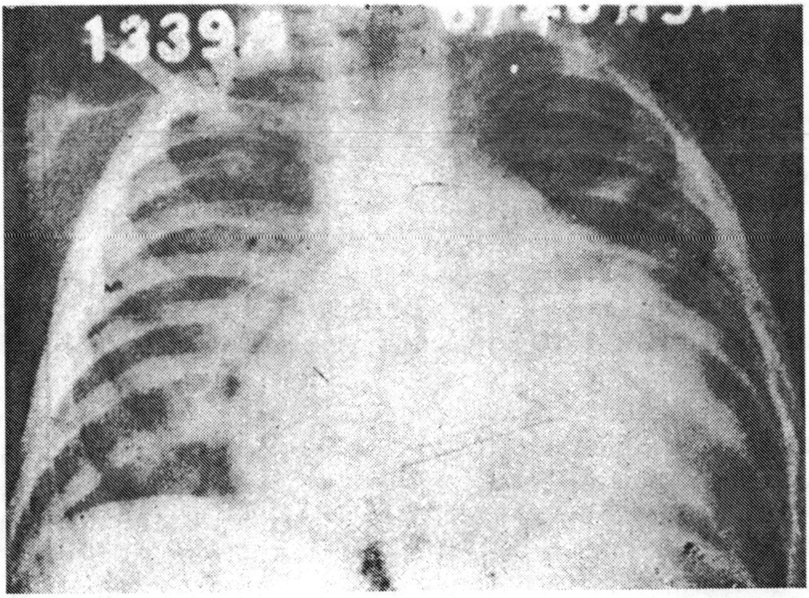

Figure 1a. Chest radiography of a Han male infant aged 6 months with PHAHD proven at necropsy. Showing pronounced cardiomegaly as a spherical heart, with the pulmonary artery enlarged.

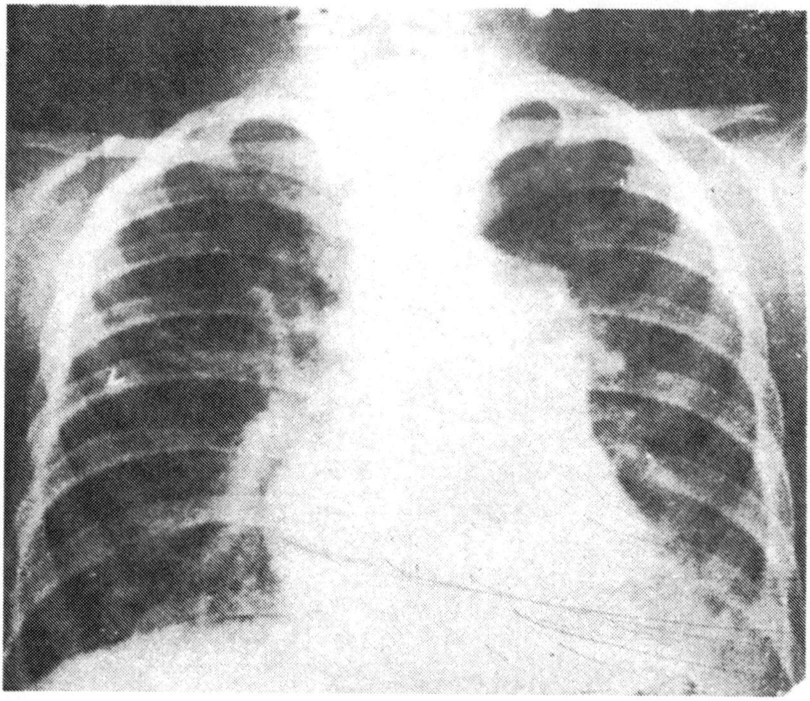

Figure 1b. Chest X-ray of a Han male child aged 4 who had been born and lived at 3400 m and presented with cough, dyspnoea, cyanosis and peripheral edema for one year. Chest X-ray reveals significant prominence of the pulmonary artery segment and prominent dilatation in the descending portion of the right pulmonary artery, with right heart enlargement.

Chest X-ray findings included prominence of the pulmonary artery or of the pulmonary conus, right ventricular hypertrophy and dilatation. In babies, always showing a spherical cardiac silhouette (Fig. 1a), enlargement of the pulmonary hilum and coarsening of the pulmonary line. In older children, X-rays reveal prominent dilatation in the descending portion of the right pulmonary artery (Figure 1 b). ECG showed a right axis deviation, clockwise rotation, right ventricular hypertrophy, right bundle branch block and /or P pulmonale (Figure 2).

Echocardiography reveals enlargement and hypertrophy of the right ventricle and normal sized left-ventricle with normal ejection fraction. Elevated right ventricular systolic pressure were estimated by measurements of the systolic regurgitated tricuspid flow velocity and an estimate of right atrial pressure.

Only a few cases (about 6–10%) had a moderate erythrocytosis, in the others their hemoglobin concentrations and hematocrit values were not increased. Conversely, about a fourth presented various degrees of anemia. The arterial oxygen saturation in cases with PHAHD is even lower than that found in normal infants at the same altitude.

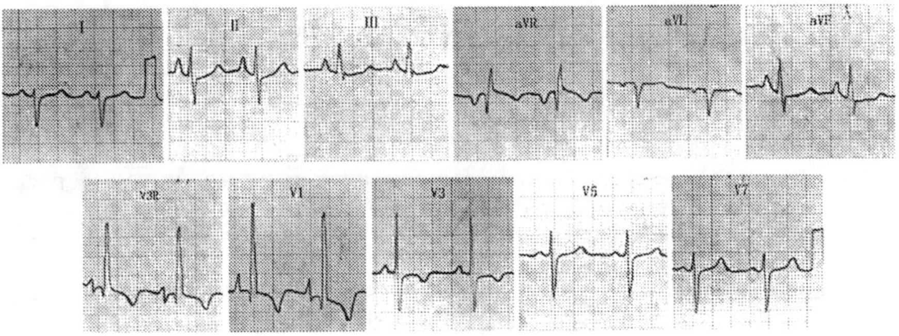

Figure 2. ECG in a Han female young child aged 14 months with PHAHD. It shows a sinus rhythm, right axis deviation, prominently peaked P-wave in lead V3R, V1 and V3. Decreased RS-T segment in Lead II, III, aVF. The R wave in the right precordial leads are of greater magnitude than the S wave and a deepened S-wave in lead V5 and V7 could be indicative of pronounced right ventricular hypertrophy with significant clockwise motion.

Hemodynamic Studies

Only a few hemodynamic studies of PHAHD or ISMS have been performed at high altitude during hospital admission. Cardiac catheterizations were performed in 15 patients. One in La Oroya (3730 m), Peru, and a repeat catheterization was performed at sea level [12]; seven cases were done in Leadville (3100 m), CO [8,17]; and eight patients developed PHAHD at altitudes between 3008m and 4280 m, while catheterizations were performed in Xining (2261 m), Qinghai, and compared with the results of 12 normal infants living at 2261 m [44]. The results are summarized in Table 2.

Pulmonary hypertension was presented in all, the mean pulmonary artery pressure (MPAP) ranging from 33±2 mmHg to 47±24 mmHg, with a normal pulmonary wedge pressure (4–8 mmHg). Pulmonary vascular resistances were increased to 686–1078 dynes/sec/cm. The administration of 100 percent oxygen rapidly lower PAP but normal values were not reached. Exercise and induced hypoxia resulted in a marked rise in pressure.

Diagnosis

Typical PHAHD is not difficult to diagnose. The infant presents a history of born or brought up to high altitude, the findings of a severe pulmonary hypertension (MPAP≥4 kPa or 30 mmHg, via noninvasive echo-Doppler, or catheterization), right ventricular hypertrophy and congestive heart failure support the diagnosis of PHAHD. However, PHAHD may be most readily confused with primary pulmonary hypertension (PPH) and congenital heart disease at high altitude.

TABLE 2. Cardiac catheterization data in infants or children with severe pulmonary hypertension in mountainous areas of the world

		Pulmonary artery pressure (mmHg)			
Altitude	Subject	Systolic	Diastolic	Mean	Reference
Leadville-Climax CO, 3360–3890m	Six white infants and Children, 6–17 months	70.8±27	30±26	47±24	(16)
Leadville, CO	One white girl, 15 yr	67	27	44	(7)
At 3100m		144	85	109*	
At sea level		33	8	17	
	After 11 months				
Qinghai-Tibet 3008–4280m	Eight Han infants	52.9±16	19.9±9	33.2±2	(41)
Xining, 2261m	12 Han healthy infants	22.5±2	7.8±2	13.4±3	
La Oroya, Peru	One American boy, 8 yr	144	104	117+	
At 3730m		76	36	57++	(11)
		56	33	47•	
At sea level		47	9	22	

*During supine cycle ergometer exercise, +: During his episode of reentry high altitude pulmonary edema, ++: After administration of oxygen for 15 minutes, •: After recovering from high altitude pulmonary edema at high altitude.

In our experience, PPH rarely occurs in Tibetan natives on the Tibetan plateau. Also, the disease appears to be rare among the Quechua Indians in the Andes [31]. But there is no clear evidence that PPH is more frequent in sojourners at high altitude compared with sea level. However, O'Neill et al. (1981) [31] reported a girl who had been born of British parents at an altitude of 3960 m in the Peruvian Andes for the first 15 months of life, subsequently developed pulmonary hypertension, which did not improve on return to sea level and proved fatal at the age of 19 years. The clinical and necropsy features were thus of PPH, based on plexogenic pulmonary arteriopathy proven on histological examination [31]. Pathologist Heath suggests that it is conceivable that the early exposure in life to hypobaric hypoxia and its effect on the pulmonary vasculature left a fateful legacy for subsequent years [11]. The relationship between PPH and altitude hypoxia needs to be explored in future studies.

Khoury and Hawes (1963)[17] reported several cases and used the term "PPH" in children at high altitude, which is a misunderstanding because their patients improved on moving to a lower altitude and did not exhibit the usual serious progressive course of PPH. In addition, the plexiform arteriopathy particularly associated with PPH was not described in one case who died suddenly. Therefore, the reported pediatric cases should be ISMS or PHAHD.

Although the diagnosis of PHAHD or ISMS can be made on the basis of the clinical, radiographic, electrocardiographic manifestations and measurement of pulmonary artery pressure, it is however, especially difficult to exclude congenital heart diseases, such as septal defect or patent ductus arteriosus. Congenital cardiovascular malformations are common at altitude and have been shown to have a higher pulmonary artery pressure than sea-level dwellers [5, 22]. Thus, a differential diagnosis based only on clinical data could not be completely excluded. Under such conditions, cardiac catheterization should be performed to establish the diagnosis and to demonstrate that a congenital abnormality is not present.

Pathology

Not as pathologically deficient as those in CMS, there are a series of pathological data obtained from post-mortems of PHAHD or ISMS [10, 11, 17, 20, 23, 35, 37, 39].

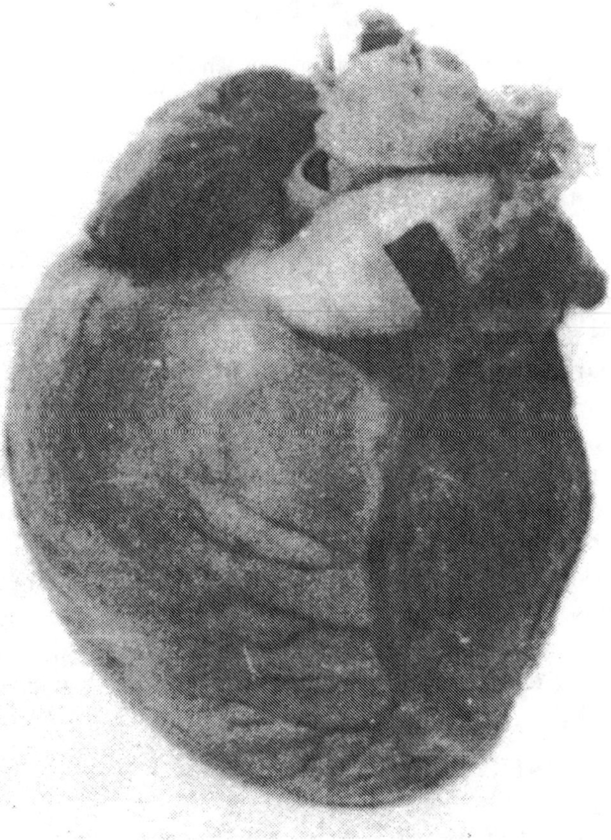

Figure 3a. Heart of a Han female infant of 5 months with PHAHD who died of congestive heart failure. There is massive right ventricular hypertrophy and dilatation of the pulmonary trunk.

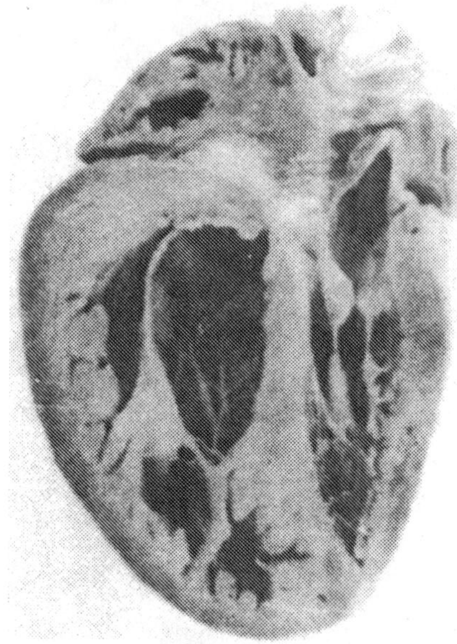

Figure 3b. Tangent plane of a heart from a Han female aged 14 months with PHAHD. Showing severe hypertrophy and dilatation of the right ventricle.

At autopsy, the right ventricle shows severe hypertrophy with pronounced dilatation of the pulmonary trunk (Figure 3, a, b). In some cases, mild hypertrophy of the left ventricle also exists. The ratio of right ventricular weight to left ventricular weight varied between 80 percent and 160 percent (normal values are 20-30 percent with a mean of 24 percent). Histologic studies revealed marked medial hypertrophy of the pulmonary arteries (Figure 4), arterioles and venules. Fresh and partially organized thrombi were found in the small pulmonary arteries (Figure 5) or venules. Peripheral edema, ascites and congestion of the liver confirmed the presence of right heart failure. The above pathological features suggest that ISMS is a pulmonary vascular disease.

We noted that at high altitude the muscularity of some Han infant pulmonary arteries fails to regress as it does at sea level [39]. However, in normal Tibetan infants over the age 4 months and up to the age of 2 years, the small pulmonary arteries are presented with thin walls [10, 35, 46]. Disruption of the normal process of cardiopulmonary transition can result in SHAPH [30].

The Nature of PHAHD

The syndrome of PHAHD fully represents the biological general character of the pulmonary circulatory adaptation at high altitude.

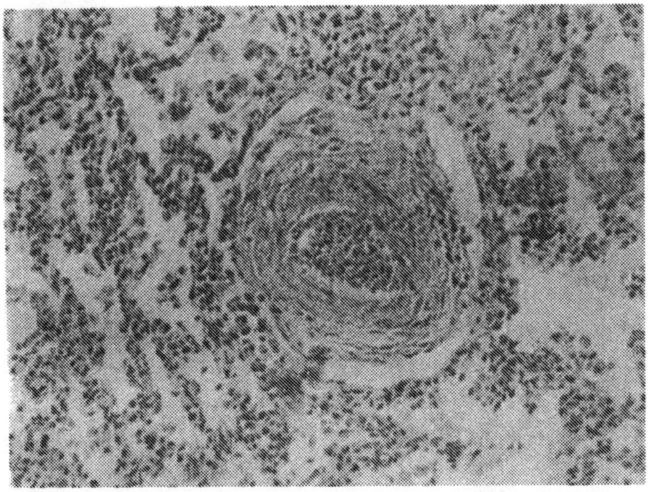

Figure 4. Transverse section of a muscular pulmonary artery from a Han male infant aged 4 months with ISMS and severe pulmonary hypertension. There is a very thick muscular media sandwich between the internal and external elastic laminae (HE× 100) (After Li and Jiao, 1983).

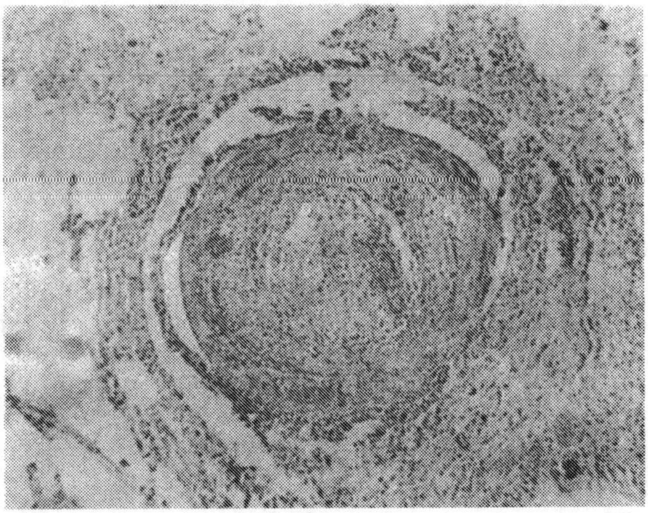

Figure 5. Transverse section of a small muscular pulmonary artery from a Han male infant with PHAHD aged 5 months. There is hypertrophy of the media and the lumen is almost totally occluded by a recent pulmonary partially organized thrombus. (HE×100). (After Wu and Lin, 1978).

In human beings, some Han infants are more susceptible to hypobaric hypoxia at high altitude, and present a syndrome of PHAHD or ISMS characterized by severe pulmonary hypertension, whereas Tibetans represented a blunted hypoxic pulmonary vasoconstrictor response [9] with the thin-walled pulmonary arteries in young children [34, 43, 46] and almost always protect against PHAHD.

Among sea-level animals, cattle are most susceptible to altitude hypoxia, it is related that cattle have a marked medial hypertrophy of the small pulmonary arteries [36]. Especially in calves, if brought up to high mountains, the altitude hypoxia renders them vulnerable to congestive cardiac failure and thus, edema occurs between the forelegs and the neck, the brisket of commerce and therefore known as “Brisket disease”.

Newborn calves exposed to a simulated 4300 m altitude in a chamber for 14 days induced a medial and adventitial thickening of the pulmonary arteries and distal muscularization [34] and developed severe pulmonary hypertension and right heart failure [18]. It is the animal model of ISMS in humans, in other words, PHAHD or ISMS is the human model of Brisket disease in cattle [3,38], actually, we can call this syndrome “human Brisket disease”.

In contrast, the yak has successfully adapted to chronically hypoxic altitude conditions by both largely eliminating the hypoxic pulmonary vasoconstrictor response [1] and thin-walled pulmonary vessels [6] and do not develop brisket disease.

PHAHD or ISMS and Brisket disease both affected the young (infants vs. calves) with a common pathogenetic basis, they are two similar forms of mammals’ poor adjustment to high altitude.

In recent years, there has been a renewed theoretical interest in the relation between ISMS and chronic mountain sickness (CMS) or Monge’s disease. The syndrome of ISMS or PHAHD is distinguished from CMS in that CMS affects adults, usually in middle age, after prolonged exposure to high altitude. It is characterized by excessive polycythemia, severe hypoxemia and alveolar hypoventilation, with moderate pulmonary hypertension and rare cardiac failure. Clearly, there are two varieties of subacute or chronic mountain sickness, one is a respiratory form – CMS, the other is a cardiovascular variety – PHAHD or ISMS.

Treatment and Prevention

PHAHD is a serious illness with a high rate of mortality in infants in Tibet. The mortality rate in the 50s of the 20th century was as high as 50%. In the 60s it was 15–23%, in the 70s it was 4.2–15% [22, 39]. In fact, the mortality rate from ISMS has declined nearly 40% over the last 50 years, due to strengthening prevention among infants. At present, however, with the mortality rate id usually at about 5% of patients with ISMS in Qinghai-Tibet, this serious disease cannot be forgotten.

Remaining at altitude and local therapy led to disastrous results, because the failing heart simply does not respond to treatment at altitude. Administration of oxygen and treatment with cardiotonics, diuretics, corticoids and antibiotics might buy time and provide temporary relief, but there is no alternative to rapid descent.

To avoid the disease, it is common practice for Han mothers to descend to their lowland homes to give birth and then entrust their child to the care of elderly relatives, because the Han mother must return to altitude and work. The child is then not brought to high altitude until is it over a year old or more. If some Han mothers must to give birth at high altitude for economic or personal reasons, the newborns should be under the care of the hospital. Establishing an oxygen enrichment room for infants is extremely necessary in Tibet. Nutritional supplements such as carbohydrates, proteins, iron and vitamins are necessary both for pregnant women and for infants. Prevention of respiratory infections is more important in children at high altitude.

Acknowledgments

This work was founded by Grants of 973 Program, No. 2006CB 504100, CB 708514 and supported in part by Grant LS-CNNSF 30393130, PRC.

References

1. Anand IS, Harris E, Ferrari R, Pearce P, Harris P (1986) Pulmonary hemodynamics of the yak, cattle, and cross breeds at high altitude. Thorax 42:696–700
2. Anand IS, Chandrashekhar Y (1992) Subacute mountain sickness syndrome: role of pulmonary hypertension. In: Sutton, JR, Coates G, Houston CS (eds) Hypoxia and Mountain Sickness, edited by advances in the Biosciences Vol. 84, Pergamon Press, Oxford, pp 241–251
3. Anand IS, Wu TY (2004) Syndromes of subacute mountain sickness. High Alt. Med. Biol. 5:156–170
4. Aparicio O, Antezana G (1992) Enfermedades cardio-vasculares en la altura. Acta Andina 1:54–55
5. Blount S Jr (1977) Comparison of patients with ventricular septal defect at high altitude and sea level. Circulation 56: Suppl. 1:79–82
6. Durmowicz AG, Hofmeister S, Kadyraliev TK, Adashev AA, Stenmark KR (1993) Functional and structural adaptation of the yak pulmonary circulation to residence at high altitude. J. Appl. Physiol. 74:2276–2285
7. Ge RL, Gaowa H, Jin GE, Yang YZ (2003) High-altitude heart disease in Qinghai-Tibet. In: Viscor G, Richar A, and Leal C (eds) Health & Height. Publicacions: Universitat de Barcelona, pp 197–204
8. Grover R, Vogel J, Voigt G, Blount SJr (1966) Reversal of high altitude pulmonary hypertension. Am. J.Cardiol. 18:928–932

9. Groves BM, Droma J, Sutton JR, McCullogh RG, McCullogh RE, Zhuang J, Rapmand G, Sun S, Janes C, Moore LG (1993) Minimal hypoxic pulmonary hypertension in normal Tibetans at 3658 m. J. Appl. Physiol. 74:312–318
10. Heath D, Harris PO, Sui GJ, Liu YH, Gosney J, Harris E, Anand IS (1989) Pulmonary blood vessels and endocrine cells in subacute infantile mountain sickness. Respir. Med. 83:77–85
11. Heath D, Williams DR (1995) High-Altitude Medicine and Pathology. Fourth Edn, Oxford University Press, Oxford, pp 213–221
12. Hultgren H, Lopez C, Lundberg E, Miller H (1964) Physiologic studies of pulmonary edema at high altitude. Circulation 29:393–408
13. Hultgren H (1964) High Altitude Medicine. Hultgren Publications, Stanford, California, USA, pp 406–412
14. Hurtado Gomez L, Calderon RG (1985) Hipoxia de altura en la insuficiencia cardiaca del lactante. Bolet. Soc. Boliv. Pediatr. IX. 11–23
15. Jiang MX (1977) [High-altitude heart disease]. J.Tib.Med. 2:160–168
16. Jones TK, Wiggins JW, Wolfe RR (1982) Symptomatic high altitude pulmonary hypertension of infancy. Circulation 66 (Suppl II): 48
17. Khoury GH, Hawes CR (1963) Primary pulmonary hypertension in children living at high altitude. J. Pediatr. 62:177–185
18. Lemler MS, Bies RD, Frid MG, Sastravaha A, Zisman LS, Bohlmeyer T, Gerdes AM, Reeves JT, Stenmark KR (2000) Myocyte cytoskeletal disorganization and right heart failure in hypoxia-induced neonatal pulmonary hypertension. Am. J. Physiol. Heart Circ. Physiol. 279:H1365–1376
19. Leòn-Velarde F, Maggiorini M, Reeves JT, Adashev A, Asmus I, Bernardi L, Ge RL, Hackett P, kobayashi T, Moore LG, Penaloza D, Richalet J-P, roach R, Wu TY, Vargas E, Zubieta-Castillo G, Zubieta-Calleja G (2005). Consensus statement on chronic and subacute high altitude diseases. High Alt. Med. Biol. 6:147–157
20. Li JB, Wang IY, Jiao HG (1966) [A pathologic observation of infantile altitude illness]. Chin J. Pathol. 10:98–99
21. Lin CP, Wu TY (1974) Clinical analysis of 286 cases of pediatric high altitude heart disease. Natl. Med. J. China (English supplement to No.6) 54:353–356
22. Miao CY, Zuberbuhler JS, Zuberbuhler JR (1988) Prevalence of congenital cardiac anomalies at high altitude. J. Am. Coll. Cardiol. 12:224–228
23. Mo LF, Jiang MX, Li JB, Jiao HG (1983) [Pediatric high altitude heart disease]. In: The People's Hospital of Tibetan Autonomous Region (ed) High Altitude Medicine. Lhasa, Tibetan People's Publisher, pp 251–259
24. Monge MC (1948) Acclimatization in the Andes: Historical confirmation of "Climatic Aggression" in the development of Andean man. Baltimore: Johns Hopkins Press
25. Moore LG, Curran-Everett L, Droma T, Groves BM, McCullough RE, McCullough RG, Sun S, Sutton JR, Zamudio S, Zhuang JG (1992) Are Tibetans better adapted ? Int. J. Sports. Med. 13 Suppl 1:S86–S88
26. Moore LG, Zamudio S, Zhuang J, Sun S, and Droma T (2001) Oxygen transport in Tibetan women during pregnancy at 3658 m Am. J. Phys. Anthropol. 114:42–53
27. Moore LG, young D, McCullough RE, Droma T, Zamudio S (2001) Tibetan protection from intrauterine growth restriction (IUGR) and reproductive loss at high altitude. Am. J. Human. Biol. 13:635–644
28. Niermeyer S,Yang P, Shanmina D, Zhuang J, Moore LG(1995) Arterial oxygen saturation in Tibetan and Han infants born in Lhasa, Tibet. N. Engl. J. Med. 333:1248–1252
29. Niermeyer S, Andrade P, Vargas E, and Moore LG (2002) Prolonged postnatal cardiopulmonary transition at 3700–4000 m. (Abst.). High Alt. Med. Biol. 3:439
30. Niermeyer S (2003) Cardiopulmonary transition in the high altitude infant. High. Alt. Med. Biol. 4:225–239
31. O'Neill D, Morton R, Kennedy JA (1981) Progressive primary pulmonary hypertension in a patient born at high altitude. Brit. Heart J. 45:725–728

32. Penaloza D, Ruiz L, Arias-Stella J, Scavino Y, Hurtado A (1977) Mal de Montana cronico: formas vascular y respiratoria. En: Jornadas Cientificas (XV Aniversario) 1961–1978. Lima: Universided Peruana Cayeytano Heredia, pp 52
33. Pollard A, Niermeyer S, et al (2002) Children at high altitude: An International Consensus Statement by an Ad Hoc Committee of the International Society for Mountain Medicine, March 12, 2001. High Alt. Med. Biol. 2:389–403
34. Stenmark KR, Fasules J, Hyde DM, Voelkel NF, Henson J, Tucker A, Wilson H, Reeves JT (1987) Severe pulmonary hypertension and arterial adventitial changes in newborn calves at 4300 m. J. Appl. Physiol. 62:821–830
35. Sui GJ, Liu YH, Cheng XS, Anand IS, Harris E, Harris P, Heath D (1988) Subacute infantile mountain sickness. J. Pathol. 155:161–170
36. Tucker A, Rhodes J (2001) Role of vascular smooth muscle in the development of high altitude pulmonary hypertension: an interspecies evaluation. High Alt. Med. Biol. 2:173–189
37. Wu DC, and Liu YR (1955) [Pediatric high altitude heart disease]. Chin. J. Pediatr. 6:348–350
38. Wu TY, Li CP, Wang ZW (1965) [Adult high altitude heart disease, an analysis of 22 cases]. Chin. intern. Med. 13:700–702
39. Wu TY, and Lin CP (1978) [High altitude heart disease: an observation in Tibet]. Chin. J. Cardiovasc. Dis. 6:186–190
40. Wu TY, Ge RL, Die TF, Ren XM, Liu H, Wang X.Z (1983) An investigation of high altitude heart disease (with English Abst.). Natl. Med. J. China 63:90–92
41. Wu TY, Die TF, Huo KS, Zang B, Jing YS, Liu PF (1987) An epidemiological study on high altitude disease at Qinghai-Tibetan plateau (with English Abst.). Chin. J. Epidemiol. 8:65–69
42. Wu TY (2000) [Tibetan populations at high altitude] Chin. J. High Alt. Med. 10:56–64
43. Wu TY (1994) Children on the Tibetan plateau. Newsletter of the International Society for Mountain Medicine. 4:5–7
44. Wu TY, Miao CY (2002) High altitude heart disease in children in Tibet. High Alt. Med. Biol. 3:323–325
45. Wu TY, Miao CY, Wang XQ (2003) High altitude heart disease in children in Tibet. In: Viscor G, Richat A, Leal C, (eds) Healthy & Height. Publicacions: Universitat de Barcelona, pp291–294
46. Wu TY, Kayser B (2006) High altitude adaptation in Tibetans. High Alt. Med. Biol. 7:193–208
47. Zhou HS, Mo If, Wang DQ (1964) [Clinical observations of 238 cases of pediatric high altitude heart disease]. Chin. J. Pediatr. 13:364–386

CHAPTER 18

CLINICAL AND FUNCTIONAL FEATURES OF CHRONIC OBSTRUCTIVE PULMONARY DISEASE IN THE HIGHLANDERS OF KYRGYZSTAN

T.M. SOORONBAEV, S.B. SHABYKEEVA, A.K. MIRZAACHMATOVA, G.K. KADYRALIEV, M.M. MIRRAKHIMOV

National Centre for Cardiology and Internal Medicine, Bishkek, Kyrgyzstan

Abstract: A 3-year long prospective study was carried out with the aim to investigate clinical and functional features of COPD in 46 patients with severe stable COPD living at high altitude in Kyrgyzstan (At-Bashi and Aksai valleys, 2,400 to 3,600 meters above sea level). The control group included 34 patients with severe stable COPD who lived at low altitude (Chui valley, Bishkek, 760 meters above sea level). The COPD patients were randomized by sex, age, body mass index (BMI) and FEV1 values. We found a difference between the clinical characteristics and functional status of COPD in patients living at high and low altitudes. Highlanders with COPD showed a greater degree of breathlessness, significant decline of life quality and physical performance. At the same time, background values of FEV1 were similar in mountain and valley inhabitants. It is important to note that after 3 years, COPD symptoms in patients from high altitude areas became more progressive compared with patients from low altitude areas. This could be caused by a great increase of bronchial obstruction and a significant alteration of oxygen saturation (SaO2) in highlanders with COPD.

Keywords: chronic obstructive pulmonary disease, lung function, quality of life, high altitude

Chronic obstructive pulmonary disease (COPD) is one of the greatest problems of modern medicine because of its broad spread, frequent deterioration of working ability and significant influence on the death rate [11, 12, 20]. COPD is the 4th most prevalent cause of death in the world [12, 18]. It is reported that COPD caused 2.74 million deaths in 2000 and further expansion of the morbidity and mortality from COPD is expected in the future.

A. Aldashev and R. Naeije (eds.), Problems of High Altitude Medicine and Biology, 249–257.

The WHO has reported that the COPD will become the fifth most prevalent disease worldwide by 2020 [18].

COPD is a real problem in healthcare in the mountainous regions of the world [5, 22]. Some investigations have revealed a negative influence of short stays at low altitudes (lower than 2,500 meters above sea level) on COPD [6, 9, 13, 19].

For mountainous Kyrgyzstan, COPD is a very real problem in view of the fact that half of the territory is situated at 3,000 meters above sea level or higher and the main part of the population lives in extreme conditions of the mountains, which may cause pulmonary diseases and sometimes cause deterioration in them [17, 23].

AIM: to research the clinical and functional features of chronic obstructive pulmonary disease in people living in high altitude areas of Kyrgyzstan in a 3-year prospective study.

Patients and Methods

PATIENTS

The research was carried out on 46 patients (men) aged 56.2 ± 5.6, with severe stable COPD who permanently resided in high-altitude areas (At-Bashi and Aksai valleys, 2,400 to 3,600 meters above sea level). The control group included 34 patients (men) aged 50.6 ± 6.8, with severe stable COPD, permanently residing in low-altitude areas (Chui valley, Bishkek, 760 meters above sea level). The disease was diagnosed and its severity was determined by the criteria of the Global Initiative for COPD [11], where besides the clinical symptoms, the main criterion is the limitation of reversibility of bronchial obstruction during bronchodilator testing with a short-acting B2-agonist.

STUDY DESIGN

COPD patients were randomized by sex, age, spirometric indicators, body mass index (BMI) and groups of high and low-altitude mountaineers did not differ from each other. The studies were carried out during the same season. In the established groups of patients the studies were repeated after 3 years in the same way and under the same conditions for a prospective analysis.

METHODS

For the quantitative estimation of the severity of breathlessness and its influence on daily activities, we used the 5-point Medical Research Council (MRC) Dispnea Scale [24], which was recommended for COPD [11] where the breathlessness is categorized as follows: grade 1, "I only get breathless with strenuous exercise"; grade 2, "I get short of breath when hurrying on the level or up a slight hill"; grade 3, "I walk slower than people of the same age on the level because of breathlessness or have to stop for breath when walking at my own pace on the level"; grade 4, "I stop for breath after walking 100 yards or after a few minutes on the level"; grade 5, " I am too breathless to leave the house".

The quality of life of COPD patients was estimated with the help of the Russian version of the St George's Respiratory Questionnaire (SGRQ) [14], which is based on appraisal of the three following criteria: symptoms (ailing because of respiratory symptoms); activity (low physical activity and limited agility because of breathlessness); influence (psychosocial consequences of the disease). We studied the value of certain life quality criteria by using the total points according to the SGRQ, which characterized the overall impact of the disease on fitness status.

The 6-minute walk test was carried out by the standard protocol [8]. Patients were asked to walk as far as possible in 6 minutes. Before and at the end of the test the heart rate, breath rate and SaO2 were measured. The distance in meters walked during 6 minutes (6MWD) was measured to estimate physical activity.

The lung function was tested by portable spirometer "Spiro-Pro" (Jager, Germany), which could automatically gather the data and compare them with normal values in accordance with the BTPS system. The spirometric study was carried out by the standard method recommended by the American Thoracic Society [1]. The following indicators were estimated: forced vital capacity (FVC), forced expiratory volume in one second (FEV1) and FEV1/FVC. Indicators were estimated by comparing them with normal values, taking into consideration the sex, age and height of the tested person. When comparing the results of the repeated tests, an appraisal of ventilation disorders and process dynamics was held, with consideration of degrees of deviation over certain indicators.

The test of oxygen saturation of arterial blood (SaO2) was performed on calmly sitting patients. A skin electrode was fixed to the tip of the forefinger. As is well known, heating the skin produces a diffusion of carbon dioxide and oxygen into the electrodes through the skin. The measurement was fully automated.

STATISTICS

The data were processed using standard statistical software. The reliability of the differences was calculated through the application of non-parametric criteria χ^2 and Z as well as parametric Student t-criterion with Bonferroni correction. The difference was considered reliable at $p<0.05$.

Results

One of the best known COPD factors is smoking [2]. The main part of the observed COPD patients residing at both high and low altitudes, were heavy smokers. The percentage of COPD patients who had given up smoking or had not smoked was significantly smaller in both groups (Figure 1).

The basic data in the compared groups of COPD patients living in high and low areas are shown in Table 1. It is well known that breathlessness is the main reason for limited physical activity of COPD patients [16]. Our study has shown that breathlessness was more clearly expressed in COPD patients living at high altitude. The quantitative estimation by the MRC Scale showed 3.4 ± 0.3 in mountaineers and not more than 2.4 ± 0.5 in patients from low altitude regions. Breathlessness is an important factor that impacts the quality of life of COPD patients. The quality of life is an integral indicator, which demonstrates human adaptability to the disease and a capability for routine activities in accordance with the socioeconomic status of subject [15]. The life quality is estimated by standard questionnaires, where the St George's Respiratory Questionnaire (SGRQ) is one specially used for COPD patients. The study of the quality of life by the SGRQ tool has proved that COPD patients from high altitude areas are prone to underestimating their own health condition, which resulted in a clinically significant (>4 points) increase of values on the scales of the questionnaire. It becomes most evident during the analysis of total points. Thus, among COPD patients from high altitude, the average values reached 72.6 ± 6.3 by the SGRQ scale, while in the low altitude patients group, the changes were not so high. The investigation of the breathlessness and the quality of life in COPD patients is closely related with appraisal of the functional status – the physical performance. Some studies have displayed a direct relation between the breathlessness

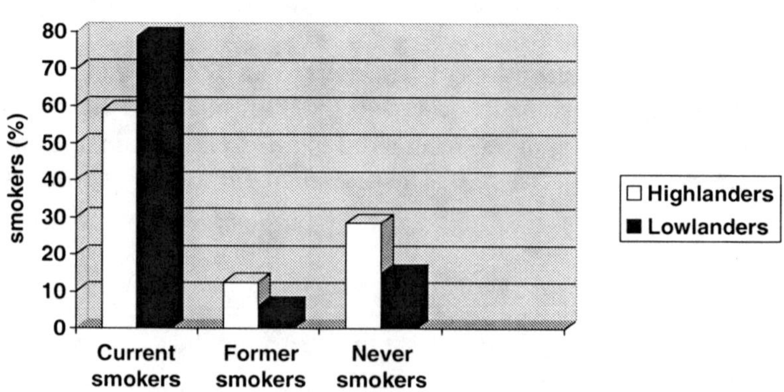

Figure 1. Quantity of smokers highlanders and lowlanders with COPD (men).

TABLE 1. Clinical and functional parameters of severe COPD in highlanders and lowlanders

Parameters	Highlanders (n=46)	Lowlanders (n=34)
Dispnea, MRC (balls)	3,4 ± 0,3	2,4 ± 0,5[1]
Quality of life, SGRQ Total Score	72,6 ± 6,3	57,8 ± 5,8[1]
Six-min.walk test (6MWD,m)	108,2 ± 19,0	139,8 ± 13,6[1]
FEV1 (L)	1,68 ± 0,6	1,7 ± 0,4
FVC (L)	1,48 ± 0,5	1,54 ± 0,6
SaO2 (%)	71,9 ± 5,6	78,4 ± 4,8

[1]p<0,05 vs compared groups
MRS: Medical Research Council Dispnea Scale; SGRQ: St George's Respiratory Questionnaire Scores; FEV1: forced expiratory volume in one second;
FVC: forced vital capacity; SaO2: oxygen saturation

intensity, the life quality and the physical performance of COPD patients [4]. In practice, the 6-minute walk test has become the most popular and provides the 6-minute walking distance as the main criterion of physical activity. We have discovered that COPD patients from high altitude areas walk significantly shorter distances during 6 minutes than lowlanders – 108.2 ± 19.0 meters and 139.8 ± 9.6 meters, respectively.

The background spirometric research has shown that FEV1 values in both groups depended on the degree of severity of COPD, but did not differ from each other. It is important that the reliable values for SaO2 were lower (71.9 ± 5.6%) in the highlanders group than in patients from low mountain areas (78.4 ± 4.8%) at comparable FEV1 values.

To analyze the course of the disease and its progressive rate, we monitored the observed indicators after 3 years. The results showed the steady progress of COPD in both groups of patients (Table 2) and the changes were seen more clearly in COPD patients from high mountain regions. The estimation of the breathlessness intensity degree by the MRC scale has revealed a significant increase of breathlessness in patients from high mountain areas, producing a strong decline of physical activity in this group of patients: the 6-minute walking distance value decreased to 68.9 ± 8.6 meters and to 98.9 ± 18.4 meters in the group of patients from low mountain areas. It is especially important to note the drastically increased negative impact of the disease on the quality of life of COPD patients (Figure 2), which is more evident for patients from high mountain areas. Moreover, the alteration of FEV1 after 3 years is important, as FEV1 represents the "golden standard" for appraising the severity of COPD because it characterizes the degree of bronchial obstruction. There is no doubt that the progressive course of the disease that was revealed by the prospective 3-year long study, is related with

TABLE 2. Clinical and functional parameters of severe COPD in highlanders and lowlanders (prospective 3-year study)

Parameters	Highlanders (n=26)	Lowlanders (n=24)
Dispnea, MRC (balls)		
Baseline	3,4±0,3	2,4±0,5[1]
After 3 years	3,9±0,2[2]	2,8±0,3
Quality of life, SGRQ		
Total Score Baseline	72,6±6,3	57,8±5,8[1]
After 3 years	97,9±5,2[3]	69,9±4,6[2]
Six-min.walk test (6MWD,m)		
Baseline	108,2±19,0	139,8±13,6[1]
After 3 years	68,9±8,6[3]	98,9±18,4[2]
FEV1 (L)		
Baseline	1,68±0,3	1,7±0,3
After 3 years	1,36±0,2[2]	1,49±0,3[2]
SaO2 (%)		
Baseline	71,9±5,6	78,4±6,8
After 3 years	58,9±9,6[3]	69,6±9,8

[1]p<0,05 vs compared groups; [2] p<0,05 vs into groups; [3] p<0,001 vs into groups
MRS: Medical Research Council Dispnea Scale; SGRQ: St George's Respiratory Questionnaire Scores; FEV1: forced expiratory volume in one second;
SaO2: oxygen saturation

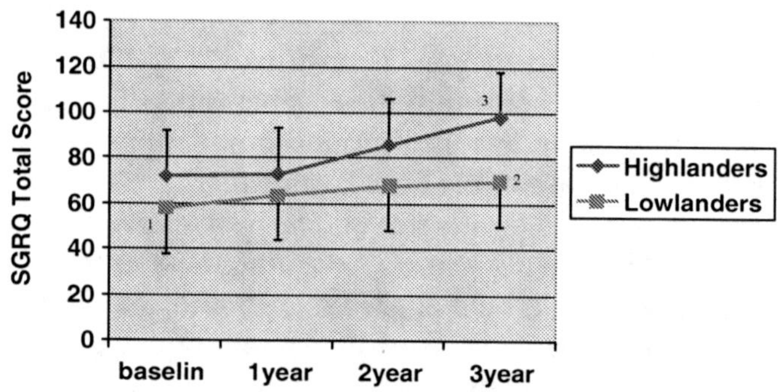

Figure 2. Life quality in highlanders and lowlanders with severe COPD (prospective 3-year study).
[1]p<0.05 vs in compared groups; [2] p<0,05 vs into groups ; [3] p<0.001 vs into groups
SGRQ: St George's Respiratory Questionnaire Scores

progressive bronchial obstruction in patients from both groups. Yet, despite relatively similar starting indicators, the FEV1 averages in patients from high mountain areas became lower 3 years later and equal to 1.36±0.21 versus 1.49±0.31 in patients from low mountain areas. SaO2 values changed in a similar trend.

Discussion

The study has revealed differences in clinical displays and functional status of COPD in patients from high and low mountain areas, while FEV1 values and disease dynamics were relatively similar. Also, it is important to note that with time, the breathlessness intensity, the deterioration the quality of life, the decline of physical activity of patients from high mountain areas occur more intensively compared to patients from low mountain areas. It is caused by increasing bronchial obstruction and a significant decrease of SaO2, especially for patients from high mountain areas. Analysis of the more severe course and more rapid progress of COPD in patients from high mountain areas has revealed the following reasons, connected with high mountain conditions: hypoxia [3], cold [10] and dehydration [7]. In the last few years, research on the impact of pollutants inside homes on COPD development and progress has caused greater concern [21]. In this context, some features of the lifestyle and social conditions in the high mountain areas of Kyrgyzstan should be taken into consideration. When people build houses in high mountain areas, they pay special attention on the following tasks: raising the inside temperature, cutting down heat loss through convection and radiation and increasing relative humidity. That is why the houses of people in high mountain areas are erected as solid, free design structures with a small area for quite a large number of people in a family. In such situations, people normally cook and sleep in the same room, continuously exposing themselves to the impact of smoke. To warming up these houses, people from high mountain areas of Kyrgyzstan have traditionally used bioorganic material (compressed dung) during the season, which lasts for 9 to 10 months in the cold and severe climatic conditions of the high mountain areas. Sometimes furnaces do not function properly or the design of the premises does not allow for sufficient air ventilation. On the whole, these factors raise pollutants inside homes and the exposition of pollutants in the respiratory tract, which can also influence a more severe and progressive course of COPD in people in high mountain areas. The composition of pollutants inside homes in the mountains has not yet been completely researched.

Conclusion

Therefore, unlike patients from low mountain areas, COPD patients from high mountain areas have a more severe and more rapid progress of the disease, which requires the improvement of prophylactic and treatment intervention for this category of patients.

References

1. American Thoracic Society (1994). Standardization of spirometry. Am J Respir Crit Care Med 152: 1107–1136
2. Anthonisen NR, Connett JE, Kiley JP, Altose MD, Bailey WC, Buist AS, Conway Wa Jr, Enright PL, Kanner RE, O'Hara P, et al. (1994). Effects of smoking, intervention and the use of an inhaled anticholinergic bronchodilatator on the rate of decline of FEV1. The Lung Health Study. JAMA 272: 1497–1505
3. Bedu M, Giraldo H, Janicot H, Fellmann N, Coudert J. (1996). Interaction between cold and hypoxia on pulmonary circulation in COPD. Am J Respir Crit Care Med 153: 1242–1247
4. Bestall JC, Paul EA, Garrod R, Garnham R, Jones PW, Wedzicha JA. (1999). Usefulness of the Medical Research Council (MRS) dyspnoe scale as a measure of disability in patients with chronic obstructive pulmonary disease. Thorax 54: 581–586
5. Cogo AL, Fisher R, Shoene RB. (2004). Respiratory diseases and high altitude. High Alt Med Biol 5: 435–444
6. Dillard TA, Rajagopal KR, Slivka WA, Berg BW, Mehm WJ, Lawless NP. (1998). Lung function during moderate hypobaric hypoxia in normal subject and patients with chronic obstructive pulmonary disease. Aviat Space Environ Med 69: 979–985
7. Dossing M, Khan J, al-Rabiach F. (1994). Risk factors for chronic obstructive lung disease in Saudi Arabia. Respir Med 88: 519–522
8. Enricht PL, Sherill DL. (1998). Reference equations for the six-minute walk in healthy adults. Amer J Respir Crit Care Med 158: 1384–1387
9. Fisher R. (2002). Respiratory pathologies in the mountains – how high can people go? In: Health and Height. Proceedings of the 5th World Congress on Mountain Medicine and High Altitude Physiology, Barcelona: 75–79
10. Giesbrecht GG. (1996). The respiratory system in a cold enviroment. Aviat Space Environ Med 66: 890–902
11. Global Initiative for Chronic Obstructive Lung Disease (2001). NHLBI/WHO Workshop Report
12. Global Initiative for Chronic Obstructive Lung Disease (2003). NHLBI/WHO Workshop Report
13. Gracham WG, Houston CS. (1978). Short-term adaptacion to moderate altitude. Patients with chronic obstructive pulmonary disease. JAMA 240: 1491–1494
14. Jones PW, Quirk FH, Baveystock CM. (1992) The St.George's respiratory questionnaire. Respir Med 85: 25–31.
15. Karnofsky DF, Burchenal JH. (1947). The clinical evaluation of chemotherapeutic agents in cancer. In: Maclead C.M. (ed.) Evaluation of chemotherapeutic agents. Columbia University Press: 107–134
16. Killian KJ, Leblanc P, Martin DH, Summers E, Jones NL, Campbell EJ. (1992). Exercise capacity and ventilatory, circulatory and symptom limitation in patients with chronic airflow obstruction. Am J Respir Crit Care Med 146: 935–940
17. Mirrakhimov MM, Brimkulov NN, Cieslicki J, Tobiasz M, Kudaiberdiev Z, Moldotashev I, Shmidt G, Zielinski J. (1993). Effects of acetazolamide on overnicht oxygenation and acute mountain sickness in patients with asthma. Eur Respir J 4: 536–540
18. MurrayC.JL, Lopez AD. (1996). The global burden of disease: a comprehensive assessment of mortality and disability from diseases, injuries and risk factors in 1990 and projected to 2020. Cambridge, MA: Harvard University Press
19. Naughton MT, Rochford PD, Pretto JJ, Pierce RJ, Cain NF, Irving LB. (1995). Is normobaric simulation of hypobaric hypoxia accurate in chronic airflow limitation? Am J Respir Crit Care Med 152: 1956–1960
20. Postma DS, Siafakas NM. (1998). Management of chronic obstructive pulmonary disease. European Respiratory Monograph: 6–18

21. Samet JM, Marbury M, Spengler J. (1987). Health effects and sources of indoor air pollution. Am Rev Respir Dis 136: 1486–1508
22. Shoene RB. (1999). Lung diseases and high altitude. Adv Exp Med Biol 474: 47–56
23. Sooronbaev TM, Mirrakhimov EM. (2003). Clinically functional features in the course of chronic obstructive pulmonary disease in residents at high altitude. 6th Annual congress Turkish Thoracic Society (abstract):389
24. Wedzicha JA, Bestall JC, Garrod R, Garnham R, Paul EA, Jones PW. (1999). Randomized controlled trial of pulmonary rehabilitation in severe chronic obstructive pulmonary disease patients, stratified with the MRC dispnoea scale. Eur Respir J 12: 363–369

CHAPTER 19

MONITORING THE MORPHOLOGICAL AND FUNCTIONAL PARAMETERS OF PLATELETS IN PATIENTS WITH THROMBOCYTOPENIC PURPURA DURING HIGH MOUNTAIN TREATMENT

ABDUKHALIM R. RAIMJANOV, IRINA TSOPOVA, SVETLANA ASTAPOVA

Scientific Center for Hematology, Bishkek, Kyrgyzstan

Abstract: With modern techniques, 31 patients with idiopathic thrombocytopenic purpura (ITP) were investigated. All patients received high-mountain treatment in the Tuya-Ashu pass (3200 m. above sea level). It is shown that after a forty-day high-mountainous climatotherapy for patients with ITP there was a quantitative gain in the number of thrombocytes and simultaneous increase in their functional capacity.

Keywords: idiopathic thrombocytopenic purpura, high-mountain treatment, thrombocytes, hemostasis, aggregation

Introduction

ITP is a disease which most often (40% of events) is the cause of hemorrhagic symptoms and in hematological practice falls into the heavy pathology of system of the blood, which demand a permanent search for new methods of treatment [1, 14]. Perennial scientific probes and clinical observations of domestic scientists such as Mirrakhimov M.M., (1977) and Raimjanov A.R. (1988, 2002), have proved the considerable efficacy of high-mountainous climatotherapy for patients with ITP [11].

We studied the parameters of primary hemostasis, morphology platelets and megakariocytes, in patients with thrombocytopenic purpura during a 40-day stay in mountains (Tuya – Ashu, 3200 m). Conditions of hypoxia influencing bone marrow hemopoeisis and stimulating work grown factors, entail activation of part of the hemostasis system . Dynamic, positive changes are found in the morphology and functions of platelets and megakariocytes.

A. Aldashev and R. Naeije (eds.), Problems of High Altitude Medicine and Biology, 259–262.

Materials and Methods

Thirty-one patients with ITP, from the age of from 16 to 55, receiving high mountainous treatment in the hospital at Tuya-Ashu pass (3200 m above the sea level) were investigated. The control group consisted of 10 healthy people, aged from 18 to 35 years. The investigation was conducted under the schedule: background (Bishkek, 760 m), rise in mountains – for 5th, 20th, 30th, 40th days of stay in mountains (Tuya-Ashu pass, 3200 m), on 2nd day after descent to Bishkek (760 м).

Calculation of thrombocytes was made by unitized method of Phonio and megacaryocytes with the Fux-Rosental chamber [8, 9].

Processes of aggregation were studied on the evaluator of thrombocytes aggregation "Biola", method of Born [5, 12].

All quantity indicators were exposed to mathematical computerization with use of software (Statistica 5.0, Curve-Expert 1.34) [6, 10].

Discussion

In the outcomes of high mountains treatments, special changes in the quantity and structure of megacaryocytes of the bone marrow of patients with ITP are revealed. It is proven that with ITP, the quantity of active megacaryocytes is not reduced and is enlarged [2]. Two groups of patients with ITP were secured: group 1 (10 people) – with fewer megacaryocytes; group 2 (11 people) - with more megacaryocytes and also group 3 (control group) - with a normal quantity of megacaryocytes (Table 1).

As a result of the treatment, in group 1 the quantity of megacaryocytes grew by a factor of 1.2, in the second group 1.9, in the control group – 1.2. The quantity was accordingly increased 1.9, 1.15 and 1.2-fold ($p < 0.05$). Correlation analysis revealed connections between the mean size of megacaryocytes and their quantity in bone marrow.

TABLE 1. Quantity of megacaryocytes (MCC) and their size in 1 mcl of sternal punctat in patients with ITP and in control group

Groups of patients	MCC before the rise	MCC on 40th day of stay	Size of MCC before the rise	Size of MCC on 40th day of stay
1 n=10	114.8±6.5*	135.5±6.9*	51.53±2.49*	97.58±2.76*
2 n=11	50.5±3.43*	95.18±2.57*	97.38±3.61*	122.81±3.12*
3 n=10	66.8±3.28	80.5±2.86	94.52±2.55	114.9±2.85

* - $P < 0.05$ - in relation to the control.

TABLE 2. Quantity of thrombocytes (10^9/l) in patients with ITP and the healthy people

Before rise		After descent	
patients	20. ± 4.8*	patients	70.3± 6.2*
healthy	184.0 ± 7.6	healthy	226.1± 3.4

* - P <0.05 in relation to the control.

TABLE 3. The mean size of aggregators and the percentage of light-passing (%) for patients with ITP in the process high mountainous treatment

	Before rise				After descent			
	healthy		patients		healthy		patients	
Inductor	Y.e.	%	Y.e.	%	Y.e.	%	Y.e.	%
Ristomycin	11.2±1.7	66.9±2.2	3.1±3.1	21.2±4.1	11.4±2.0	67.0±3.2	7.16±4.1	38.7±3.7
Collagen	9.9 ±4.0	71.9±3.5	1.7±2.4	25.4±3.9	10.1±2.4	72.4±2.8	4.5±1.7	39.0±2.1
ADP	13.0±2.7*	66.5±4.1*	1.8±3.1*	20.8±3.9*	13.1 ±4.0*	67.1±3.4*	5.9±2.6	44.6±4.3

P <0.03 in relation to the control.

In all patients with ITP, a fall in the number of thrombocytes in peripheral blood was found [4, 8]. After 40 days of high-mountainous climatotherapy in patients with ITP, the number of thrombocytes increased 2.5-fold (Table 2).

We analyzed the aggregation of thrombocytes in high-mountainous conditions, as this shows the functions of primary hemostasis [7, 8]. Ristocetin, collagen and ADP were used to induce aggregation. These substances – agonists, interact with specific receptors on the surface of thrombocytes and activate last [3, 5, 13] (Table 3).

Conclusion

1. After 40 days staying in conditions of high mountains, patients with ITP show, that for patients with ITP there is a 2.5-fold increase in the quantity of thrombocytes and the structure of the megacaryocytes in bone marrow.
2. The aggregational function of the thrombocytes is improved. In parameters of aggregatogrammers, in patients with ITP, after descent there is a marked increase in induced aggregation and size of aggregators of thrombocytes.

References

1. Barkagan ZS. (1988) Hemorrhagic diseases and sets of syndromes. - Moscow, p. 70– 76.
2. Barkagan ZS. (2001) Diagnostics and controllable therapy of infringements of hemostasis. Moscow, p. 11 – 17.
3. Berkovskiy LV, Vasiliev SA. (2002) Manual for the study of the adhesively-aggregational function of thrombocytes. - Moscow , p. 4 – 16.
4. Doniush EK. (1999) Modern concepts about idiopathic thrombocytopenic purpura in children // Pediatrics No. 2. p. 57–61.
5. Gabbasov ZA, Popov EN., Gavrilov IU. (1989) New, a highly sensitive method for research into the aggregation of thrombocytes in vitro. - Moscow, p. 5 – 18.
6. Gubler EV. (2002) Computational methods for the analysis and definition of pathological processes. - Moscow, p. 7 – 39.
7. Hermanov EB, Piskanov ON. (1996) Erythrocytes, thrombocytes, leucocytes. - Kuibyshev, p. 79 – 104.
8. Korobova FV, Shmarova DA, Ivanova TV. (2000) Analysis of thrombocytes of peripheral blood and computer cytometry // Clinical and laboratory diagnostics. No. 7. – p. 36 – 37.
9. Menshikov VV. (1987) Laboratory methods for research in clinics. -Moscow, p. 136 – 137.
10. Nazarenko GI, Kishkun AA. (2002) Clinical estimation of results of research. - Moscow, p. 42 – 57.
11. Raimjanov AR. (2002) Aplastic anemia and mountainous climates. - Bishkek, p. 23 – 98.
12. Shen S, Castle W, Fleming R. (1994) // Science. Vol. 100. - p. 387 – 389.
13. Thompson NT, Scrutton M. (1996) Particle volume changes associated with light transmittance changes in the platelet aggregometer // Thromb. Res. V.41. - p. 615 – 626.
14. Vorobiov AI. (2002) Manual for hematology. - Moscow, V.1. – p. 50 – 53.

CHAPTER 20

ROLE OF EXOGENOUS HYPOXIA IN TREATMENT OF CHRONIC GLOMERULONEPHRITIS

R.R. KALIEV, M.M. MIRRAKHIMOV

National center for cardiology and internal medicine, Bishkek (Kyrgyzstan)

Abstract: For a long time, investigations under the initiative of academician M. M. Mirrakhimov (1964 – 2004) used exogenous (hypobaric and high-altitude) hypoxia. The most attractive features of the application of hypoxia at chronic glomerulonephritis (ChGN) are its antihyperlipidemic, antihypertensive, immunomodulating and erythropoiesis-stimulating properties. Development of the new method of treatment for hyperlipidemia in nephrotic ChGN with the separate use of exogenous hypoxia and mevacor, and also their combined application and study of the effects of high-altitude climate on ChGN patients with a urinary syndrome. Two groups of patients with ChGN were studied. In the first group, 51 patients ChGN with NS (?) were surveyed. They were divided into 4 subgroups depending on treatment (of hypobaric hypoxia training, mevacor, combination of hypoxia with mevacor and control). The second group included 17 patients with expressed urinary syndrome and was treated in a high-altitude climate. The duration of the treatment was 28 days. In the first group, the antihyperlipidemic effect of the treatment with hypobaric hypoxia and with mevacor appeared to be the same (16.1% and 20.1% respectively) and their combined application led to more a expressive effect (26.6%, $p<0.05$), when favorable shifts were observed in the greater lipid spectrum. In the second group, the treatment in high-altitude climate led to positive changes in the parameters for red blood cells and immunoglobulin G. Combined use of hypobaric hypoxia and mevacor increases the antihyperlipidemic effect of mevacor in ChGN patients with nephrotic syndrome. Treatment in a high-altitude climate stimulates erythropoiesis at ChGN.

Keywords : chronic glomerulonephritis; hypoxia; high altitude.

A. Aldashev and R. Naeije (eds.), Problems of High Altitude Medicine and Biology, 263–273.

Introduction

The increased interest in last decade in the study of primary and secondary kidney disease is stimulated by the continuing increase of end-stage renal failure (ESRF) occurrence among population. One of the main causes of ESRF is chronic glomerulonephritis (ChGN). Its clinical manifestations are rather similar; they do not depend distinctly on the cause and etiology mechanisms of the disease [31, 34]. At the same time, the progress of ChGN is predetermined by etiological factors and pathogenetic mechanisms [18, 31]. Recently in study of ChGN pathogenesis, significant successes have been achieved. Thus, besides specification and expansion of our knowledge in the field of immune manifestations, live renal morphologic changes were reflected in the corresponding WHO classification, evidence of the presence of non-immune shifts promoting ChGN progressing: anemia, intraglomerular hypertension with hyperfiltration, nephrotoxicity of hyperlipidemia (HLP) and plasma proteins excreted in the urine [3, 4, 7, 10, 11, 12, 17, 19, 21, 24, 28, 29, 33]. That is why the tactics of glomerulopathy treatment had to be reconsidered. New approaches to therapeutic interventions in different clinical-morphological variants of ChGN [19, 35] have appeared.

It is known that one of the non-immune mechanisms promoting glomerulosclerosis, the HLP is nowadays avowed. It has been discovered, that in ChGN patients with hypercholesterolemia and hypertriglyceridemia, renal failure develops twice as quickly than at a normal levels of cholesterol (ChS) in the blood [13, 26]. In this connection, development of the medical interventions directed towards correction of the raised blood lipid level proves that it can positively influence ChGN current [10, 35, 6, 21, 25, 27 , 32, 37, 38]. In this respect, thank to the statins inhibiting 3-hydroxy-3-methylglutaryl-coenzyme A-reductase development and introduction into clinical practice, new opportunities have appeared. At the same time, the direct influence of statins on mechanisms of the progress of nephritis by means of suppression of mesangium cell proliferation [23] and enhancing the vascular wall endothelial cells function are not excluded [1, 5, 10]. The lipid-lowering effect can also appear at high-altitude exercise. Thus, as reported by M.M. Mirrakhimov in 1964 [14, 15], high-altitude inhabitants have less risk of atherosclerosis development. Antiatherogenic shifts in the blood lipoprotein system of plainsman periodically rise in mountain regions [2] and in people with coronary heart diseases exposed to mountain-climatic exercise under conditions of a mid-altitude sanatorium [20] were established. A clear decrease was found in the total ChS and low-density lipoprotein (LDL) - ChS in rabbits adapted to barometric chamber hypoxia (6000 m above sea level), that three months previously were on a ChS-rich diet in comparison with non-adapted animals. In the first group, a more effective neutralization of the highly toxic products of lipid oxidation [8, 9] was revealed.

However, there are no data in the literature on the use of exogenous hypoxic exercise for HLP correction in ChGN with nephrotic syndrome (NS), which has induced the present study.

The aim of study: development of a new scheme for nephrotic ChGN treatment by the use of non-medical intervention (hypobaric hypoxia) and mevacor, and also their combined application and to study the effect of high-altitude climatic therapy (HACT) in ChGN.

Materials and Methods

Two groups of patients with ChGN were examined. The first group consisted of 51 patients (36 men and 15 women) with ChGN and NS aged 24.8 ± 1.6 years. Before treatment and on 28th day after the clinical-laboratory research was conducted. The content of total ChS was determined by photometry (Abell-Kendall method), content of triglycerides (TG) was measured by photometry (S. Gottfried), HDL- ChS was evaluated in supernatant after precipitation of other classes lipoproteins by heparin in the presence of manganese cations; LDL- ChS was calculated by W. Friedewald's formula. Creatinine content, blood protein and protein fractions and daily proteinuria were estimated by standard methods (Jaffe reaction, refractometry, electrophoresis on a paper and sulfosalicylic acid respectively). It should be noted that in 27 patients diagnosis of ChGN was confirmed by morphological study of renal biopsy samples.

According to treatment programs, the patients from group 1 were divided into 4 subgroups comparable in age, sex, indicators of renal process activity, lipid spectrum and renal function. During examination, the patients did not take the ACE-inhibitors or immunosuppressive medicines.

The first subgroup (15 persons) was exposed to hypobaric hypoxic exercise (barometric chamber PBK-53). Patients have "climbed" to an "altitude" corresponding to 3200 m above sea level for 60 minutes daily. In the first two days the rarefaction of the oxygen (pO2) in the chamber was 140 and 126 mmHg (1000 and 2000 m) respectively and for the third day and following days it was 112 mmHg (3200 m). The patients were exposed to oxygen therapy only in case of essential deterioration of their health status at the "altitude". During 28 days, every patient was exposed to hypoxic exercise.

In the second subgroup (16 persons) mevacor (Merck Sharp and Dohme IDEA) in dosages of 20 mg once a day during 4 weeks was prescribed. During treatment, possible side effects of the medicine were considered.

The third subgroup (10 persons) received combined therapy (28 "rises" in barometric chamber and 20 mg a day mevacor).

The fourth subgroup (10 persons) was on the lipid-lowering diet only (control group).

All patients were on a low-fat diet (30% of the usual caloric content) and ChS (upto 300 mg/day).

The second group was for HACT and included 17 patients with ChGN with expressive urinary syndrome. They were hospitalized for background examination in the Nephrology Department of the National Center for Cardiology and Therapy (NCCT) and were exposed to dynamic examination: background examination in Bishkek (760 m above sea level) and then on 28th day of staying at the high-altitude hospital at the Tuja-Ashuu pass (3200 m). Patients were transported to high altitude by bus (129 km). On the first day after arrival to the high-altitude hospital, patients had bed rest for 3–5 days and their motor regimen was limited to lighten the adaptation process.

The gained results were statistically analyzed. The significance of differences in the compared parameters was determined by the Student-t test and also the Wilcoxon T-pairs non-parametric test.

Results and Discussion

The effect of hypoxic barometric chamber exercises, mevacor and their combination on clinical-functional manifestations of ChGN. It is necessary to note that such a comparative study was undertaken for the first time. Clinical data showed good or satisfactory endurance of barometric chamber hypoxia by patients.

In patients who were exposed to barometric chamber hypoxic exercise (table 1), the tendency was to increase the blood protein concentration, whereas in the control group – a disposition towards its decrease was revealed. Sufficiently expressed growth of the serum albumin content in these patients appeared. It is possible that with more patients included in the sample and/or longer terms of hypobaric therapy, these changes will appear more significant.

The collected data testify that the course of hypoxia exercise causes a significant decrease in total ChS levels (16.1%, $P<0.05$), very low-density lipoprotein (VLDL) – ChS and TG (32.2 and 32.8 %, $P<0.01$, respectively, table 1), which correspond with publications [16, 36] received on practically healthy people and in the presence of other pathology forms. We have simultaneously revealed a tendency to lower the LDL- ChS level (14.9%, $P>0.05$). At the same time, high-density (HDL) - ChS had a tendency to increase (8.8 %, $P>0.05$). In the control group adhering only to the diet, all the parameters of the lipid spectrum showed no essential changes.

TABLE 1. Dynamics of clinical-laboratory parameters (M±m) in patients with ChGN under barometric chamber hypoxic exercises

	subgroup I (n = 15)		Control (n = 10)	
Parameters	Back ground	After 28 days	Back ground	After 28 days
S.B.P (mmHg)	125.0±3.1	126.0±4.8	108.0±3.8	107.1±1.8
D.B.P (mmHg)	84.0±4.5	87.0±5.2	73.0±2.1	75.7±2.9
ESR (mm/hour)	28.5±4.4	29.9±6.3	35.4±6.0	41.6±6.9
Proteinuria (g/day)	7.1±1.1	7.7±1.1	6.4±0.9	6.3±1.1
Total serum protein (g/l)	54.0±1.2	56.5±3.7	50.9±2.5	48.4±5.0
Serum albumins (%)	30.2±2.8	37.1±2.1	22.2±3.5	23.6±3.0
A_2-globulins of serum (%)	22.9±1.4	21.5±1.3	26.5±2.9	23.8±1.9
γ-globulins of serum (%)	20.8±1.6	21.6±1.0	23.5±1.4	27.6±2.4
Serum creatinine (mkmol/l)	94.9±3.0	58.6±3.5	68.0±4.9	76.4±11.0
Total serum ChS (mmol/l)	9.3±0.7	7.8±0.9*	9.9±0.9	9.9±1.4
LDL-ChS of serum (mmol/l)	6.8±0.5	5.8±0.8	7.4±0.8	7.0±1.4
HDL-ChS of serum (mmol/l)	0.8±0.03	0.9±0.04	0.9±0.08	0.9±0.07
VLDL-ChS of serum (mmol/l)	1.4±0.2	0.9±0.1**	1.5±0.3	1.8±0.5
Serum TG (mmol/l)	3.2±0.4	2.1±0.3**	3.4±0.8	4.1±1.2

* -Pt <0.05, **-Pt<0.01 – differences are significant compared to background data.

Thus, our research results testify that the 28days barometric chamber hypoxic exercise was accompanied by significantly favorable shifts in an initially disturbed blood lipid spectrum: basically the total ChS, VLDL-ChS and TG. Though an essential decrease in the parameters of the activity of ChGN was not observed.

The four-week lipid-lowering therapy by mevacor (Merck Sharp and Dohme IDEA) was taken well by patients. There was no reason to cancel the medicine because of any side effects. In this group of patients, a disposition to severe reduction of proteinuria and an increase in total blood proteins content (table 2) were observed. Such positive shifts have both a lipid-lowering effect and influence the activity of the inflammatory process of the vascular endothelium.

Our data have proved a high lipid-lowering efficacy of mevacor in secondary nephrotic HLP: the content of total serum ChS decreased by 20.1% (from 11.3±0.6mmol/l to 9.0±0.7mmol/l, P<0.01) and LDL- ChS - by 26.7 % (from 9.0±0.6 to 6.6±0.7mmol/l, P>0.01). However, levels of VLDL- ChS and TG had, on the contrary, a disposition towards growth (to 15.3 and 14.2 % respectively, p>0.1), and the concentration of HDL- ChS was not exposed to any significant changes. The concentration of serum creatinine practically stood still, at the initial level.

TABLE 2. Dynamics of clinical-laboratory parameters (M±m) in patients with ChGN under mevacor treatment

Parameters	subgroup II (n = 16)		Control (n = 10)	
	Background	After 28 days	Back ground	After 28 days
S.B.P (mmHg)	125.0±5.3	121.0±2.3	108.0±3.8	107.1±1.8
D.B.P (mmHg)	81.0±4.3	81.0±4.0	73.0±2.1	75.7±2.9
ESR (mm/hour)	38.4±3.9	48.1±5.1	35.4±6.0	41.6±6.9
Proteinuria (g/day)	13.2±2.4	7.6±1.6**	6.4±0.9	6.3±1.1
Total serum protein (g/l)	52.6±1.8	59.4±2.2**	50.9±2.5	48.4±5.0
Serum albumins (%)	27.2±2.1	29.5±4.2	22.2±3.5	23.6±3.0
A_2-globulins of serum (%)	30.3±3.2	32.9±3.4	26.5±2.9	23.8±1.9
γ-globulins of serum(%)	18.3±1.2	19.4±2.3	23.5±1.4	27.6±2.4
Serum creatinine (mkmol/l)	80.0±8.1	101.6±21.9	68.0±4.9	76.4±11.0
Total serum ChS (mmmol/l)	10.8±0.7	8.4±0.8**	9.9±0.9	9.9±1.5
LDL-ChS of serum (mmol/l)	8.4±0.7	6.0±0.7**	7.4±0.9	7.0±1.4
HDL-ChS of serum (mmol/l)	1.0±0.03	0.9±0.05	0.9±0.08	0.9±0.07
VLDL-ChS of serum (mmol/l)	1.2±0.1	1.3±0.1	1.6±0.3	1.8±0.6
Serum TG (mmol/l)	2.7±0.3	3.0±0.4	3.4±0.8	4.1±1.2

** - significant differences (P<0.05) compared to background data.

Hence, in NS caused ChGN, the mevacor treatment positively affects indicators of disease activity by influencing lipid metabolism and also by some reduction of proteinuria. This effect is probably caused by both the essential lipid-lowering and anti-inflammatory properties of this medicine.

Combined application of hypobaric hypoxia exercise and mevacor at ChGN with NS increased the albumin concentration in blood serum (table 3). The ESR and proteinuria had the disposition to decrease, which indirectly testifies to the positive influence of the combined therapy on ChGN activity.

The evaluation of lipid spectrum reaction in patients with ChGN after combined application of barometric chamber hypoxic exercise and mevacor has shown a decrease in total ChS content of on average 26.6%, LDL- ChS - of 35.8%, VLDL- ChS - of 19.4%, TG - of 28.9%. It is necessary to consider a moderate increase of HDL- ChS of 10.2%, though also insignificant, as a tendency (table 3). Expressiveness of the revealed shifts in the wide lipid spectrum appeared to be essentially higher than with the application of each of the treatment methods separately. Hence, it is possible to believe that there is some synergism in the applied methods of therapy.

A comparative study of the efficacy of each of the treatment programs on the active ChGN has confirmed the benefit of the combined application of barometric chamber hypoxic exercise and mevacor. Thank to this, the effect of intervention appears to be more pronounced. Here, we once again

TABLE 3. Dynamics of clinical-laboratory parameters (M±m) in patients with ChGN under combined therapy by barometric chamber hypoxic exercise and mevacor

	III subgroup (n = 10)		Control subgroup (n=10)	
Parameters	Background	After 28 days	Background	After 28 days
S.B.P (mmHg)	117.0 ± 3.9	120.0 ± 2.6	108.0 ± 3.8	107.1 ± 1.8
D.B.P (mmHg)	73.0 ± 2.1	81.0 ± 2.2	73.0 ± 2.1	75.7 ± 2.9
ESR (mm/hour)	28.4 ± 4.5	22.8 ± 8.3	35.4 ± 6.0	41.6 ± 6.9
Proteinuria (g/day)	7.7 ± 1.5	7.3 ± 2.2	6.4 ± 0.99	6.3 ± 1.1
Total serum protein (g/l)	56.1 ± 1.9	55.4 ± 3.0	50.9 ± 2.5	48.4 ± 5.0
Serum albumins (%)	31.5 ± 2.6	37.2 ± 4.8	22.2 ± 3.5	23.6 ± 3.0
A_2-globulins of serum (%)	21.1 ± 3.1	19.5 ± 3.7	26.5 ± 2.9	23.8 ± 1.9
γ-globulins of serum(%)	20.4 ± 1.1	20.8 ± 2.2	23.5 ± 1.4	27.6 ± 2.4
Serum creatinine (mkmol/l)	56.7 ± 3.0	70.2 ± 12.1	68.0 ± 4.9	76.4 ± 11.0
Total serum ChS (mmmol/l)	10.0 ± 1.7	7.4 ± 1.4*	9.9 ± 0.9	9.9 ± 1.5
LDL-ChS of serum (mmol/l)	7.3 ± 1.1	4.7 ± 1.3*	7.4 ± 0.9	7.0 ± 1.4
HDL-ChS of serum (mmol/l)	0.9 ± 0.06	1.0 ± 0.1	0.9 ± 0.08	0.9 ± 0.07
VLDL-ChS of serum (mmol/l)	1.8 ± 0.3	1.4 ± 0.4*	1.6 ± 0.3	1.8 ± 0.6
Serum TG (mmol/l)	3.9 ± 0.8	2.8 ± 0.9*	3.4 ± 0.8	4.1 ± 1.2

* - $P_T < 0.05$ significant differences compared to background data.

pay attention to the fact that levels of total ChS in patients who received combined treatment decreased by 26.6%, whereas in the subgroup exposed only to the influence of barometric chamber hypoxia it was 16.1%. In the subgroup of patients treated with mevacor – by 20.1%. The LDL-ChS concentration in the first group decreased by 35.8%, whereas in the second - it was 26.7%. Application of the barometric chamber hypoxic exercise did not cause any significant decrease in the analyzed parameter level (only by 14.9%). At the same time, the reduction of the VLDL-ChS level in the subgroup exposed to the influence of exogenous (barometric chamber) hypoxia was 32.2% compared to 19.4% in the "combined" subgroup. At the same time, in the subgroup treated with mevacor, the concentration of the studied parameters had a contrary tendency towards growth (by 15.3 %).

Similar regularity is established concerning the dynamics of TG concentration. In the subgroup treated by hypoxic exercise the TG level decreased by 32.8%, in the "combined" subgroup - by 28.9%. In the "mevacor" subgroup, the disposition to increase (by 14.2 %) was marked. The revealed decrease of the total ChS, LDL- ChS levels testifies to the antiatherogenic orientation of the interventions we applied. In this respect, hypoxic exercises have a special advantage.

The greater efficacy of combined applications of exogenous hypoxia and mevacor on clinical-functional parameters are explained by their synergist and lipid-lowering effects. Undoubtedly, hypoxic exercises are more preferable for the reduction of increased TG and VLDL- ChS levels, which often happen in diabetic nephropathy.

High-altitude adaptation and ChGN. Having revealed the positive results of the barometric chamber hypoxic exercises, we have decided to evaluate the exercises efficacy in ChGN under natural hypoxic conditions (high altitude). Analysis of the collected data (Table 4) has shown that patients exposed to a28-day intervention (adaptation at the "Tuja-Ashuu" pass, 3200m) have statistically significant shifts of the red blood parameters (increase in erythrocytes from 4.59 ± 0.13 to 4.84 ± 0.12 × 10^{12}/l, $P<0.05$; hemoglobin concentration from 135.3 ± 3.53 g/l to 147.8 ± 4.37 g/l, $P<0.01$) connected with the stimulation of erythropoietin production [30]. It should not be excluded that the results achieved with the help of barometric chamber hypoxic exercises are not connected with effect of erythropoietin concentration increase in the blood. An important fact was also the decrease in immunoglobulin G levels (from 1.7 ± 0.2 to 1.0 ± 0.01 g/l, $P<0.05$), which confirms the decreasing pathological immune process activity. As a probable consequence, a tendency of the following parameters to decrease was observed: ESR (from 15.24 ± 3.96 to 12.69 ± 4.21 mm/hour), daily proteinuria (from 2.4 ± 0.8 to 1.9 ± 0.8 g) and also the serum A_2-globulins level (from 14.45 ± 3.15 up to 12.85 ± 2.31%). An insignificant increase in total blood proteins level (from 66.92 ± 4.13 to 68.05 ± 2.96 g/l) and albumins (from 47.11 ± 3.61 to 48.75 ± 2.95%) was simultaneously observed.

Thus, 28-day HACT has rendered an essential positive influence on the red blood parameters and immunoglobulin G concentration in patients with ChGN accompanied by a disposition to decreasing ESR, proteinuria and dysproteinemia.

TABLE 4. Influence of 28-day stay at the "Tuja-Ashuu" pass (3200 m) on some laboratory parameters of ChGN with expressed urinary syndrome

Parameters	Background	After 28 days
Total serum protein (g/l)	66.92 ± 4.13	68.05 ± 2.96
Serum albumins (%)	47.11 ± 3.61	48.75 ± 2.95
α_2-globulins (%)	14.45 ± 3.15	12.85 ± 2.31
γ-globulins (%)	20.02 ± 0.99	19.8 ± 1.51
Proteinuria (g/day)	2.4 ± 0.8	1.9 ± 0.8
ESR (mm/hour)	15.24 ± 3.96	12.69 ± 4.21
Erythrocytes × 10^{12}/l	4.59 ± 0.13	4.84 ± 0.12*
Hemoglobin (g/l)	135.3 ± 3.53	147.82 ± 4.37*
Serum IgA (g/l)	0.2 ± 0.03	0.2 ± 0.03
Serum IgM (g/l)	0.1 ± 0.01	0.1 ± 0.02
Serum IgG (g/l)	1.7 ± 0.2	1.0 ± 0.01*

* - $P< 0.05$.

Conclusions

1. Hypobaric hypoxic exercises, mevacor and their combined application in nephrotic ChGN lead to an essential decrease in blood lipid levels.
2. Exercises by means of hypobaric (barometric chamber) hypoxia are accompanied by a more vigorously expressed decrease of very low density lipoproteins and triglycerides.
3. Mevacor in ChGN in greater doses reduces the total cholesterol and the low density lipoproteins levels.
4. Combined application of hypoxic exercises and mevacor lead to a more clearly expressed reduction of the total cholesterol, the low-density lipoproteins and the very low-density lipoproteins levels.
5. High-altitude adaptation of patients with ChGN is accompanied by both an essential increase in erythrocytes numbers and blood hemoglobin concentration and a decrease in immunoglobulins G content. It is also accompanied by a tendency for the ESR to decrease, proteinuria, increase of the total blood protein and albumins levels.
6. Non-medical intervention by means of barometric chamber hypoxia exercises and high-altitude adaptation is advisable for ChGN treatment, especially in the presence of nephrogenous hyperlipidemia.

References

1. Afzalli B, Haydar AA, Vinen K, Goldsmith DJA. (2004) From Finland to Faterland: Beneficial effects of statins for patients with chronic kidney disease. J. Am. Soc. Nephrol. 15: 2161 – 2168.
2. Aitbaev KA, Madaminov I, Meimanaliev TS, Shleifer EZ, Kim NM. (1990) Study of influence of migration to mountain regions on the blood lipoproteins system. Cosm. biol. and aviacosm. med. 6; C. 45 – 46. (In Rus).
3. Baud L, Fouqueray B, Belocq A. (2001) Cytokines and hormones with anti-inflammatory effects: new tools for the therapeutic intervention. Curr. Opin. Nephrol. Hypert. 10: 49 – 54.
4. Brenner BM, Meyer TW, Hostetter TH. (1982) Dietary protein intake and progressive nature of kidney disease: the role of hemodinamically mediated glomerular injury in the pathogenesis of progressive glomerular sclerosis on aging, renal ablation and intrinsic renal disease. N. Engl. J. Med. 307: 652 – 659.
5. Campese VM, Nadim MK, Epstein M. (2005) Are 3-hydroxy-3-methylglutaryl-CoA reductase inhibitors renoprotective? J. Am. Soc. Nephrol. 16: 11 – 17.
6. Diamond JR, Hanchack NA, McCarter MD, Karnovsky MJ. (1990) Cholestyramine resin ameliorates chronic aminonucleoside nephrosis. Am. J. Clin. Nutr. 51: 606 – 611.
7. Iseki K, Ikemiya Y, Iseki C, Takishita S. (2003) Proteinuria and the risk of developing end-stage renal disease. Kidney int. 4: 1468 – 1474.
8. Kitaev MI, Aitbaev KA, Lyamzev VT. (1999) Influence of hypoxic hypoxia on atherosclerosis development. Aviacosm. med and ecol. med. 5: 54 – 57. (In Rus).

9. Kitaev MI, Lyamzev VT, Aitbaev KA, Mainazarova ES, Titeeva GR. (2000) Development features of experimental atherosclerosis in animals adapted to interrupted barometric chamber hypoxia. Cardiology 5: 54 – 58. (In Rus).
10. Kolina IB, Stavrovskaya EV, Shilov EM. (2004) Dyslipemia and chronic progressive kidney diseases. Ther. Arch. 9: 75 – 78.
11. Locatelli F, Del Vecchio L. (2001) Prevention of progress of chronic renal insufficiency. Successes of nephrology / Edition of N.A. Mukhin, S.V. Grachev, L.V. Kozlovskaya and others – M.: «The Russian doctor», 81 – 93.
12. Locatelli F, Del Vecchio L, Pozzoni P, Manzoni C. (2006) Nephrology: Main advances in the last 40 years. J. Nephrol. 19: 6 – 11.
13. Mashio O, Oldrizzi L, Rugiv C, Loschiavo C. (1989) Serum lipids in patients with chronic renal failure on long-term, protein-restricted diets. Am. J. Med. 87: 51 – 54.
14. Mirrakhimov MM. (1964) About peripheral blood picture in the Tyan-Shan and Pamir high-altitude conditions. – Frunze, 128. (In Rus).
15. Mirrakhimov MM. (1977) Treatment of internal diseases by mountain climate. – L.: Medicine. –208 p. (In Rus).
16. Mirrakhimov MM, Aitbaev KA, Murataliev TM, Kim NM. (1991) Study of opportunity of atherogenic dyslipoproteinemia correction by mountain climate treatment. Cardiology. 3: 8 – 11. (In Rus).
17. Moorhead J, Chan M, El- Nahas M, Varghese Z. (1982) Lipid nephrotoxicity in chronic progressive glomerular disease. Lancet 2: 1309 – 1311.
18. Mukhin NA. (2001) Chronic progressive kidney diseases and modern nephroprotective strategy – statements, opportunities and prospects. Successes of nephrology / Edition of N.A. Mukhin NA, Grachev SV, Kozlovskaya LV, et al. (2001) M.: "The Russian doctor", 66 – 80.
19. Mukhin NA, Kozlovskaya LV, Kutyrina IM, Shvetsov Miu, Fomin VV. (2002) Proteinuric remodeling of tubulointerstitium is target of nephroprotective therapy in chronic renal diseases Ther. arch. 6: 5 – 11.
20. Murataliev TM, Mirrakhimov MM, Aitbaev KA, Kim NM. (1991) Study of opportunities of atherogenic dyslipoproteinemia correction by mountain climate. Cardiology 3: 27 – 31. (In Rus).
21. Neverov NI. (1994) The role of lipids in progressing of nephropathies Authoassay of dissertation … of doctor of medical sciences: 14. 00. 05. – M., 35p.
22. Neverov NI, Polyakov AN. (1995) Antihyperlipidemic influences in treatment of nephropathies. Materia Medica 1995; 2: 51 – 56.
23. O'Donnel MP, Kasiske BL, Kim Y, Atluru D, Keane WF. (1993) The mevalonate pathway: importance in mesangial cell biology and glomerular disease. Miner. Electrolyte Metab. 19: 173 – 179.
24. Ryan XZ, Varghese Z, Moorhead JF. (2003) Inflammation modifies lipid-mediated renal injury. Nephrol. Dial. Transplant. 18: 27 – 32.
25. Sahadevan M, Kasiske BL. (2002) Hyperlipidemia in kidney disease: causes and consequences. Curr. Opin. Nephrol. Hypertens. 11: 323 – 329.
26. Samuelsson O, Mulec H, Knight-Gibson C, Attman PO, Kron B, Larsson R, Weiss L, Wedel H, Alaupovic P. (1997) Lipoprotein abnormalities are associated with increased rate of progression of human chronic renal insufficiency. Nephrol. Dialysis Transplant. 12: 1908 – 1915.
27. Shah S, Paparello J, Danesh FR. (2005) Effects of statin therapy on the progression of chronic disease. Adv. chr. kidney dis. 12: 187 – 195.
28. Serov VV, Varshavsky VA, Ivanov AA. (2000) Morphology of glomerulonephritis Nephrology / Edition I.E. Tareyeva. – M., Medicine. 211 – 224. (In Rus).
29. Shilov EM. (2001) Immunopathology of renal diseases. Successes of nephrology / Edition of N.A. Mukhin, S.V. Gracheva, Kozlovskaya et al., – M.: «The Russian doctor», 132 – 145.

30. Tan C.C, Eckardt K.U, Firth J.D, Ratcliffe P.J. (1992) Feedback modulation of renal and hepatic erythropoietin mRNA in response to graded anemia and hypoxia. Am. J. Physiol. 26: 474 – 481.
31. Tareyev EM. (1983) Glomerulonephritis // Clinical Nephrology / Edition of E.M. Tareyeva. - M.: Medicine, 2: 5 – 99. (In Rus).
32. Tareyeva IE, Neverov NI, Androsova SA. (1995) Mevacor and antihyperlipidemic diet at chronic nephritis. Clin. Pharmacol. and Ther. 1995; 4: 36 – 38.
33. Tareyeva IE. (1996) Mechanisms of glomerulonephritis progression. Ther. arch. 6: 5 – 10.
34. Tareyeva IE. (2000) Clinical features of separate morphological forms of glomerulonephritis. Nephrology. Guidance for doctors / Edition of I.E. Tareyeva. - M.: Medicine, 239 – 245. (In Rus).
35. Tareyeva IE, Kutyrina IM, Neverov NI. (2000) Hemodynamic and metabolic mechanisms of progression of glomerulonephritis. Nephrology. Guidance for doctors / Edition of I.E. Tareyeva. – M.: Medicine, 2000: 229 – 234. (In Rus).
36. Tinkov AN, Aleshin IA, Kots Ya I, Makshantsev SS, Farberov VN, Nikonorov AA. (1999) Dynamics of blood lipid spectrum in patients with ischemic disease of the heart under adaptation influence to periodic barometric chamber hypoxia. Cardiology 1: 31 – 33. (In Rus).
37. Vogt L, Laverman GD, Dullaart RP, Navis G. (2004) Lipid management in the proteinuric patient: do not overlook the importance of proteinuria reduction. Nephrol. Dial. Transplant. 19: 5 – 8.
38. Wheeler DC, Fernando RL, Gillet MPT, Zaruba J, Persaud J, Kingstone D, Varghese Z, Moorhead JF. (2001) Characterization of the binding of low-density lipoproteins to cultured rat mesangial cells. Nephrol. Dial.Transplant. 6: 701 – 708.

CHAPTER 21

ATHEROGENESIS OF BRAIN VESSELS IN CONDITIONS OF HYPOXIA IN KYRGYZ HIGHLANDERS

T.K. KADYRALIEV, J.K. RAYIMBEKOV,
N.K. RAYIMBEKOV

Institute of molecular biology and medicine, Bishkek, Kyrgyzstan

Abstract: In the complex climatic and geographical conditions of Kyrgyzstan (high-altitude hypoxia, sharp fluctuations of atmospheric pressure, and varying conditions of nutrition), the prevalence of vascular pathologies remains high. The development of new concepts for pathogenesis and atherosclerosis remain insufficient. We have studied the role of structural changes in the vascular wall in conditions of hypoxia.

Keywords: Atherosclerosis of vessels of the brain; atherosclerotic angioencephalopathy; tissue hypoxia; ischemic insult.

Introduction

In studying the problem of diseases of the brain on the basis of our knowledge of the laws and interrelationships of metabolism, blood circulation and functions of the brain, the presence of atherosclerosis is actually well timed. The most widespread and heavy consequences still result in insult. In the Kyrgyzstan, the number of cerebral thrombosis cases becoming lethal is growing such that it is greater than death due to heart attack. In the past few years, cellular and molecular mechanisms of the development of atherosclerosis have been intensively studied. According to many researchers [6], the features of development of atherosclerosis in humans cannot be explained from the point of view of the lipoproteid theory. Within the limits of the insufficiently studied given problem, there is the role of changes in the vascular wall, especially in conditions of natural hypoxia, which can lead to the proliferation of cell intimae, because of the development of a high degree of tissue hypoxia.

The purpose of the research is to study the features of pathomorphogenesis, a vascular pathology of the brain in atherosclerosis in inhabitants of various heights in Kyrgyzstan.

A. Aldashev and R. Naeije (eds.), Problems of High Altitude Medicine and Biology, 275–279.

Materials and Methods

Victims of casual reasons (seven highlanders and nine lowlanders) were used as sample group for research puposes (the general artery, an internal artery, basilar arteries, and interbrain arteries). The sites of the brain from the zone of an ischemic insult, and uninjured zones of nine patients who died from an ischemic insult were also investigated. The tissues of the brain and the main vessels were fixed in a buffering solution of 10% formalin. They were then dehydrated in spirit at a rising concentration with enlightenment in xylene and filled-in paraffin. For light optical and morphometrical study, slices of 5–7 μm were painted with hematoxylin – eosine, picrophycsin – phycsillin, and creosilviolet. Morphometry microvessels were exposed defining the diameters of their shafts of light and the area of the vascular channels.

Results

The study of structural changes in the arterial system of the brain during atherosclerosis allows the designation of all complexes of the observed, interconnected and diverse processes in the vascular system of the brain. Displays of atherosclerotic angiopathies in our study are shown at three structurally-functional levels. The first is the main arteries of the brain (carotid and vertebral arteries), whose basic function is the delivery of blood to the brain. The second is extracerebral arteries, i.e., the arteries of the base of the brain. The third type of microcircular channels provides exchange processes in the brain.

Research into vessels of the brain during morphological changes in the wall of an internal carotid artery reveals the proliferation of cells in an internal environment. These processes of proliferation are more pronounced in the vessels of highlanders (Figure 1a, b). It is necessary to note that hyperplasia is of essential value in the development of stenosed atherosclerotic plaques as intimae. Another promoting factor in the development of atherosclerosis is the increase of cellular intimae due to lymphocytes and monocytes (Figure 1a, b).

Hyperplasia of intimae leads to infringement of the process of plasma perfusion in the walls of vessels and promotes delays in lipids, small muscle cells and monocytes. In our opinion, the expressiveness of proliferation cells in internal carotid arteries in highlanders is connected to a great extent with the action of fabric hypoxia. In extracranial portions of an internal carotid artery, both in the lowlands and in conditions of high altitude, the development of atherosclerosis to various degrees was marked (Figure 2).

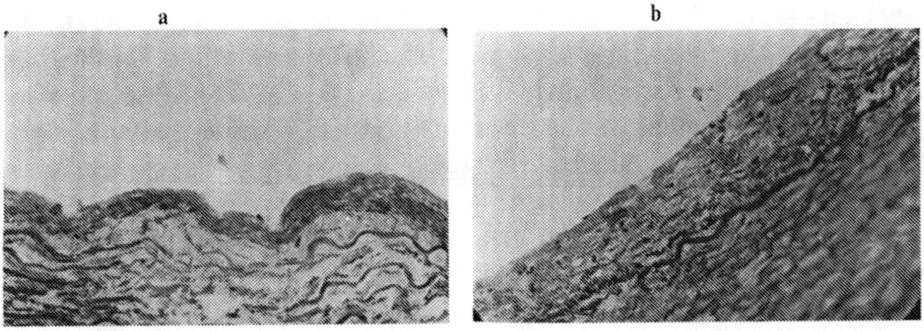

Figure 1. **(a)** The wall of an internal carotid artery in an inhabitant of lowland N. The membrane is visibly beaded in internal elastic. Proliferation of internal cells is absent. Painting picrophycsin – phycsillin. Panel a × 480. **(b)** The wall of an internal carotid artery of the radical mountaineer D is marked with a proliferation of cells for internal elastic membrane and increased cellularity due to lymphocytes and monocytes. Painting picrophycsin – phycsillin. Panel b × 480.

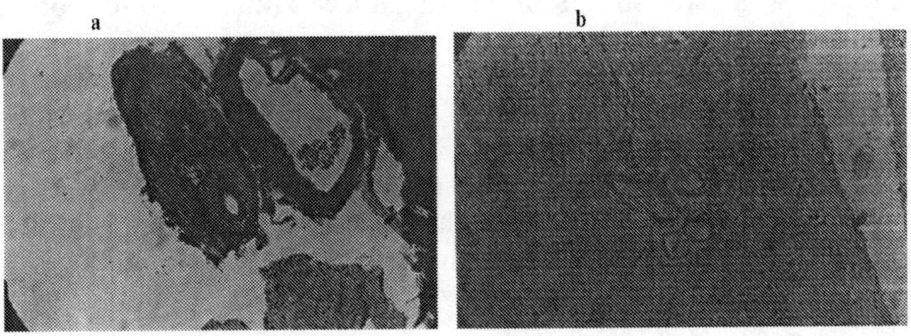

Figure 2. **(a)** Stenosed atherosclerotic plaque in extracranial arteries. Painting on Van-Gizon. Panel a × 120. **(b)** New growth as angiomatosis. Painting hematoxylin – eosine. Panel b × 120.

The definition of a degree of expressiveness of atherostenosis in extracranial portions of an internal carotid artery has exclusive value for the estimation of its role in cerebral hemodynamic infringement and in the choice of an adequate method of treatment. Nowadays, a stenosis is considered to be of pathogenetic significance in 70% or more of internal carotid arteries. Thus, there are quantitative and qualitative changes in a blood channels, leading to an insufficiency of the blood supply to the brain.

In extracranial arteries, atherosclerotic changes often develop in an area of bifurcating arteries. In intracerebral arteries, atherosclerotic angiopathy was expressed in the form of remodeling arteries as a result of the reduced blood channel caused by atherostenosis of the extracranial and intracranial arteries and at the same time, the growth of new vessels as angiomatosis became more marked (Figure 2a, b).

Such changes are characteristic of brain hypoxia. In the brain, the substance of the bark of the hemispheres of the brain has been defined and expressed as pericellular and perivascular hypostases. It is necessary to note that early stages of ischemic defeat of the brain are characterized by original changes in the form and maintenance of vessels and microvascular channels in the form of nonfibrin blood clots, plenty of the plasmatic capillaries and sharply expressed nonuniformity of the gleam of vessels. These changes can have an important diagnostic role when other attributes of necroric tissue of the brain do not reach sufficient morphological expressiveness for a pathological diagnosis.

Conclusion

Results have shown that in inhabitants of Kyrgyzstan, both in lowland conditions and at high-altitude, atherosclerotic angiopathy of vessels of the brain develops at three structural functional levels (main, extracerebral and microcircular). In highlanders, the tendency to express more proliferational reactions in the cells of an internal environment of the carotid artery is marked, which is probably caused by the increased development of tissue hypoxia. It is also noted that hyperplasia is of essential value in the development of stenosed atherosclerotic plaques in the arteries of the brain, with the formation of a powerful fibrous elastic layer, limiting opportunities for expansion of the arteries which can have intimae.

References

1. Anestiadi V., Nagorzev V. (1982) Morphogenesis of Atherosclerosis. Kishinev.
2. Anichkov N.N. (1965) Atherosclerosis, pp. 14–21.
3. Anichkov N.N., Volkova K.G., and Zahareva M.A. (1948) Pathological anatomy of hypertonic illness. 18–29.
4. Avtandilov G.G. (1970) Dynamics of the atherosclerotic process in humans. M.
5. Barnett H., Barnes R.W., Clagett G.P., Ferguson G.G., Robertson J.T., Walker P.M. (1992) Symptomatic carotid artery stenosis: a solvable problem: North American Symptomatic Carotid Endarterectomy Trial. Stroke 23(8):1048–1053.
6. Ficher M. (1992) Cellular basis of atherosclerosis. In: Norris J. and Hachinski V. (eds) Prevention of stroke. Spinger-Verlag, Berlin, pp. 19–36.
7. Gannushkina I.V. (1996) Pathomorphological mechanisms of infringements of brain blood circulation and new directions in their preventive maintenance and treatment. No. 1, 14–18.
8. Nogornev V.A. and Maltseva S.Y. (1996) Atherosclerosis 51:245–251.
9. Raines E.W., Rosenfeld M.E., and Ross R. (1996) The role of macrophages. In: Fuster V., Ross R., and Topol E.J. (eds) Atherosclerosis and Coronary Artery Disease. Lippincott-Raven Publishers, Philadelphia, pp. 539–555.

10. Ross R. (1997) Atherosclerosis 131(Suppl.):3–4.
11. Vereshagin N.V. (1980) Deformations of the main arteries of the head and their value in the development of infringement of brain blood circulation in advanced age. No. 12., 7–12.
12. Vereshagin NV, Morgunov VA, Gulevskaya TS. (1997) Pathology of a brain at an atherosclerosis and an arterial hypertension, Moscow, 287.
13. Vihert A.M., Jdanov V.S., Matova E.E., Aptekar C.G. (1981) Geographical pathology of atherosclerosis. M.

CHAPTER 22

PARTICULARITIES OF NEUROPSYCHOTROPIC EFFECTS OF MEXIDOL IN VARIOUS ALTITUDE CONDITIONS

U.M. TILEKEEVA, A.Z. ZURDINOV, T.A. VORONINA

Kyrgyz State Medical Academy, Clinical and Basic Pharmacology Department, Scientific Research Institute of Pharmacology, Russian Academy of Medical Sciences

Abstract: In conditions of adaptation to natural high mountains, Mexidol has a positive neuropsychotropic action. It represents an interesting prospective means for the further research as an indicator during medical interventions during adaptation to high mountains. Summarizing the obtained data, Mexidol can be defined as a promising stress protective medicine in mid-mountains but it requires further comprehensive research for high altitudes.

Keywords: Altitude; mexidol; central nervous system; antioxidant.

Introduction

Pharmacological correction of the negative influences of complex of high-altitude climatic factors on the human organism is an actual problem for Kyrgyzstan, because of intensified development of a raw-material base for industrial and agricultural production, expansion of tourism, development of monitoring methods of work, etc. It leads to increasing of number of people who are temporarily living in this territory and are exposed to regular horizontal and vertical migration.

It is known that the influence of adverse climatic and geographical factors of high mountains leads to a decrease in the reserves of an organism and the development of disadaptation, which is accompanied by various pathological conditions. Vital activity and, furthermore, the professional activity of some categories of specialists, who are engaged in manufacturing, demand an optimum level of functional adaptation not only by the vitally important organs and systems, but with preservation of the cognitive functions of the Central Nervous System (CNS) [1, 4, 5].

A. Aldashev and R. Naeije (eds.), Problems of High Altitude Medicine and Biology, 281–284.

On this basis, searching for means of adaptation to high mountains should be based on modern views on the mechanisms of its formation. It is thus important to achieve a desirable effect, but not by any cost, rather due to influencing key pathogenetic parts of the development of the damage and its significance. In this regard there is scientific and practical interest in Mexidol, an original medical preparation. It is a representative of the membrane-active antioxidants, a structural analogue of Pyridoxine with a metabolic type of action and with the original spectrum of pharmacological activities. It is widely applied in various areas of clinical medicine [4, 7, 8].

MATERIALS AND METHODS

All animals and experimental procedures were authorized and approved by the Local Ethics Committee; procedures were performed in compliance with the NIH Guide for the Care and Use of Laboratory Animals. All behavioral tests were randomly run during the light phase from 10.00 a.m. to 2.00 p.m. Food and water were available ad lib (except for conflict test, see below).

All trials were done at different natural altitudes above sea level: mid-mountains – Bishkek – 760 m; high mountains – Tuya-Ashu research base – 3200 m above sea level. Two periods of adaptation were studied: periods of urgent (3 days) and long-term adaptation (30 days). Experiments were carried out with white inbred mice – males, with body weights of 18 – 24 g and white inbred rats – males, with body weights of 160 – 180 g. The tested compound mexidol was injected intraperitoneally in doses of 20.50 and 100 mg/kg. In order to discover the antiamnestic action of Mexidol, conditioned reflex of passive avoidance (CRPA) was used 24 h after training. Skopolamin was used as an amnesic actor in doses of 2.5mg/kg, the maximum electroshock (MES), which was carried out immediately after a session of training [2, 3, 6].

The stress protective effect of Mexidol was studied in strict 12-hour immobilization models. Tests on stomach mucosal ulceration in rats had been chosen as an indicator for the emotional stress morphological signs and the assessment of its pharmacological prevention rate.

Results and Discussion

Experimental research on the influence of Mexidol on cognitive functions and its stress protective effect have shown variability in the pharmacological effect depending on high altitude.

Mexidol has shown a marked protective effect in all the used dosing regimens (20, 50, and 100 mg/kg) by all registered indicators in the mid-mountains. In the high mountain conditions, during periods of urgent and long-term adaptation to the natural hypoxia, Mexidol demonstrated a significant protective effect in one of the checked indicators – the number of ulcers in average / per rat / per group, regardless of the dosing regimen. The stress protective effect of Mexidol retains distinctly qualitative and quantitative parameters during various terms of adaptation, in a dose of 50 mg/kg, whereas in mid-mountain conditions, such parameters were obtained with a dose of 100 mg/kg (Figures 1–4).

It is established that in conditions of natural high altitude hypoxia, a conditioned reflex of passive avoidance, serves as a neurogenic marker of the adaptation of an organism to a new environment and the action of stress, its change serves as an index of disturbance of the integrative activity of the brain and restoration means the formation of an adaptation. In the beginning, high altitude is accompanied by retrograde amnesia in 25% of cases.

Research into the mnemotropic effect of Mexidol in a dose of 100 mg/kg, while using an MES and scopolamine as amnesic actors, has revealed a distinctive antiamnestic effect of the preparation. In the control group, MES had a distinctive amnestic action and obliterates trained experience. Introducing Mexidol before the training session prevents the development of amnesia and retains a memorable trace. In this group, the latent period of going a "dangerous compartment" was considerably (3.2-fold) prolonged, and the period staying in a "safe compartment" of the experimental chamber - by 2.1 times. Thus, animals remember the electric shock and painful irritation and prefer to stay in a light, "safe" compartment (Figures 5, 6).

Research into the influence of Mexidol on short-term memory during short-term adaptation was done on the 3rd day of stay in mountains in the same dosage and on the same models of amnesia. Preservation of the antiamnestic effect of the preparation has been shown in cases of short-term adaptation to natural high altitude conditions. The comparative analysis of efficiency has shown that the antiamnestic activity of the preparation was more expressed in shock amnesia, than the scopalaminic one.

Thus, research conducted on the mnemotropic activity of Mexidol on traditional models attests the distinctive antiamnestic effect of the preparation. The preparation has an antiamnestic effect under middle altitude conditions, which is retained during short-term adaptation to high mountains. However, in extreme conditions of high mountains, the ability of Mexidol to prevent amnesia, which is caused by scopolamine, considerably decreases in expressiveness of a similar effect in conditions modeling electroshock amnesia.

On the basis of the analysis of the given references on the mechanisms of realization of the pharmacological properties of Mexidol, it may be assumed that the mnemotropic effect of Mexidol is caused by its membrane modulating action, which may promote the formation of certain conformational changes in protein molecules, causing an optimization of the process of formation, fixing and saving of the angram [3].

Cerebral and vascular activity, optimization of the microcirculation system, decreasing thrombocyte aggregation, increasing erythrocyte plasticity, increasing adhesion to the endothelium of vessels and viscosity of the blood also play an important role in the realization of the neurometabolic and antihypoxic effects of mexidol. Many articles can be found confirming this [3, 7].

Thus, in conditions of adaptation to natural high mountains, Mexidol has a positive neuropsychotropic action. It represents an interesting prospective means for further research as an indicator for medical interventions during adaptation to high mountains. Summarizing the obtained data, Mexidol can be defined as a promising stress protective medicine in mid-mountains, but requires further comprehensive research for use at high altitudes.

References

1. Agadjanyan NA. (2001) Problem of adaptation and survival strategy. // Ecology-physiological problems of adaptation: materials of X International symposium. - M.
2. Bures J, Buresova O, Houston JP. (1983) Techniques and basic experiments for the study of brain and behavior. Amsterdam. New York, 398 p.
3. Hickenbottom Sl, Glotta J. (1998) «Neuroprotective therapy» // Semin Neurol; 18(4), 485–92.
4. Lukyanova LD. (2000) Modern problems of hypoxia // Bulletin RAMS - 9.-p.3–12
5. Novikov VE., Katunina NP. (2002) Pharmacology and biochemistry of hypoxia // Reviews on clinical pharmacology and medicinal therapy. - v.1.-p.73–87.
6. Voronina T. (2000) Methods of nootropic activity investigation in experimental (preclinical) investigation of novel pharmacological substances. "Remedium", P. 153, Moscow.
7. Voronina TA, Smirnov LD. (2000) Dyumaev K.M. Possibilities of mexidol application in extreme situations. // The human and remedy: Thesis of report of 7th Russian national congress - M.- p.483.
8. Zurdinov AZ, Atanaev TB, Nanaeva MT, Tilekeeva UM, Seitalieva Ch T. (1999) Comparative examination of the antioxidizing activity of some pharmacological means by the method of hemiluminiscence. // Medicine and pharmacy. - 1. - P.19–23.

CHAPTER 23

INFLUENCE OF HIGH-ALTITUDE HYPOXIA ON ADAPTIVE AND NON-ADAPTIVE STRUCTURAL CHANGES IN THE VESSELS OF THE PULMONARY CIRCULATION

T.K. KADYRALIEV, N.K. RAIYMBEKOV, A.A. ALDASHEV

Institute of Molecular Biology and Medicine, Bishkek, Kyrgyzstan

Abstract: The aim of this study was to investigate the adaptive and non-adaptive structural changes of the pulmonary vessels during the development of high-altitude pulmonary hypertension (HAPH) and their characteristics in patients with COPD at high altitude. Histological, morphometrical and electron microscopy methods were applied. In native highlanders, due to long (chronic) adaptation, regional morphofunctional changes of the pulmonary vessels develop, which are caused by strengthening of the upper and medial zones of the lungs, increase in the capacity of the capillary channel and the extent of working zones of the air haematic barrier. The following characteristics are revealed in patients with chronic obstructive pulmonary diseases (COPD) at high altitude: remodeling of pulmonary arteries and arterioles, substantial expressed arterializations of the finest arterioles by diameter from 30 to 40 microns, with simultaneous increase in their quantity, reduction of terminal arteries and arteriole lumens as a result of endothelial and smooth muscle cell proliferation towards a vessel lumen from the internal elastic membranes, formation of multichannel arteries due to endothelial and smooth muscle cell proliferation with simultaneous growth of collagen and elastic fiber and development of the angiomatosis foci, which represent closely located vessels with different diameters. During rapid ascent to high altitude, more than 3000м above sea level, pulmonary edema develops in people who are not adapted to high altitude.

Keywords: altitude; pulmonary circulation.

Introduction

It is known that high altitude results in a hypoxic form of pulmonary arterial hypertension. Despite numerous investigations devoted to vascular remodelling of pulmonary arterioles during HAPH, [10,1,18,7,8,9,15,5,6]

A. Aldashev and R. Naeije (eds.), Problems of High Altitude Medicine and Biology, 285–294.

the structural changes in the cellular elements of the vessel wall remain unknown. Because of the simultaneous influences of cold and hypoxia at high altitude, people develop chronic obstructive pulmonary diseases (chronic obstructive bronchitis, chronic emphysema). It is therefore of interest to study the characteristics of vascular remodelling of the pulmonary circulation in these conditions.

The aim of study was to investigate the adaptive and non-adaptive structural changes of the pulmonary vessels during the development of HAPH and their characteristics in patients with COPD at high altitude.

Tasks:

1. To reveal the characteristics of the morphology of the pulmonary vessels in native highlanders of Tien-Shan and Pamir.
2. To reveal the characteristics of structural changes in vessels of the pulmonary circulation in patients with some nosologic forms of COPD.
3. To determine the structural mechanisms of development of high altitude pulmonary edema as disadaptive state at high altitude.

Materials and methods. The lungs and hearts of 16 accidentally killed highlanders without pulmonary-related pathology were investigated. As a control the lungs and hearts of 5 health lowlander aboriginals were used. To study the structural changes of the pulmonary vessels the lungs and hearts of 10 deceased highlanders with COPD were investigated. As a control the lungs and hearts of 10 deceased lowlanders with COPD were used. Also, in 3 cases, the lungs and hearts of patients who died from high altitude pulmonary edema and in 2 cases – from high altitude pulmonary edema with COPD were investigated.

Volume of the right lung. For this, into the main bronchial tube was injected about 100 ml of 10% formalin solution. Then the lungs were submerged in formalin and after 2–3 days sections were cut from 3 zones of the right lung 2,5 × 3 × 1 cm in size. The lung sections were stained by hematoxylin-eosin and picrofuchsin-fuchselin.

For transmission electron microscopy, the sections were fixed in a 2.5% solution of glutaraldehyde in 0.1 M phosphate buffer. After additional fixing by 1% solution of four oxides of osmium, the sections were put into epoxy embedding medium. Ultra thin sections were examined by electron microscope PEM-100 after staining with citrate lead.

For scanning electronic microscopy, the pulmonary vessels were longitudinally dissected, dehydrated in ethanol of increasing concentration, dried up to transition of critical point and, after processing by palladium, examined on a scanning electron microscope "Philips-500".

Morphological methods: the method of separate weighing of heart by Muller, as updated by Kruchkova, was used. Thirty arteries and 30 arterioles from each zone of the lung were measured. For morphometry of the air haematic barrier, the negative components were used for electronogram by magnification × 20,000 on the basis of 25 measurements from each block.

Morphometrical ultrastructures were conducted according to the principles of stereologic analysis (Veibell, 1970; G.G.Avtandilov, 1981).

Statistical analysis. All quantity data were processed by methods of variational statistics.

Results and discussion. Characteristics of structural adaptive changes in the lungs of native highlanders, as result of the influence of chronic high altitude hypoxia, have been revealed. The expressiveness of adaptive morphological changes of the pulmonary vessels and right ventricular hypertrophy amplifies with increasing altitude. The weight of the right ventricle in native highlanders living over 3000 m above sea level was 10.1 ± 1.4 g (control - 6.8 ± 0.3 g, $P \leq 0.002$). Ventricle index reached 0.70 ± 0.03 (control- 0.42 ± 0.02, $P \leq 0.002$). This rate of right ventricular hypertrophy was close to the level of right ventricular hypertrophy in patients in the initial stages of COPD.

The morphometry of vessels in three zones of the right lung of native highlanders has detected redistribution of the bloodstream due to an increase in the upper and medial lobes. Though the morphometry of intralobular and terminal pulmonary arteries in the upper and medial lobes has shown an increase in the volumetric speed of the bloodstream, there was an increase pulmonary-vascular resistance, due to an increase of pulmonary arterioles tone in all zones of the lungs. The functional parameter of vessels tone – the percentage of media to lumen (%) decreases in the central intralobular and terminal arteries, especially in the upper and medial zones of the lungs, except for arterioles where the visible increase of this parameter in all zones of the lungs is noted.

Development of a longitudinal muscular layer is marked in the walls of the intralobular and terminal arteries of the upper and medial lung lobes in highlanders group living over 3000 m above sea level. These changes of the vessels level of resistance', in the form of lumen expansion and development of a longitudinal muscular layer, also have some similarity to changes in the pulmonary vessels in COPD.

In mechanisms of human adaptation to high altitude, the estimation of the phenomenon of the increase in capacity of the capillary bed of the alveolus has great value. The average diameter of the alveolar capillaries reached 13.0 ± 0.8 microns (control - 8.1 ± 0.4, $P \leq 0.002$). The increase in capacity of the capillary bed follows the primary expansion of their lumen and frequent occurrence of capillaries bulging adjoining to lumen with two alveoli.

Studying the endothelium ultrastructure of the alveolar capillaries has shown a twofold increase in the volumetric density of mitochondria, granules, granular endoplasmatic reticulum, microtubules and ribosomes. The hypertrophy of the pulmonary endothelium can be considered as a compensative adaptive reaction, which is a new qualitative level of functioning (figure 1).

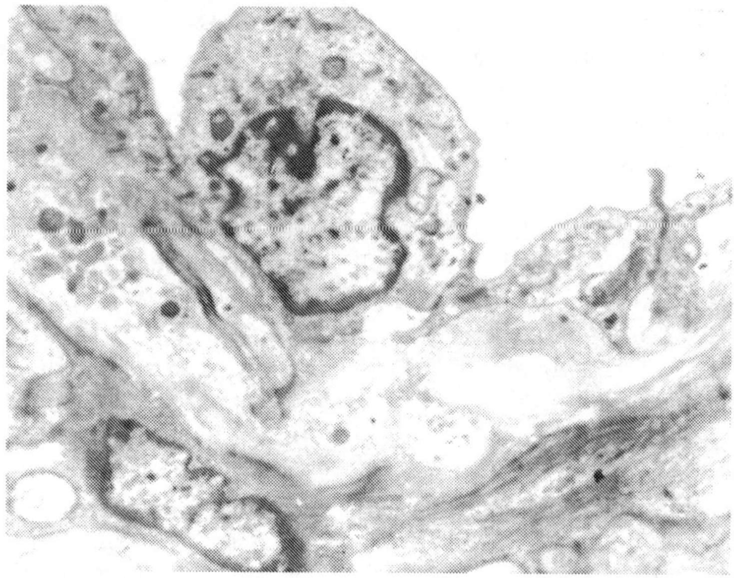

Figure 1. Electronogram. Pulmonary artery of a highlander. The endothelial (E) cell. Magnification × 6 000

At the present time, an increasing volume of experimental data indicate that the influence of vasoactive agents results in the endothelium expression of regulators modulating the effects of these agents on vessels [17,2,16,13,14]. Vasoactive substances synthesized by endothelial cells and circulating in the blood channel can penetrate into smooth muscle cells through mioendothelial contacts (figure 2).

The adaptable sense of the pulmonary capillaries capacity for growth consists in an increase of blood volume directly in the zone of gas diffusion.

The revealed changes of the air haematic barrier (AGB) ultrastructure concern basal membranes, alveocytes I type and the endothelium. Thickening of the air haematic barrier basal membranes is noted in highlanders living over 3 000 m above sea level reached 0.6 ± 0.095 microns (control 0.3 ± 0.071 microns, $P \leq 0.001$). Thickening of the basal membranes in these conditions is, in our opinion, an adaptive process in reply to increased intracapillary pressure. As is known, the basal membrane of the vessels serves not only for exchange processes, but also like a "micro-skeleton" of vessels, which thicken when intracapillary pressure increases. According to West et al. (1991) the increase in intracapillary pressure can be used as an essential reason for the occurrence of high-altitude pulmonary edema. Obviously, in cases of hyperreactivity of the cardio-vascular system to hypoxia proceeded with a significant increase in heart rhythm and cardiac output, the arterial contraction in the

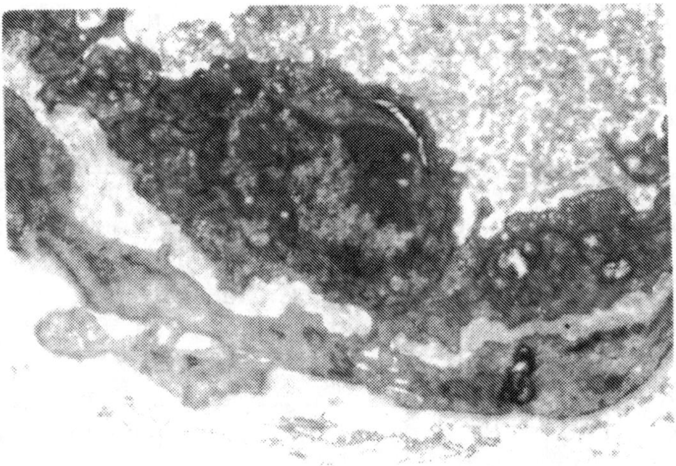

Figure 2. Electronogram. Pulmonary arterioles of a highlander. Mioendothelial contacts. Magnification × 6 000

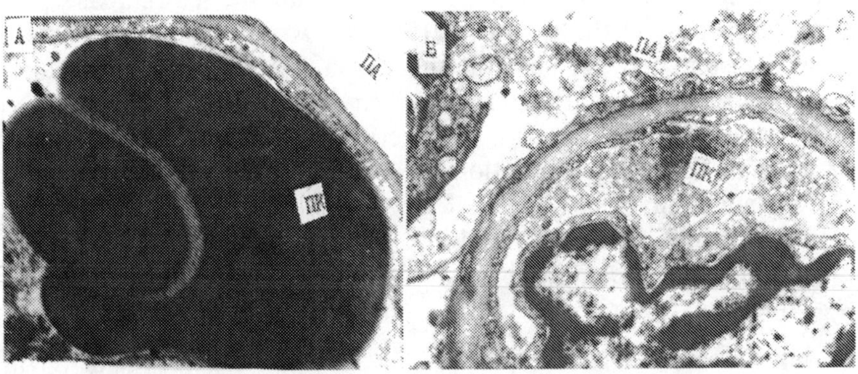

Figure 3. Characteristics of air haematic barrier ultrastructure in native highlanders and lowlanders. A) air haematic barrier in native highlanders (Murghab, 3600 m above sea level). There is marked thickening of the basal membrane of the air haematic barrier. Electronogram: magnification × 20000. air haematic barrier of native lowlander. Basal membranes have less thickness in comparison with basal membranes of air haematic barrier in native highlanders. Electronogram: magnification × 20000.

pulmonary circulation does not compensate the increase of the blood pressure in alveolar capillaries, which can promote a liquid filtration over its absorption and the development of pulmonary edema. In this connection the thickening of the air haematic barrier basal membranes of the lung in native highlanders can be considered as a protective, adaptive phenomenon against the development of pulmonary edema (figure 3).

Thus, strengthening the long-term adaptive reactions of the pulmonary circulation in native highlanders is a result of structural reorganization of the pulmonary vessels and right heart directed towards increasing the diffuse abilities of the lungs.

COPD at high altitude in the pulmonary vessels brings thickening of media terminal arteries and arterioles (Table.1), developments in the longitudinal muscular layer in a wall of intralobular arteries, which is formed towards a vessel lumen from internal elastic membranes of cambial elements, developing mioelastofibrosis, which leads to a substantial increase in pulmonary-vascular resistance and to the development of pulmonary hypertension.

The above-stated morphological changes occur in COPD both in high- and lowlanders and lead to the development of cor pulmonale. It is known, that cor pulmonale makes the prognosis gloomier and is one of the major factors defining the survival rate of patients with COPD. However, at the same time, highlanders with COPD also had distinctive characteristics in the development of morphological changes of arterializations of small arterioles in diameter from 30 to 40 microns, with a simultaneous increase in their quantity (30 to 100 alveoli) (control 10 to 100). Arterializations of arterioles occurs as a result of hyperplasia of the media smooth muscle cells and the appearance of an external elastic layer. Arterialization of the pulmonary arterioles makes adaptive sense in connection with a new level of regulation by perfusion and ventilation relationship in reply to a decreased partial pressure of oxygen in alveolar air. The following difference was the occurrence of the foci of angiomatosis in the lungs of highlanders with COPD. These plural angiomas represent closely located arteries of different diameters from 100–400 microns (figure 4).

TABLE 1. Comparison of regional characteristics of resistance of pulmonary terminal arteries in highlanders and lowlanders with COPD (M ± m).

Pulmonary lobes	Lowlanders		Highlanders		Percentage of media to lumen (%)	
	Altitude above sea level (m)					
	760 Media area (μm)	760 Lumen area (μm)	2700–3000 Media area (μm))	2700–300 Lumen area (μm)	760	2700–3000
Upper	6422 ± 11	10801 ± 82	5821 ± 191	15204 ± 168	31,0 ± 2,1	50,9 ± 1,7
Medial	5588 ± 24	10292 ± 67	6124 ± 276	16936 ± 62	36,0 ± 1,1	54,2 ± 1,6
Basal	6021 ± 56	9334 ± 51	6487 ± 77	14783 ± 92	40,3 ± 1,7	64,0 ± 0,7

In highlanders with COPD, we can note the sharp narrowing and obliteration of terminal arteries and arterioles lumens, owing to proliferation of endothelial and smooth muscle cells towards a vessel lumen from internal elastic membranes, with formation of multichannel arteries (figure 5).

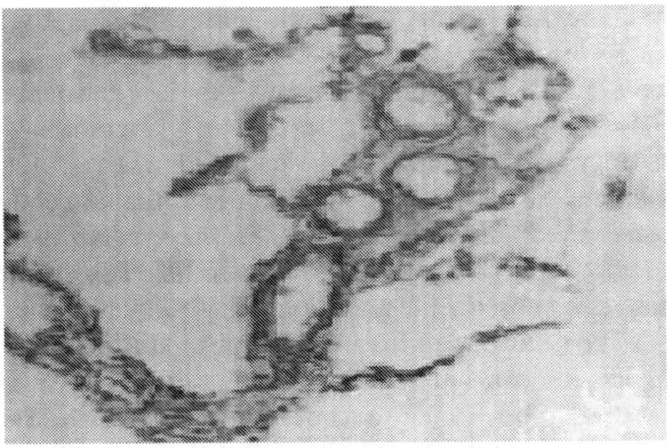

Figure 4. Lung of patient with COPD at high altitude (2700–3000 m above sea level). Foci of small pulmonary arteries with diameters of 70–80 microns are found. Capillaries have wide lumens. Magnification × 480. Stained by picrofuchsin-fuchselin.

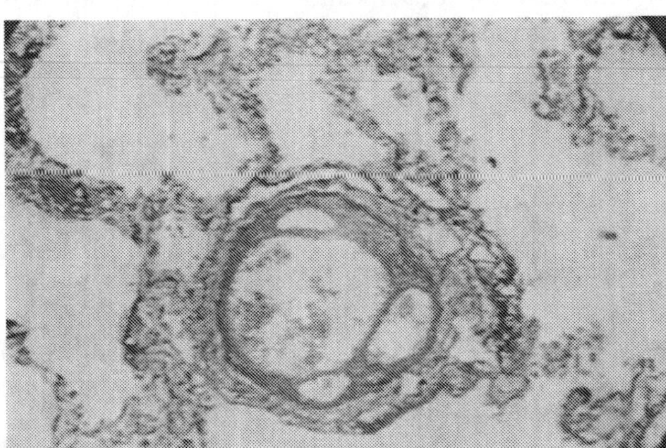

Figure 5. Lung of patient with COPD at high altitude (2700–3000 m above sea level). A pulmonary artery with a diameter of 200 microns. Growth of intims due to proliferation of endothelial and smooth muscle cells with formation of new intravascular channels is marked. There is also a marked thickening of the pulmonary artery wall, due to the growth of collagenic fiber of the adventitial layer. Among the collagen fibers are found lymphatic capillaries with wide lumens. Magnification × 480. Stained by picrofuchsin-fuchselin.

These characteristics of structural changes in the pulmonary vascular bed are caused by strongly expressed tissue hypoxia, developing in patients with COPD at high altitude hypoxia.

In our studies there were also cases of the development of a severe alveolar edema in highlanders with COPD during physical load and ascension of a small heights and also cases of the development of high-altitude severe pulmonary edema in healthy people during rapid ascent to heights over 4,000 m above sea level.

In both cases, irrespective of the reasons for the occurrence of a severe alveolar edema, 3 stages are passed: intramural, interstitial and alveolar. In intramural stages the spasm of alveolar capillaries is observed, loosening argirophylic and elastic skeleton, swelling endothelial cells and I and II type alveolocytes. Because alveolar cells are connected to themselves more strongly than endothelial cells, edematic liquor is held back in the intermediate tissue. There is a subsequent interstitial stage, which is characterized by development of stasis in the capillaries. In these conditions there is a further swelling of collagenic fiber, significant accumulation of a serous liquor in the interalveolar septum, perivascular and peribronchial spaces. Such a congestion of edematic liquor with hyperplasia of the connective tissue is regarded as an anatomic substratum of X-ray symptoms of the pulmonary edema. In the alveolar stage of the pulmonary edema the collagenic fibers are vacuolated and also split, which are considered to be morphological attributes of the increased permeability. Thus, endothelial and epithelial cells are exposed to a dystrophy and thinning occurs and breach of the air hematic barrier (figure 6).

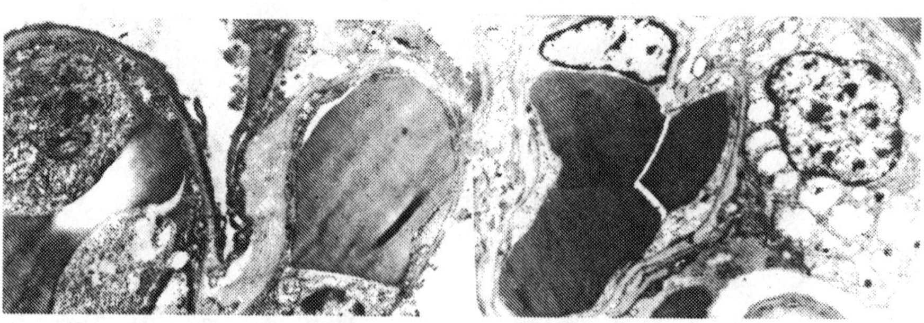

Figure 6. Lungs of a patient with EDEMA. A) Vacuolar dystrophy of the endothelium. Swelling of the mitochondria. Thinning of the air haematic barrier. Electronogram: magnification × 5 000. Vacuolization of alveolocyte cytoplasm type II. Osmophylic granules were not detected. erythrocytes are seen in a lumen of a capillary. Thinning of the air haematic barrier. Electronogram: magnification × 5 000.

Conclusions:

1. In native highlanders, due to long (chronic) adaptation, regional morphofunctional changes of the pulmonary vessels develop, caused by strengthening of the upper and medial zone of lungs, increase in capacity of the capillary channel and the extent of the working zones of the air haematic barrier.
2. The hypertrophy of the endothelium is provided by increasing of volume of cell, nucleus and also the volumetric density of mitochondria, ribosomes and the endoplasmic reticulum.
3. The revealed thickening of the basal membranes of the air haematic barrier in native highlanders provides increased durability of the capillaries, which allows one to consider this fact as a protective - adaptable phenomenon, reducing the development of pulmonary edema.
4. The following characteristics are revealed in patients with COPD at high altitude: remodelling of the pulmonary arteries and arterioles, substantially expressed arterializations of the finest arterioles by diameter from 30 to 40 microns, with a simultaneous increase in their quantity, reduction of terminal arteries and arterioles lumens, as a result of endothelial and smooth muscle cells proliferation towards a vessel lumen from internal elastic membranes, formation of multichannel arteries due to endothelial and smooth muscle cells proliferation, with simultaneous growth of collagen and elastic fiber and development of the angiomatosis foci, which represent closely located vessels of different diameters.
5. During rapid ascent to high altitude 2500–3000м above sea level, pulmonary edema develops in people who are not adapted to high altitude. In patients with COPD, high altitude pulmonary edema develops during the ascent of small heights (2000 m above sea level), which is connected with a chronic pulmonary hypertension, which results quite often in the development of interstitial edema with rapid transition in these conditions into high altitude alveolar pulmonary edema.

References

1. Arias-Stella I., Saldane M.(1962) Pulmonary circulation in man at high altitude.- Med. Thorac. 19:484–493.
2. Botney MD, Liptay MJ, Kaiser LR, Cooper JD, Parks WC, Mecham RP.(1993) Active collagen synthesis by pulmonary arteries in human primary pulmonary hypertension. Am J Pathol 143: 121–129.
3. Hurtado A.(1966) Man and altitude. -Am. Instr. Hyg. Associat. v.29,N4,p.313–320.
4. Kadyraliev T.K.(1990) Morphological changes of pulmonary vessels of resistance in development of high-mountainous pulmonary arterial hypertension - archive a stalemate. WITH. 36–40.

5. Kadyraliev T.K., Rajymbekov N.K.(2001) Remodeling of vessels of a small diameter . Blood circulation under the influence of high-mountainous hypoxia – Bishkek. The international symposium on mountain medicine.
6. Kadyraliev T., Gaparov B/G., Rajymbekov N.K.(2001) Morphology of featured Myocardium and vessels of minor blood circulation in animals - native to high mountains, the 2001.international symposium on mountain medicine.
7. Mirrahimov M.M. (1971) Diseases, illness of heart and mountains. - Frunze.
8. Mirrahimov M.M., (1978) Goldberg P.N. Mountain medicine. - Frunze.
9. Mirrahimov M.M. (1988) All-Union, a symposium on pulmonary arterial to hypertensia: material.-M. of Frunze48–52.
10. Monge C.(1942) Life in the Andes and chronic mountain sickness// Science l.95: 79–82.
11. Morrel N.W. Yang X., Sheares K.K., Davie N., Upton P.D., Taylor G.W.. Wharton j. Stimulation and inhibition of distal pulmonary artery smooth muscle cell growth b\ hypoxia : role of COX – 2.
12. Morrell NW, Atochina EN, Morris KG, Danilov SM, Stenmark KR.(1995) Angiotensin converting enzyme expression is increased in small pulmonary arteries of rats with hypoxia-induced pulmonary hypertension. J Clin Invest 96: 1823–1833.
13. Morrell NW, Morris KG, Stenmark KR.(1995) Role of angiotensin-converting enzyme and angiotensin II in the development of hypoxic pulmonary hypertension. Am J Physiol 269: H1186–H1194.
14. Morrell NW, Upton PD, Higham MA, Yacoub MH. Polak JM, Wharton J.(1998) Angiotensin II stimulates proliferation of human pulmonary artery smooth muscle cells via the ATI receptor. Chest 114: 90–91.
15. Rabinovitch M, Gamble W, Nadas AS, Miettinen OS. Reid L.(1979) Rat pulmonary circulation after chronic hypoxia: hemodynamic and structural characteristics. Am J Physiol. 236: H818–H827.
16. Stenmark KR, Dempsey EC, Badesch DB, Frid M, Mecham TP. Parks WC. (1993) Regulation of pulmonary vascular wall cell growth: developmental and site-specific heterogeneity. Eur Respir Rev 3: 629–637.
17. Vanhoutte P.M., Luscher T.T. (1989) Endothelium-derived contracting factors .-In : International symposium on endothelium-derived vasoactive factors. Philadelphia, 117.
18. Wagenvoort C.A.(1982) High altitude pulmonary hypertension // Pulmonary Arterial Hypertension.Transactions of the International Symposium. June 28–30, Frunze. 1985: 344–348.
19. Weibell E.R. (1966) Morphometry of human lung. Philadelphia.

CHAPTER 24

ACUTE OXYGEN SENSING MECHANISMS

E. KENNETH WEIR[1], JESUS. A. CABRERA[2], ANDREA OLSCHEWSKI[3], MARIA OBRETCHIKOVA[1], ROSEMARY F. KELLY[2], RAJAT JHANJEE[1], ZHIGANG HONG[1]

[1]Department of Medicine & [2]Surgery Minneapolis VA Medical Center and University of Minnesota
[3]Medical University of Graz, Austria

Abbreviations: PA: Pulmonary artery; DA: Ductus arteriosus; HPV: Hypoxic pulmonary vasoconstriction Potasssium channels; Kv: Voltage-gated; KCa: Calcium-sensitive; TASK: Two-pore, acid-sensitive; PVR: Pulmonary vascular resistance; SMC: Smooth muscle cell; SOC: Store-operated current; TRP: Transient receptor potential; ROS: Reactive oxygen species; DTT: Dithiothreitol.

Abstract: At birth, associated with the rise in oxygen levels, the resistance pulmonary arteries (PA) dilate and the ductus arteriosus (DA) constricts. In neonatal and adult life, hypoxia in the small airways causes pulmonary vasoconstriction (HPV) which helps to direct mixed venous blood away from poorly ventilated alveolae. HPV and normoxic contraction of the DA both involve at least three different mechanisms that combine to cause smooth muscle cell contraction. These are: Inhibition of the outward potassium current across the cell membrane, resulting in membrane depolarization and calcium entry through L-type calcium channels; release of calcium from the sarcoplasmic reticulum and repletion through the store-operated channels; and calcium-sensitization, in both PA and DA, the change in oxygen tension stimulates Rho kinase, which inhibits myosin light-chain phosphatase and potentiates contraction.

However, there is no consensus on the initial sensing mechanism by which changes in oxygen tension are recognized. In both the resistance PA and the DA a decrease in oxygen tension may reduce the production of reactive oxygen species, such as hydrogen peroxide, from the mitochondria and NAD(P)H oxidase. Consequently, the smooth muscle cell is more reduced during hypoxia and more oxidized during normoxia. This change in cytoplasmic redox status may be signaled through small G-proteins, such as RhoA, to the executive arm. This chapter reviews the evidence for both the oxygen sensing and executive components.

A. Aldashev and R. Naeije (eds.), Problems of High Altitude Medicine and Biology, 295–304.

Introduction

Over the last 300 million years, oxygen has varied between 15 and 35% of the Earth's atmosphere. For most organisms, oxygen poses a dilemma, we cannot survive with too much and we cannot live without it. In the course of evolution many adaptations have occurred, which optimize the transfer of oxygen to the tissues. This chapter examines the mechanisms by which different organs in the body, particularly the pulmonary arteries and ductus arteriosus, detect acute changes in oxygen tension and initiate responses. Specialized tissues that sense the local oxygen tension include the type 1 cells of the carotid body, the neuroepithelial bodies in the lungs, the chromaffin cells of the fetal adrenal medulla and the smooth muscle cells of the resistance pulmonary arteries, systemic arteries, placenta and the ductus arteriosus [32].

The Carotid Body

The carotid body provides a classic model of oxygen sensing; "sensing" the level of oxygen in the arterial blood from its vantage point adjacent to the carotid artery. Hypoxemia in the blood (< 60 mm Hg O_2 pressure) causes exocytosis of vacuoles from the type 1 (glomus) cells of the carotid body. The release of acetylcholine and ATP from the vacuoles stimulates the sensory nerve endings of the carotid sinus nerve, increasing nerve traffic and activating the respiratory center. This gives rise to the sense of breathlessness noticed at high altitude. Although the immediate sensing mechanism is still debated, hypoxia inhibits potassium channels in the type 1 cells, resulting in membrane depolarization and influx of calcium through the voltage-gated L-type calcium channels [10]. The rise in cytosolic calcium, which signals the exocytosis, does not occur in the absence of membrane depolarization, indicating the importance of this component of the hypoxia-sensing mechanism [4]. The potassium channels inhibited by hypoxia can be voltage-gated (K_v), calcium-sensitive (K_{Ca}) or two-pore, acid-sensitive (TASK) channels, depending on factors such as maturity (fetal vs adult) [6] [34] [3]. The mechanism that determines the oxygen-sensitive gating of the K^+ channels in the type 1 cell is still uncertain.

Hypoxic Pulmonary Vasoconstriction

In the fetus, partially oxygenated blood returning from the placenta, flows through the right side of the heart. Because of the high resistance of the unexpanded lungs, the blood is diverted from the right atrium and pulmonary artery, across the foramen ovale and ductus arteriosus to the left atrium and aorta respectively. The high pulmonary vascular resistance (PVR) in utero can be demonstrated to be due in part to hypoxic pulmonary vasoconstriction (HPV), as when a maternal animal is ventilated with high concentrations of oxygen, the fetal PVR falls. At birth as the oxygen tension rises, the small, resistance pulmonary arteries dilate and the ductus arteriosus contracts. The opposite response of these vessels to the increase in oxygen is a fascinating conundrum.

After birth, HPV may occur as a result of a localized area of alveolar hypoventilation (e.g., atelectasis). This HPV diverts the flow of relatively desaturated, mixed venous blood to better ventilated areas of the lung. If HPV is inhibited, there is a reduction in systemic arterial oxygen tension, even in normal subjects, but particularly in patients with small airways disease [7]. Thus HPV in the presence of localized hypoxia is beneficial but generalized hypoxia can lead to pulmonary hypertension and remodeling. Acute HPV predominantly affects small pulmonary arteries and veins ($<500\,\mu$ in diameter) [23]. The "executive" mechanism of HPV has three components. The first requires hypoxic inhibition of K^+ channels in the cell membrane of the pulmonary artery smooth muscle cells (PASMCs), membrane depolarization and calcium entry through the L-type calcium channel, just as occurs in the carotid body type 1 cell [18] [13]. The second involves release of calcium from the sarcoplasmic reticulum of PASMCs into the cytoplasm and its repletion by calcium entry through store-operated calcium (SOC) channels [21] [27]. The third mechanism exploits calcium sensitization [20], which can sustain smooth muscle contraction when cytosolic levels of calcium are decreasing [25]. Myosin light-chain phosphatase normally dephosphorylates myosin light-chain and ends the interaction between actin and myosin that is responsible for calcium-calmodulin mediated smooth muscle contraction. During hypoxia there is an increase in the activated form of the small G protein, RhoA, in PASMCs. Active RhoA stimulates Rho kinase which then inhibits myosin light-chain phosphatase and prevents dephosphorylation, thus prolonging and augmenting HPV. In the presence of localized areas of acute alveolar hypoxia these three mechanisms result in localized HPV.

Chronic Hypoxic Pulmonary Hypertension

Chronic hypoxic pulmonary hypertension is the consequence of both pulmonary vasoconstriction and remodeling. The importance of each component is still disputed. It is usually considered that proliferation (or decreased apoptosis) of cells in the intima, media and adventitia causes the vessel wall to intrude upon the lumen and pose a "fixed" resistance to flow through the lungs. Supporting this contention is the repeated observation that after

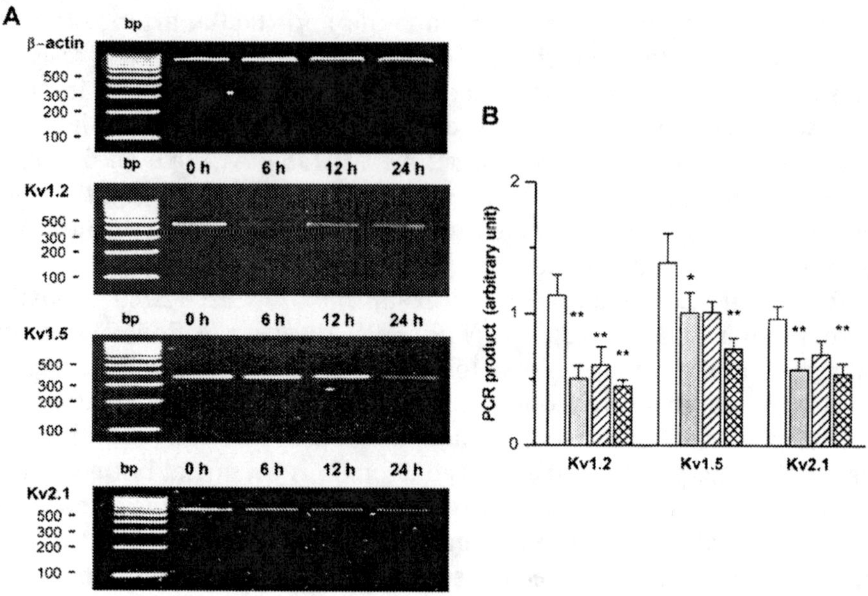

Figure 1. Effect of short-term (6 h [shaded bars], 12 h [striped bars], and 24 h [cross-hatched bars]) hypoxia on mRNA levels of Kv1.2, Kv1.5, and Kv2.1 -subunits in PASMCs. (A) PCR amplified products are displayed in agarose gel for Kv1.2, Kv1.5, Kv2.1 and β-actin transcripts. Lane 1 shows the molecular weight marker used to indicate the size of the PCR fragments. (B) Data were normalized to the amount of β-actin in PASMCs in normoxia (0 h) or after 6, 12, and 24 h moderate hypoxia. Values are means ± SEM (experiments were repeated 6 times independently). $^{*}P < 0.05$, $^{**}P < 0.01$ versus normoxic controls (0 h, open bar). (From Hong Z, Weir EK, Nelson DP, Olschewski A. Sub-acute hypoxia decreases Kv channel expression and function in pulmonary artery myocytes. Am J Respir Cell Mol Biol. 2004; 31: 337–343).

several weeks of hypoxia, return to normoxia or to hyperoxia does not rapidly restore pulmonary vascular resistance to pre-hypoxic levels. However, it has recently been reported that the compound Y-27632, which inhibits Rho kinase and calcium sensitization, will acutely reverse chronic hypoxic pulmonary hypertension. Thus, chronic hypoxia sets in play a signaling cascade causing vasoconstriction that persists when the hypoxic stimulus is removed. This signaling cascade can be rapidly interrupted by Y-27632, (but not immediately by oxygen), indicating that after a few weeks of hypoxia, although cell proliferation occurs, it is not the principal reason for pulmonary hypertension. It remains to be seen whether hypoxic pulmonary hypertension that has been present for several years can be so quickly reversed.

The effect of the Y-27632 compound indicates a role for calcium sensitization in the increased pulmonary vascular tone seen in chronic hypoxia. There is also evidence for the involvement of SOC and K^+ channels. The expression of TRPC1 and 6 genes (which code for SOC channels) is increased in the PASMCs of both rats and mice exposed to hypoxia (10% O_2) for three weeks [28]. The functional corollary of these observations is that capacitative (SOC) calcium entry is enhanced in PASMCs from the resistance pulmonary arteries of rats exposed to chronic hypoxia. The increased expression of TRPC 1 and 6 during hypoxia is absent in mice partially deficient for HIF-1α and, as a consequence, the resting cytosolic calcium is not elevated. The conclusion is that the stabilization of H1F-1α that occurs in hypoxia, leads to increased expression of TRPC1 and 6, which results in increased calcium entry [28].

Chronic hypoxia, over 12 hours in duration, results in decreased expression of oxygen-sensitive K^+ channels (e.g. K_v 1.5 and 2.1) in the PASMCs and membrane depolarization [24] [16] [8] (Figure 1). The decreased expression of K^+ channels in chronic hypoxia again involves H1F-1α [22]. In view of the decreased expression of K^+ channels in chronic hypoxia and the role of K^+ channels in acute HPV, it is not surprising that exposure to chronic hypoxia reduces acute HPV [11]. The finding that transfection of K_v 1.5 by aerosol can restore acute HPV indicates the importance of K^+ channels in the pulmonary vascular response to hypoxia [19]. The K^+ channels involved, include not only voltage-gated K^+ channels but also two-pore acid-sensitive K^+ channels (TASK channels) [15].

The Ductus Arteriosus

As described earlier, the ductus arteriosus constricts in response to a rise in oxygen tension, the opposite reaction to that of the resistance pulmonary arteries. However, the tripartite executive mechanism that causes constriction in response to the change in oxygen is the same: K^+ channel inhibition, membrane depolarization and calcium entry through L-type channels [26], calcium entry through store-operated channels, and calcium sensitization [9]. As acute HPV is lost after a few days of chronic hypoxia, so acute normoxic contraction of the ductus is selectively lost and mRNA for K_v 1.5 and 2.1 is reduced after several days in culture under normoxic conditions [12]. Ex vivo transfection with K_v 1.5 or 2.1 restores much of the normoxic contraction, thus emphasizing the importance of these K^+ channels in the response to changes in oxygen. Interestingly, the fact that the transfection of the same K_v 1.5 channel can restore oxygen sensitivity in both HPV and normoxic ductal contraction, indicates that the opposite behavior of pulmonary arteries and ductus does not derive from the channel protein itself.

The release of calcium from the sarcoplasmic reticulum of the ductus arteriosus smooth muscle cells (DASMCs) stimulated by normoxia leads to influx of calcium through store-operated calcium channels. These SOC channels are encoded by the transient receptor potential (TRP) superfamily of genes. We have identified mRNA for TRPC 1, 3, 4 and 6 and protein of TRPC 1 and 4 in DASMCs [9]. Contraction of the ductus in response to switching from 0 to 2mM calcium in the tissue bath, in the presence of nifedipine to block L-type channels, is greatly enhanced in normoxia compared to hypoxia. The increase in calcium in DAMSC, elicited by switching from 0 to 2 mM calcium in the presence of cyclopiazonic acid, (used to release calcium from the SR), can be inhibited by incubation of the cells with an antibody to TRPC 1. This study demonstrates the functional importance of the SOC channels in DASMCs.

The third mechanism involved in normoxic contraction of the ductus is calcium sensitization. In the mirror image of what occurs in the pulmonary artery, it appears that an increase in oxygen activates rho kinase and leads to inhibition of myosin light-chain phosphatase, thus prolonging the interaction of actin and myosin. Two structurally dissimilar inhibitors of rho kinase, Y-27632 and fasudil, both prevented normoxic contraction of the ductus [8] (Figure 2). It is possible that an increase in Rho A, the step in calcium sensitization before rho kinase, may also potentiate the mechanism of oxygen sensing involving the K^+ channels. RhoA has been reported to

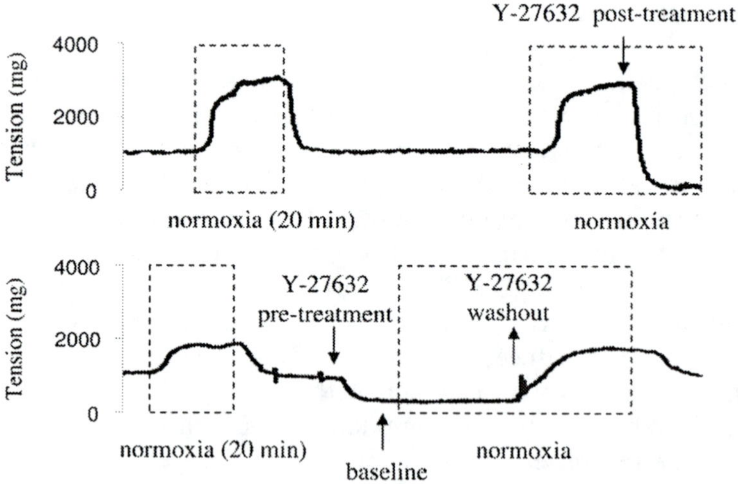

Figure 2. Representative DA ring tension tracing shows the experimental protocol and illustrates that 3 μmol/L Y-27632 completely reverses (post-treated, top) or prevents (pretreated, bottom) normoxia-induced contraction. The prevention is rapidly lost after Y-27632 is washed out (pretreated, bottom). (From Hong Z, Hong F, Olschewski A, Varghese A, Nelson DP, Weir EK. Store-operated calcium channels and calcium sensitization are involved in normoxic contraction of the ductus arteriosus. Circulation 2006;114: 1372–1379).

inhibit K_v 1.2 [5] and to facilitate inward current passing through L-type calcium channels [35]. The latter observation was made in cardiac myocytes but if it also occurs in vascular SMCs and signals through rho kinase, it could explain the ability of rho kinase inhibitors to ablate normoxic contraction of the ductus.

Sensing of Oxygen

At birth the resistance pulmonary arteries dilate in response to the rise in oxygen tension, while the ductus arteriosus contracts. The sensing mechanism responsible for this opposite behavior is still uncertain. The executive mechanisms, described above, seem to be present in both vessels but are triggered differently. Given that K^+ channels are involved, perhaps they are gated in an opposite manner in these vessels, in response to a change in oxygen tension. An elegant experiment by Platoshyn et al makes this unlikely [17]. K_v 1.5 is a potassium channel which is known to be "oxygen-sensitive." The gene for this channel was over-expressed in rat PASMCs and in mesenteric artery SMCs, markedly increasing K^+ current in both. However, only in the PASMCs was the K^+ current inhibited by hypoxia [17]. This study indicates that there is another component, besides the channel protein, that confers oxygen sensitivity. This conclusion is in keeping with the observations, cited earlier, that transfection of the same K^+ channel (K_v 1.5), can partially restore HPV and normoxic contraction of the DA. Again, the opposite behavior of the vessels did not lie in the channel protein.

The role of reactive oxygen species (ROS) in oxygen sensing has sparked considerable interest. While it seems likely that redox changes signal changes in oxygen tension, the importance of ROS per se is unresolved. It is not even agreed whether ROS go up or down during hypoxia in the pulmonary vasculature [29] [Weir and Archer 2006]. Recent papers continue the debate [30] [2]. If ROS were to be the key difference between PA and DA, then they should go in opposite directions in the two vessels in response to a specific change in oxygen tension, such as going from normoxia to hypoxia. There is no report that this is the case. Why then the emphasis on redox changes? The PA and DA both constrict in response to agents such as KCl, phenylephrine and endothelin and relax in response to vasodilator prostaglandins. They differ in their response to oxygen and to redox agents. In the presence of a reducing agent, such as dithiothreitol (DTT), the PA constricts, while the DA relaxes, mimicking hypoxia [14]. In the presence of an oxidizing agent, such as DTNB, the PA relaxes, while the DA constricts, mimicking normoxia. DTT and DTNB also behave like hypoxia and normoxia in terms of their effects on K^+ current, membrane potential and cytosolic calcium; each having opposite effects in the PA and DA. These observations suggest that the difference in the response of the PA and DA to hypoxia, for instance, involves a step where the addition of electrons to the signaling pathway achieves diametrically opposite vasoactive results. This step has yet to be identified.

The small Rho GTPases, such as RhoA, Rac 1 and Cdc 42, play a part in the signaling of changes in oxygen tension. In cultured PA endothelial cells from adult pigs acute hypoxia increases RhoA and Cdc 42, while decreasing Rac 1 [33]. The changes in RhoA and Rac 1 increase endothelial permeability. In the case of PASMCs taken from conduit PA, the responses of RhoA and Rac1 activity to acute hypoxia vary, depending on the developmental age of the animal and whether the PASMCs are taken from the inner or outer media of the vessel [1]. Increased actin stress fiber formation occurs in PASMCs from the fetus in response to hypoxia and is dependent upon RhoA activity. How do the small GTPases relate to HPV and normoxic contraction of the ductus? As discussed earlier, calcium sensitization appears to be involved in both HPV and normoxic contraction of the ductus as the rho kinase inhibitor, Y-27632, can markedly diminish both. Assuming that Y-27632 is specific for rho kinase and that the activity of rho kinase is increased by RhoA, this would indicate that hypoxia increases RhoA activity in the PA and normoxia increases RhoA activity in the DA. The upstream signaling responsible for this difference remains to be resolved but likely involves the redox step outlined above.

References

1. Bailly K, Ridley A, Hall S, Haworth SG (2004) Rho A activation by hypoxia in pulmonary arterial smooth muscle cells is age and site specific. Circ Res 94:1383–91
2. Bonnet S, Michelakis E, Porter CJ, Andrade-Navarro MA, Thebaud B, Bonnet S, Harmony A, Harry G, Moudgil R, McMurtry MS, Weir EK, Archer SL (2006) An abnormal mitochondrial - HIF1α – K_v channel pathway disrupts oxygen-sensing and triggers pulmonary arterial hypertension (PAH) in fawn-hooded rats: similarities to human PAH. Cir 113(22):2630–41
3. Buckler K (1997) A novel oxygen-sensitive potassium current in rat carotid body type I cells. J Physiol 498:649–62
4. Buckler K and Vaughan-Jones R (1994) Effects of hypoxia on membrane potential and intracellular calcium in rat neonatal carotid body type I cells. J Physiol 476:423–8
5. Cachero T, Moreilli A, Peralta E (1998) The small GTP-binding protein RhoA regulates a delayed rectifier potassium channel. Cell 93:1077–85
6. Ganfornina M, Lopez-Barneo J (1992) Potassium channel types in arterial chemoreceptor cells and their selective modulation by oxygen. J Gen Physiol 100:401–26
7. Hales C, Westphal D (1978) Hypoxemia following the administration of sublingual nitroglycerin. Am J Med 65:911–8

8. Hong Z, Weir EK, Nelson, DP, Olschewski A (2004) Subacute hypoxia decrease voltage-activated potassium channel expression and function in pulmonary artery myocytes. Am J Respir Cell Mol Biol 31:1–7
9. Hong Z, Hong F, Olschewski A, Cabrera JA, Varghese A, Nelson DP, Weir EK (2006) Role of store-operated calcium channels and calcium sensitization in normoxic contraction of the ductus arteriosus. Circulation 114:1372–9
10. Lopez-Barneo J, Lopez-Lopez J, Urena J, Gonzalez C (1988) Chemotransduction in the carotid body: K+ current modulated by PO2 in type I chemoreceptor cells. Science Wash DC 242:580–2
11. McMurtry I, Petrun M, Reeves J (1978) Lungs from chronically hypoxic rats have decreased pressor response to acute hypoxia. Am J Physiol 235:H104–H109
12. Michelakis E, Rebeyka I, Wu X (2002) O2 sensing in the human ductus arteriosus regulation of voltage-gated K+ channels in smooth muscle cells by a mitochondrial redox sensor. Circ Res 91:478–86
13. Olschewski A, Hong Z, Nelson D, Weir EK (2002) Graded response of K^+ current, membrane potential and $[Ca2^+]i$ to hypoxia in pulmonary arterial smooth muscle. Am J Physiol 283:L1143–L1150
14. Olschewski A, Hong Z, Peterson, D, Nelson DP, Porter V, Weir EK (2004) Opposite effects of redox status on membrane potential, cytosolic calcium, and tone in pulmonary arteries and ductus arteriosus. Am J Physiol 286:L15–L22
15. Olschewski A, Li Y, Tang B (2006) Impact of TASK-1 in human pulmonary artery smooth muscle cells. Circ Res 98:1072–80
16. Osipenko O, Alexander D, MacLean M, Gurney A (1998) Influence of chronic hypoxia on the contributions of non-inactivating and delayed rectifier K currents to the resting potential and tone of rat pulmonary artery smooth muscle. Br J Pharmacol 124:1335–7
17. Platoshyn O, Brenova E, Burg E, Yu Y, Remillard C, Yuan J (2006) Acute hypoxia selectively inhibits KCNA5 channels in pulmonary artery smooth muscle cells. Am J Physiol 290:C907–C916
18. Post J, Hume J, Archer SA, Weir EK (1992) Direct role for potassium channel inhibition in hypoxic pulmonary vasoconstriction. Am J Physiol 262:C882–C890
19. Pozeg Z, Michelakis ED, McMurtry M, Thebaud B, Wu XC, Dyck, JR, Hashimoto K, Wang S, Moudgil R, Harry G, Sultanian R, Koshal A, Archer SL (2003) In vivo gene transfer of a. the O2-sensitive potassium channel Kv1.5 reduces pulmonary hypertension and restores hypoxic pulmonary vasoconstriction in chronically hypoxic rats. Circulation 107:2037–44
20. Robertson T, Aaronson P, Ward J (1995) Hypoxic vasoconstriction and intracellular Ca^{2+} in pulmonary arteries: evidence for PKC-independent CA^{2+} sensitization. Am J Physiol 268:301–7
21. Salvaterra C, Goldman W (1993) Acute hypoxia increases cytosolic calcium in cultured pulmonary arterial myocytes. Am J Physiol 264:L323–L328
22. Shimoda L, Sylvester J, Booth G (2001) Inhibition of voltage-gated K^+ currents by endothelin-1 in human pulmonary arterial myocytes. AJP Lung 281:1115–22
23. Shirai M, Sada K, Niromiya I (1986) Effects of regional alveolar hypoxia and hypercapnia on small pulmonary vessels in cats. J Appl Physiol 61:440–8
24. Smirnov S, Robertson T, Ward J, Aaronson P (1994) Chronic hypoxia is associated with reduced delayed rectifier K+ current in rat pulmonary artery muscle cells. Am J Physiol 266:H365–H70
25. Somlyo A, Somlyo A (2003) Ca^{2+} sensitivity of smooth muscle and non-muscle myosin II: modulated by G proteins, kinases, and myosin phosphatase. Physiol Rev 83:1325–58
26. Tristani-Firouzi M, Reeve H, Tolarova S, Weir EK, Archer SL (1996) Oxygen-induced constriction of rabbit ductus arteriosus occurs via inhibition of a 4-aminopyridine-, voltage-sensitive potassium channel. J Clin Invest 98:1959–65
27. Wang J, Shimoda L, Weigand L, Wang W, Sun D, Sylvester JT (2005) Acute hypoxia increases intracellular [Ca2+] entry. Am J Physiol Lung Cell Mol Physiol 288:L1059–L69

28. Wang J, Weigand L, Lu W, Sylvester J, Semenza G, Shimoda L (2006) Hypoxia inducible factor 1 mediates hypoxia-induced TRPC expression and elevated intracellular $Ca2^{+}$ in pulmonary arterial smooth muscle cells. Circ Res 98:1528–37
29. Ward J (2006) Hypoxic pulmonary vasoconstriction is mediated by increased production of reactive oxygen species. J Appl Physiol 101:993–5
30. Waypa G, Guzy R, Mungai P, Mack MM, Marks JD, Roe MW, Schumaker PT (2006) Increases in mitochondrial reactive oxygen species trigger hypoxia-induced calcium responses in pulmonary artery smooth muscle cells. Circ Res 99:970–8
31. Weir E and Archer S (2006) Hypoxic pulmonary vasoconstriction is/is not mediated by increased production of reactive oxygen species. J Appl Physiol 101:995–8
32. Weir E, Lopez-Barneo J, Buckler K, Archer SL (2005) Acute oxygen-sensing mechanisms. N Engl J Med 353:2042–55
33. Wojciak-Stothard B, Yen Fen Tsang L, Haworth S (2005) Rac and Rho play opposing roles in the regulation of hypoxia/reoxygenation-induced permeability changes in pulmonary artery endothelial cells. Am J Physiol Lung Cell Mol Physiol 288:L749–L60
34. Wyatt C, Peers C (1995) $Ca^{2\pm}$ activated K^{+} channels in isolated type 1 cells of the neonatal rat carotid body. J Physol 483:559–65
35. Yatani A, Irie K, Otani T, Abdellatif M, Wei L (2005) RhoA GTPase regulates L-type Ca2+ currents in cardiac myocytes. Am J Physiol 288:H650–H9

INDEX

Printed in the United States
91329LV00002B/241-255/A